HEALTHCARE TECHNOLOGIES SERIES 38

Healthcare Monitoring and Data Analysis Using IoT

Other volumes in this series:

Volume 1	**Nanobiosensors for Personalized and Onsite Biomedical Diagnosis** P. Chandra (Editor)
Volume 2	**Machine Learning for Healthcare Technologies** D.A. Clifton (Editor)
Volume 3	**Portable Biosensors and Point-of-Care Systems** S.E. Kintzios (Editor)
Volume 4	**Biomedical Nanomaterials: From design to implementation** T.J. Webster and H. Yazici (Editors)
Volume 6	**Active and Assisted Living: Technologies and applications** F. Florez-Revuelta and A.A. Chaaraoui (Editors)
Volume 7	**Semiconductor Lasers and Diode-Based Light Sources for Biophotonics** P.E. Andersen and P.M. Petersen (Editors)
Volume 9	**Human Monitoring, Smart Health and Assisted Living: Techniques and technologies** S. Longhi, A. Monteriù and A. Freddi (Editors)
Volume 13	**Handbook of Speckle Filtering and Tracking in Cardiovascular Ultrasound Imaging and Video** C.P. Loizou, C.S. Pattichis and J. D'hooge (Editors)
Volume 14	**Soft Robots for Healthcare Applications: Design, modelling, and control** S. Xie, M. Zhang and W. Meng
Volume 16	**EEG Signal Processing: Feature extraction, selection and classification methods** W. Leong
Volume 17	**Patient-Centered Digital Healthcare Technology: Novel applications for next generation healthcare systems** L. Goldschmidt and R.M. Relova (Editors)
Volume 19	**Neurotechnology: Methods, advances and applications** V. de Albuquerque, A. Athanasiou and S. Ribeiro (Editors)
Volume 20	**Security and Privacy of Electronic Healthcare Records: Concepts, paradigms and solutions** S. Tanwar, S. Tyagi and N. Kumar (Editors)
Volume 23	**Advances in Telemedicine for Health Monitoring: Technologies, design and applications** T.A. Rashid, C. Chakraborty and K. Fraser
Volume 24	**Mobile Technologies for Delivering Healthcare in Remote, Rural or Developing Regions** P. Ray, N. Nakashima, A. Ahmed, S. Ro and Y. Soshino (Editors)
Volume 26	**Wireless Medical Sensor Networks for IoT-Based eHealth** F. Al-Turjman (Editor)
Volume 29	**Blockchain and Machine Learning for e-Healthcare Systems** B. Balusamy, N. Chilamkurti, L.A. Beena and P. Thangamuthu (Editors)
Volume 33	**Electromagnetic Waves and Antennas for Biomedical Applications** L. Wang
Volume 34	**The Internet of Medical Things: Enabling technologies and emerging applications** S.K. Pani, P. Patra, G. Ferrari, R. Kraleva and H. Wang (Editors)
Volume 39	**Digital Tools and Methods to Support Healthy Ageing** P.K. Ray, S.-T. Liaw and J.A. Serano (Editors)

Healthcare Monitoring and Data Analysis Using IoT

Technologies and applications

Edited by
Vishal Jain, Jyotir Moy Chatterjee,
Pardeep Kumar and Utku Kose

The Institution of Engineering and Technology

Published by The Institution of Engineering and Technology, London, United Kingdom

The Institution of Engineering and Technology is registered as a Charity in England & Wales (no. 211014) and Scotland (no. SC038698).

First published 2022

The Institution of Engineering and Technology
Michael Faraday House
Six Hills Way, Stevenage
Herts, SG1 2AY, United Kingdom

www.theiet.org

British Library Cataloguing in Publication Data
A catalogue record for this product is available from the British Library

ISBN 978-1-83953-437-9 (hardback)
ISBN 978-1-83953-438-6 (PDF)

Typeset in India by MPS Limited

Contents

About the editors

Vishal Jain is an associate professor at the Department of Computer Science and Engineering, Sharda University, India. He was awarded Young Active Member Award (2012–13) from the Computer Society of India, Best Faculty Award (2017), and Best Researcher Award (2019) from BVICAM, New Delhi. He has published over 70 peer-reviewed papers and 10 books. His research areas include information retrieval, semantic web, ontology engineering, data mining, ad hoc networks, and sensor networks.

Jyotir Moy Chatterjee is an assistant professor in the Information Technology Department at Lord Buddha Education Foundation (LBEF), Nepal. He has been a member of the organizing committee of various international conferences (IEEE, Springer, Elsevier) and serves as a reviewer for numerous international journals. His research interests include the Internet of Things, machine learning, and deep learning. He has published 22 research papers, 3 international conference papers, 28 books, and 16 chapters.

Pardeep Kumar is a professor and the head of the Software Engineering Department, QUEST University, Nawabshah, Pakistan. He is also the director for the Office of Research, Innovation and Commercialization (ORIC). His research interests include wireless communication, wireless sensor networks, distributed and embedded systems and IoT technologies. Dr. Kumar has been an author/editor of 4 books, several book chapters, and more than 50 research publications.

Utku Kose is an associate professor at the Department of Computer Engineering of Süleyman Demirel University, Turkey. He has published more than 200 journal papers, conference presentations, keynote speeches and book chapters. His research interests include artificial intelligence, machine ethics, artificial intelligence safety, optimization, chaos theory, distance education, e-learning, computer education, and computer science.

Preface

Increasingly healthcare service providers are employing Internet of Things (IoT)–enabled devices for monitoring patient healthcare, but their diagnosis and prescriptions are often instance-specific only. However, these IoT-enabled healthcare devices are generating a huge volume of data that could be analyzed for more accurate diagnosis and prescriptions.

This book concerns new and innovative ways in which such data can be collected, stored and analyzed using IoT and Big Data technologies. It addresses aspects of how "smart" healthcare can be used to detect and analyze diseases. It will also cover the underlying methodologies and related security concerns that work with patient data brings.

IoT-enabled healthcare technologies are suitable for remote health monitoring, including rehabilitation, assisted ambient living. In turn, healthcare analytics can be applied to the data gathered from different areas to improve healthcare outcomes at minimum expense.

The book is designed to be a reference to those using, designing, modeling, and analyzing intelligent healthcare services. Some of the features of this book were as follows:

- This book is aimed at showing the technologies available to make a better use of healthcare informatics.
- We aimed to show that improved outcomes can be realized through efficient and effective techniques (these include AI, machine learning, and other Big Data analytical techniques) being used to process medical data in real time.
- The intended audience includes healthcare informatics researchers, post-graduate students, developers, professionals, practitioners, and people who are interested in the personalized healthcare sector.
- Other projected audiences are the researchers and academicians who identify and develop methodologies, frameworks, tools, and applications for working with medical Big Data. These will be in computer engineering, healthcare electronics, and device design.

In Chapter 1, a model that may be useful for forecasting the distribution of COVID-19 is presented. Using support vector machine (SVM), linear regression, and naïve Bayes technique, we have conducted straight relapse. SVM with minimal mean absolute error and R^2 scores of 0.99599 for confirmed, 0.99429 for expired, and 0.97941 active cases are the best models completed. The outcome is seen and is equally consistent with the true one.

Chapter 2 discusses how the m-health technology helped patients as well as healthcare workers. Due to this, real-time monitoring of the patient from his/her place is easily possible. The chapter comprises what is m-health, the working of m-health technology, the impact of the m-health technology on the society.

The fundamental target of Chapter 3 is to numerically display the information created by an EEG acquisition method. The utilization of Big Data in dealing with an immense measure of information is proposed to investigate. Furthermore, we explore the utilization of Big Data in epileptic EEG assessment.

Chapter 4 concluded that the most dangerous part of coronavirus COVID-19 is the human-to-human transmission. It can also transmit from the contaminated surfaces of steel, aluminum, metal, wood, plastic, PVC, papers, disposable gowns, etc. to human beings. This chain is continuously increasing.

In Chapter 5, the main purpose of the study can be summarized as obtaining patient's health information via IoT, collection and evaluation of information, and providing IoT-based health solutions.

An exhaustive survey on the technologies and wearable devices used on the Internet of Medical Things (IoMT) to combat COVID-19 is done in Chapter 6.

Chapter 7 proposed an IoT-based system for a volumetric estimation of human brain morphological features from magnetic resonance images.

Chapter 8 aimed to open up the techniques and advantages of IoT in personalized healthcare and it also opens up the challenges and possible solutions that can be adopted in tracking and monitoring health status.

In Chapter 9, unstructured datasets available for research and development in E-health NLP will be discussed. In addition to the details related to unstructured datasets, challenges to tackle these unstructured information and methods and applications that have been developed for the identification and classification of important information from unstructured medical narratives will be elaborated.

Chapter 10 discussed the application of combining IoT and blockchain technologies into a solution to address challenges in the healthcare sector.

In Chapter 11, a preview of artificial intelligence's application in cardiac medical care is discussed with its latent role in simplifying precision cardiac treatment.

Chapter 12 discusses the various deep analytics applications and how they can be used specifically for COVID-19 data.

Chapter 13 looked at how deep learning computational methods can influence a few key areas of medicine as well as how to construct end-to-end systems.

Chapter 14 discussed the new development and techniques in the interpretation of signals and machine learning for biological brain signals.

Chapter 15 discusses about the classification of the interference associated with the WBAN networks and a comparative study on existing mutual interference mitigation approaches in each use case.

Chapter 16 demonstrates the potential of ML models to forecast the quantity of forthcoming patients plagued by COVID-19 that is presently thought of as a possible threat to human kind.

The accuracy of different algorithms for the diagnosis of various diseases has been compared in Chapter 17. Drug development using SVM and random forest is compared. The differences between the electronic medical record and electronic health record (EHR) are discussed, and case studies are discussed to understand the use of EHR.

Chapter 18 offers a brief introduction to the IoMT, and its impact on improving the quality of healthcare system. This chapter also provides insights into the emerging issues, i.e., security, privacy, trust, and risk due to deployment of IoMT at large scale.

Chapter 19 Internet of Unmanned Aerial Vehicle (IOU) plays an important role in the delivery of emergency medicine to remote locations. This chapter presents the use of Internet of Drones to the medical transport application.

Chapter 20 proposes a blockchain-based IoT system that might be applied to healthcare systems to fight against COVID-19 pandemic through consequently recognizing dark tainted cases similarly as predicting and evaluating the risk of COVID-19 pandemic in the networks.

Chapter 21 briefs the different AI algorithms carried out in diverse health disease detection and diagnosis. Further, it provides a review of such used algorithms.

Finally, we would like to thank all the chapter contributors for their valuable contributions as without their support this book would never have been possible.

Vishal Jain, India
Jyotir Moy Chatterjee, Nepal
Pardeep Kumar, Pakistan
Utku Kose, Turkey

Acknowledgments

I would like to acknowledge the most important people in my life, i.e., my grandfather Late Shri Gopal Chatterjee, grandmother Late Smt. Subhankori Chatterjee, my father Shri Aloke Moy Chatterjee, my Late mother Ms. Nomita Chatterjee, and my uncle Shri Moni Moy Chatterjee. This book has been my long-cherished dream that would not have been turned into reality without the support and love of these amazing people. They continuously encouraged me despite my failure to give them the proper time and attention. I am also grateful to my friends, who have encouraged and blessed this work with their unconditional love and patience.

Jyotir Moy Chatterjee
Department of IT
Lord Buddha Education Foundation
(Asia Pacific University of Technology & Innovation)
Kathmandu 44600, Nepal

Acknowledgments

I would like to acknowledge the most important people in my life, i.e., my grandfather Late Shri Gopal Chatterjee, grandmother Late Smt. Subhankori Chatterjee, my father Shri Aloke Moy Chatterjee, my Late mother Ms. Nomita Chatterjee, and my uncle Shri Moni Moy Chatterjee. This book has been my long-cherished dream that would not have been turned into reality without the support and love of these amazing people. They continuously encouraged me despite my failure to give them the proper time and attention. I am also grateful to my friends, who have encouraged and blessed this work with their unconditional love and patience.

Jyotir Moy Chatterjee
Department of IT
Lord Buddha Education Foundation
(Asia Pacific University of Technology & Innovation)
Kathmandu 44600, Nepal

Chapter 1

COVID-19 pandemic analysis using application of AI

Pawan Whig[1], Rahul Reddy Nadikattu[2] and Arun Velu[3]

Abstract

COVID disease (COVID-19) is a disease with aggravation due to added infection. The infection triggers breathing infirmity through symptoms such as unruffled, flunky, and high temperature, for example, and the problem of relief in consistently genuine cases. Coronavirus 2019 takes as an overall pandemic, and multiple evaluations are being performed to forecast the fair development of this epidemic using different statistical models. The predicted pattern involves these mathematical models focused on different components and examinations. In this chapter, a model that may be useful for forecasting the distribution of COVID-19 is presented. Using support vector machine (SVM), linear regression, and naïve Bayes technique, we have conducted straight relapse. SVM with minimal mean absolute error and R^2 scores of 0.99599 for confirmed, 0.99429 for expired, and 0.97941 active cases are the best models completed. The outcome is seen and is equally consistent with the true one.

Keywords: COVID; Machine learning; Algorithms; Statistical models; Coronavirus; Linear regression; Support vector machine; Naïve Bayes; Epidemic; Fever; Temperature; Deep learning; Classifiers; Regression coefficient; Pandemic; Infectious; Artificial intelligence; Simulation

1.1 Introduction

As of now, 2.8 crore persons are confirmed COVID-19 across the world with more than 2% mortality. The expiry rate is rising, which is a troubling factor. Based on the form of spread and time, the transmission is categorized into four stages [1,2]. Different nations are imposing separate methods such as staying at home, using

[1]Department of IT, Vivekananda Institute of Professional Studies, New Delhi, India
[2]Department of IT, University of the Cumberlands, Williamsburg, USA
[3]Equifax, Atlanta, USA

wraps, constraints on movement outside home, preventing get-togethers, washing hands regularly, and disinfecting affected spots constantly due to a traditional attempt to combat the outbreak of infection. Several countries enforced lockdown declaration that would forestall the growth of the cases [3]. The stability and economy of the numerous nations are at risk due to this social division aspect and growth constraints [4]. The GDP of many countries plunged aggressively. A person is isolated when found infected, and appropriate care is provided [5,6]. Yet, it would cause damage in terms of severity and even people left with a higher degree of sufferings [7].

It is expected that the continuing epidemiological information investigations will create stronger activity plans against infection for general population [8]. This planet has been grappling fretfully with its inspiration since the introduction of the novel COVID-19. Through the severe acute respiratory syndrome (SARS) and Middle East respiratory syndrome (MERS) coronavirus community, coronavirus has a position with the underlying side-by-side signs of the communal cold to the extreme degree of breathing challenges causing breathing problems, sleepiness, high temperature, and dry hack. Many researchers have shown that imaging using immunoelectron microscopy techniques can enhance the detection of the infection. Itemized anatomy and ultrastructure of this virus are not well known to date and no explicit antibodies or medications are active for COVID-19. Nonetheless, several concurrent research preliminaries are testing probable medications [9].

Man-made logic (artificial intelligence (AI)) will allow us to cope with the problems posed by the COVID-19 pandemic [10]. In any case, it is not the only innovation that can change the data and imaginativeness of the people who use it, but also those who do not. In fact, a portion of the crucial shortcomings of AI will most likely be exposed by the COVID-19 crisis. AI (and machine learning (ML)) functions from the interpretation of chronicled data planning plans. Individuals have a favourite scenario over AI. We should consider one case from many and adapt them to new situations, building on our complex data to make the right decisions about what can succeed or what can happen. Then again, PC-based information structures need to start up even marginally without any preparation at some stage the context or mission shifts.

Consequently, the COVID-19 crisis would illustrate all that is reliably legitimate about AI: it is a gadget, and the estimation of its use under any situation is driven by the people who structure and use it. Human intervention and change would be especially important in the current crisis of leveraging the strength of what AI can do. One solution to managing the challenge of the new scenario is to compile new preparatory data under existing circumstances [11]. Each new piece of knowledge about our current situation is especially enormous in exhorting our decisions to continue, with both human explorers and AI systems the equivalent. The more realistic we are in exchanging details, the quicker our situation is not, now novel and we can start seeing a path ahead. Man-made intelligence will assist us in coping with the challenges posed by the COVID-19 pandemic [12]. In any case, it is not only the progress that would impact, but also the knowledge and imaginative minds of the people who use it [13].

In undeniable data processing, AI, the new kind of AI, operates by perceiving plans. Individuals have a favourite scenario over AI. We should take practices from one environment and adapt them to different contexts, building on our hypothetical evidence to allow the strongest speculations about what could or may occur [14]. Interestingly, mimicked information structures ought to be picked up even to some degree without some preparation at any stage of setting or undertaking changes. Thus, the COVID-19 crisis would contain something that has been substantial regarding AI reliably: it is a system, and the estimation of its use, in any case, is driven by the people who prepare and use it. Human intervention and development would be especially important in the current crises of leveraging the power of what AI can do. One solution to managing the challenge of the new scenario is to compile new preparatory data under existing circumstances. For the equivalent of both human bosses and AI systems, any new piece of data on our current situation is especially critical in clarifying our decision-making process [15]. The more convincing we are in exchanging details, the sooner our situation is not, the new now, and we can start seeing a road forward.

1.2 Literature survey

Computerized developments have assumed fundamental components in critical well-being field challenges, including infection counteraction; over the last decade, the latest overall well-being epidemic is still calling for mechanical support to cope with COVID-19 [16]. In a report, developers outlined the thinkable submissions of advanced know-hows, such as the Internet of Things, massive knowledge analysis, counterfeit intelligence (AI), in-depth learning, and blockchain engineering to establish procedures for pandemic observation, identification, and avoidance; and also, to understand the effects of the scourge on the field of medical services (Figure 1.1). Writers recommended an autoregressive integrated moving normal model in an examination paper sponsored by Boldog *et al.* to anticipate the distribution of COVID-19 [17].

Deb *et al.* recommended a time-arrangement approach to analyse the rate trend and the COVID-19 flare-up multiplication number evaluated. In order to illustrate the current epidemiological process of a district, they carried out measurable examinations to analyse the patterns of the flare-up with the aim of distinguishing various methods to solve the COVID-19 pandemic in different countries. It is important, according to the current circumstances, to consider the early spread dynamics of pollution in order to schedule and monitor persuasive protection steps. Sujath *et al.* suggested a logical model of simple SARS family propagation towards this direction by means of dissimilar datasets to analyse the COVID flare-up within and out of Wuhan [18].

As of late, in the light of numerous open datasets, there are a few reviews targeted at the epidemiological epidemic of COVID using experimental facts investigation. In Wuhan and the rest of the country, the inquiries essentially focus on the occurrence of affirmed, demise, and improved cases to understand the

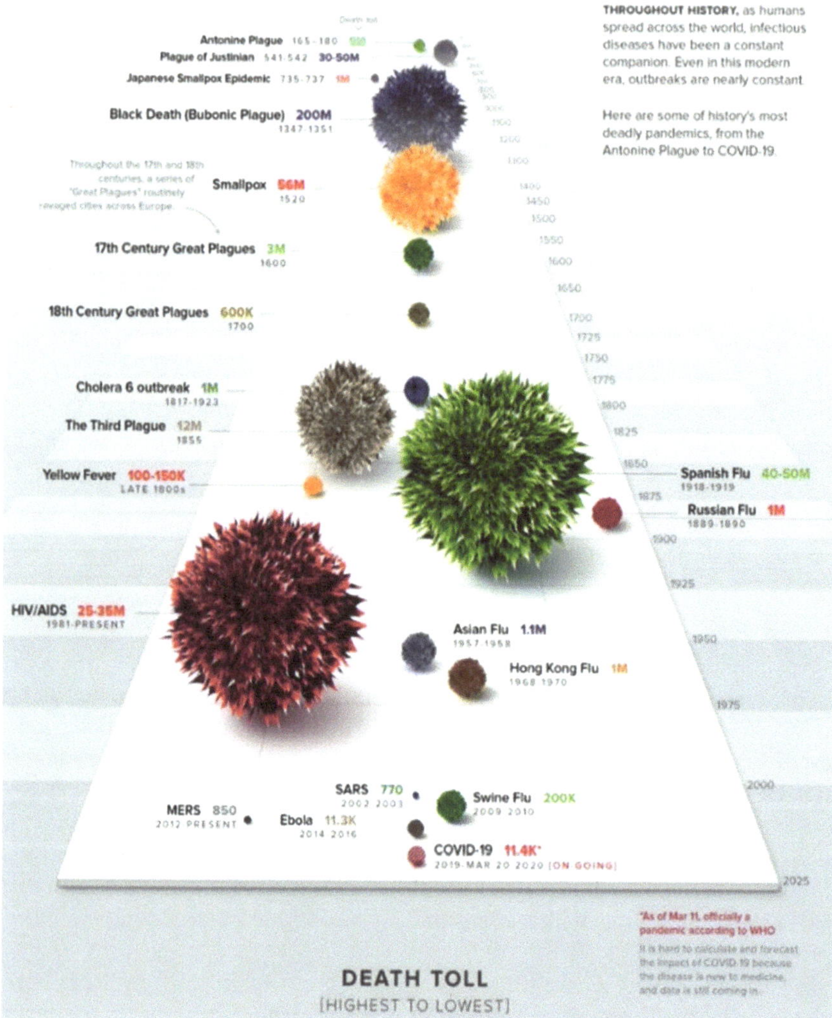
THROUGHOUT HISTORY, as humans spread across the world, infectious diseases have been a constant companion. Even in this modern era, outbreaks are nearly constant.
Here are some of history's most deadly pandemics, from the Antonine Plague to COVID-19.
Antonine Plague 165-180
Plague of Justinian 541-542 30-50M
Japanese Smallpox Epidemic 735-737 1M
Black Death (Bubonic Plague) 200M 1347-1351
Throughout the 17th and 18th centuries, a series of "Great Plagues" routinely ravaged cities across Europe.
Smallpox 56M 1520
17th Century Great Plagues 3M 1600
18th Century Great Plagues 600K 1700
Cholera 6 outbreak 1M 1817-1923
The Third Plague 12M 1855
Yellow Fever 100-150K LATE 1800s
Spanish Flu 40-50M 1918-1919
Russian Flu 1M 1889-1890
HIV/AIDS 25-35M 1981-PRESENT
Asian Flu 1.1M 1957-1958
Hong Kong Flu 1M 1968-1970
SARS 770 2002-2003
Swine Flu 200K 2009-2010
MERS 850 2012-PRESENT
Ebola 11.3K 2014-2016
COVID-19 11.4K* 2019-MAR 20 2020 (ON GOING)
*As of Mar 11, officially a pandemic according to WHO
DEATH TOLL
(HIGHEST TO LOWEST)

Figure 1.1 History of pandemic

related hazards and subsequent regulatory exercises. The question of the severity of the hatching time period for COVID was posed by Lauer *et al.* in their analysis work. A total of 181 affirmed cases were considered and found that the brooding cycle can fluctuate from 5 to 14 days and can be arranged on the basis of better observation and control exercises. Singer investigated evidence from 25 polluted districts in continuing examination work to meet transient assumptions regarding the 2019 episode of COVID-19. The study found that with different scaling instances, the clear speed of sickness spread of areas follows either consistent or unstable force law growth. The developers explored the influence of lockdown in many parts of the creation with this agreement [19–21]. In view of the previous writing, it is evident that adequate work on exploratory knowledge examination is available to grasp the existing pestilence trend, but at the same time, there are a lot of degrees to build and evaluate proficient AI-based forecast models such that constructive methodologies can be separated to cook the immediate necessities [22–24].

1.3 Dataset used for analysis

From 22 January 2020 to 20 December 2020, the COVID-19 regular popular knowledge was retrieved from the Johns Hopkins official archive. The dataset consists of regular case notes and overview tables for day-by-day time arrangements. In the current investigation, we needed some serious energy structure outline tables in comma-separated values (CSV) architecture that have three tables for COVID-19 affirmed, demise, and recovered instances with six ascribes, such as territory/state, nation/district, last change, affirmed, passing, and recovered instances, where the dataset update recurrence is once a day [25]. The following figure shows the circulation of COVID confirmed, recovered, and demise cases worldwide since the information was registered. The extraordinary production of the spread that should be monitored is anything but difficult to note. The web links of the dataset used are given in the following:

```
confirmed_df = pd.read_csv('https://raw.githubusercontent.com/CSSEGISan
dData/COVID19/master/csse_covid_19_data/csse_covid_19_time_series/time_
series_covid19_confirmed_global.csv')
deaths_df = pd.read_csv('https://raw.githubusercontent.com/CSSEGISandDa
ta/COVID19/master/csse_covid_19_data/csse_covid_19_time_series/time_ser
ies_covid19_deaths_global.csv')
recoveries_df = pd.read_csv('https://raw.githubusercontent.com/CSSEGISa
ndData/COVID19/master/csse_covid_19_data/csse_covid_19_time_series/time
_series_covid19_recovered_global.csv')
latest_data = pd.read_csv('https://raw.githubusercontent.com/CSSEGISand
Data/COVID-19/master/csse_covid_19_data/csse_covid_19_daily_reports/11-
15-2020.csv')
```

1.4 Various machine learning libraries

The COVID blowout has taken the earth under the threshold of destruction of lives because of which most extreme importance to break down the spread growth at the earliest and predict approaching prospects of the spread. The Python packages like ‘scikit-learn’ and ‘Keras’, respectively, AI, and deep learning methods are revised to anticipate the cumulative number of affirmed, restored, and moving cases worldwide. Following are numerous ML libraries used for conducting research (Figure 1.2).

ML is the science of software design a computer, as its name implies, by which they can learn from various data types. Arthur Samuel’s more general definition is

```
import numpy as np
import matplotlib.pyplot as plt
import matplotlib.colors as mcolors
import pandas as pd
import random
import math
import time
from sklearn.linear_model import LinearRegression, BayesianRidge
from sklearn.model_selection import RandomizedSearchCV, train_test_split
from sklearn.preprocessing import PolynomialFeatures
from sklearn.svm import SVR
from sklearn.metrics import mean_squared_error, mean_absolute_error
import datetime
import operator
plt.style.use('fivethirtyeight')
%matplotlib inline
import warnings
```

Figure 1.2 Various machine learning libraries

'machine learning is the area of research, which gives computers the ability to learn without explicit programming' [26–28]. Typically, they are used to solve different kind of life issues.

In the past, people have been using all the algorithms and mathematical and statistical formulas for the performance of master learning tasks manually. The process was tedious, inefficient, and time-consuming [29–31]. But today, compared to the past, Python libraries, frameworks, and modules are now very easy and efficient. Python is nowadays one of the most popular languages in the programming industry and has replaced many languages, a cause of which is the extensive library collection. In ML, Python libraries are as follows.

1.4.1 NumPy

NumPy is a popular Python library for processing large arrays and multi-dimensional arrays with a large number of advanced mathematical functions. It is well suited for basic scientific computing in ML [32]. It is particularly useful in linear algebra, Fourier transform, and random number generation. High-end libraries like TensorFlow use NumPy internally to manipulate Tensor.

1.4.2 SciPy

Because it includes optimization, linear algebra, integration, and statistics modules, SciPy is a popular Python library among ML enthusiasts [33]. There are differences between the SciPy library and the SciPy stack. SciPy is the basic package that constitutes the SciPy stack. SciPy can also perform image processing.

1.4.3 Scikit-learn

Scikit-learn is a popular ML library. It is built on top of NumPy and SciPy, the two basic Python libraries [34,35]. Scikit-learn supports most supervised and unsupervised learning algorithms. Scikit-learn can also be used for data mining and data analysis, making it a great tool for ML beginners.

1.4.4 Theano

ML is essentially math and statistics. Theano is a popular Python library for defining, evaluating, and optimizing the efficiency of mathematical expressions with multidimensional arrays [36,37]. The optimization of use of CPU and GPU is achieved. It is widely used to detect and diagnose various types of bugs for unit testing and self-verification. Theano is a powerful library which has been used for a long time in extensive scientific research in a computer-intensive manner but is simple and accessible enough for its own projects by individuals.

1.4.5 TensorFlow

TensorFlow is a popular open-source computer library developed by Google Brain's high-performance numerical computers team. TensorFlow is, as the name indicates, a frame that involves the definition and operation of tensor computations. It can develop and operate profound neural networks to develop multiple AI applications. TensorFlow is widely used in research and application in the field of deep learning [38].

1.4.6 Keras

Keras is a popular library for Python ML. The neural network API is a high-level network that works on TensorFlow, CNTK, or Theano. You can run both on CPU and GPU seamlessly. Keras is making the creation and design of a neural network for ML beginners. One of the best performances of Keras packages is that it makes prototyping simple and fast [39].

1.4.7 PyTorch

PyTorch is a popular library based on the open source and Lua wrapper learning machine library, which is developed in C. It has a lot of computer vision, natural language processing, and other ML techniques and libraries. It enables programmers to compute GPU-accelerated tensors and aids in the creation of computer graphs [40].

1.4.8 Pandas

Pandas is a well-known Python data analysis library. ML is not directly related. As we know, before training, the dataset needs to be prepared. Pandas comes handy in this case, because it was specially developed for data extraction and preparation. It offers high-level data structures and a broad range of data analytical tools. It offers numerous embedded methods to tap, mix, and filter data.

1.4.9 Matplotlib

Matplotlib is a Python library that is very popular for viewing data. Like Pandas, ML does not have a direct connection. It is especially useful if a programmer wishes to visualize data patterns. It is a library for the 2D plotting of 2D graphs and images. A pyplot module facilitates plotting for programmers because it provides control features for styling lines, font properties, axes for formatting, etc. It provides different types of diagrams and images to view data, for example, histograms, error diagrams, bar chats, etc.

1.5 Training and testing

The training observations are the experience used for learning in the algorithm. Each observation involves an output variable and more than one key input variable when learning issues are monitored.

The testing procedure is a series of findings used to assess the model's piece using a performance metric. There is refusal evidence of the exercise set in the test set. It is important. It will not be easier to review whether the procedure has become generalized by or merely memorized by the training set if the test set contains examples from the training package.

A programme that stores training information through an overwhelmingly composite model could accurately forecast the standards of the training set reply variable but does not predict the assessment of the reply variable for a new example. It is called overfitting that memorizes the training set. A programme which memorizes its observations cannot do its job properly, because it can memorize noise or coincidence relations and structures. Memorizing and generalizing, or overfitting and fitting, is a common issue for many algorithms for machine training. In order to reduce overfitting, regularization can be applied in many models. A third group of observations, known as validation or stoppage, is sometimes necessary in addition to the training and test data. The validation set is used to tune hyperparameters, which control the learning of the model. The programme remains assessed in the test set to assess its performance in the real world; its validation set performance should not be used to estimate the performance of the model in the real world since this programme is based on validation data in specific detail. The only group of supervise remarks is commonly divided keen on training, justification, and test set.

The size of the partitions is not required and may vary depending on the amount of data available. In the training set, 50% or more of the data are usually allocated, 25% are allocated to the test set, and the rest are validated. Certain training sets may contain only a few hundred observations. Unfavourable storage and network connectivity have all contribute to the current status of information or preparation groups with many examples. Smartphones with sensor packages and changing attitudes towards private lives have all contributed to this.

However, ML algorithms chase the basket inside, with the maximum wastage missing. A scholar who studies a large, puzzling error model will probably not become better than a scholar who reads a short but well-written book. In the same way, a trained algorithm for a large collection of ruined, irrelevant, or wrongly labelled data is not better than a more representative algorithm based on a smaller dataset which represents real problems.

Many controlled training sets are manually or semi-automated. In some fields, it may be expensive to create a large collection of supervised data. Luckily, quite a lot of datasets are bundle by means of scientists so that developers can concentrate instead on experiment on model.

A practise called cross-validation may be used for the development and validation of an algorithm on the same data, especially where training is limited. The training data are partitioned for cross-validation. The algorithm is taught with all other than one clock and experienced in the rest of the clock.

A well-generated programme can perform a task with new data effectively.

One of the most important mechanisms for mechanical learning is to develop the algorithm on a separate and separate training set for the test set. If this is not done, a model that cannot generalize unseen data is generalized. Sadly, this principle is not understood by all research teams.

Training and research were carried out using the scikit-learning library with a 20:80 ratio split ratio of training and testing. The relapse approach intended for scourge investigation is planned and checked on constant data by means of the number of cases of affirmed, rescued, and demise as the name for the day concerned. As a measuring work to test the relapse models, the mean squared error is the most commonly used target power and root mean square error.

1.6 Bias and variance

Many measures can be used to determine if a programme has learned more effectively to accomplish its task. Many performance measurements measure the number of prediction errors for supervised learning problems. Presently, there are two foremost causes of a model: bias and variance prediction error. Suppose you have training courses that are all exceptional to the population but similarly spokesperson. A highly biased representation will produce similar error for the effort regardless of the preparation set with which it was trained; it prefers its own assumptions about the true relationship with the training data. On the other hand, depending on the training set, a model with high variance produces various errors in the input.

In an ideal world, a representation will have both low partiality and difference, but the attempt to reduce one will often increase the extra – also called trade-off between bias and variance. Perhaps someone must take an account of the differences between different models introduced in this chapter. Uncontrolled knowledge troubles do not have an error signal to measure, as an alternative presentation metrics measure certain structural characteristics found within the data for uncontrolled study problems. Only for a specific type of task can most performance measures be developed.

ML systems should be assessed using performance measures which represent real-world error cost. The following example, while trivial, shows the make use of a presentation compute that is generally accurate for the task but not for its precise submission.

1.7 Result

The full details of the outcomes obtained are described in this section. Using the technique mentioned in the previous section, these findings were obtained. The consequences are examined after the analysis of the conclusions (Figures 1.3–1.7).

```
bayesian_confirmed = bayesian_search.best_estimator_
test_bayesian_pred = bayesian_confirmed.predict(bayesian_poly_X_test_co
nfirmed)
bayesian_pred = bayesian_confirmed.predict(bayesian_poly_future_forcast
)
print('MAE:', mean_absolute_error(test_bayesian_pred, y_test_confirmed)
)
print('MSE:',mean_squared_error(test_bayesian_pred, y_test_confirmed))
```

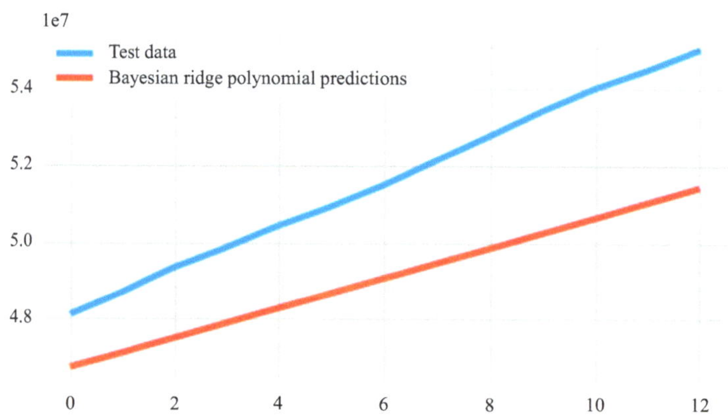

Figure 1.3 Bayesian polynomial prediction

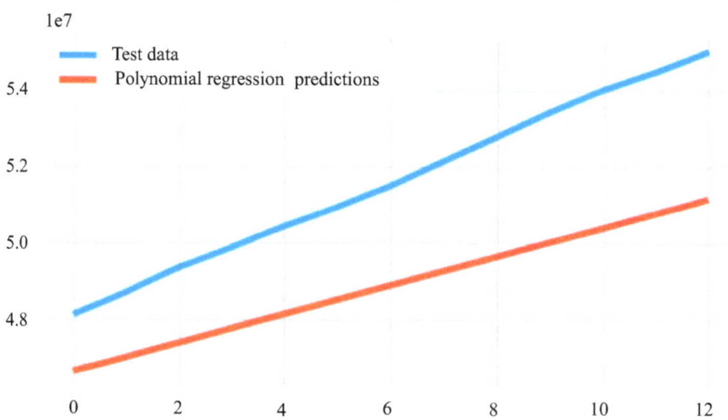

Figure 1.4 Polynomial regression prediction

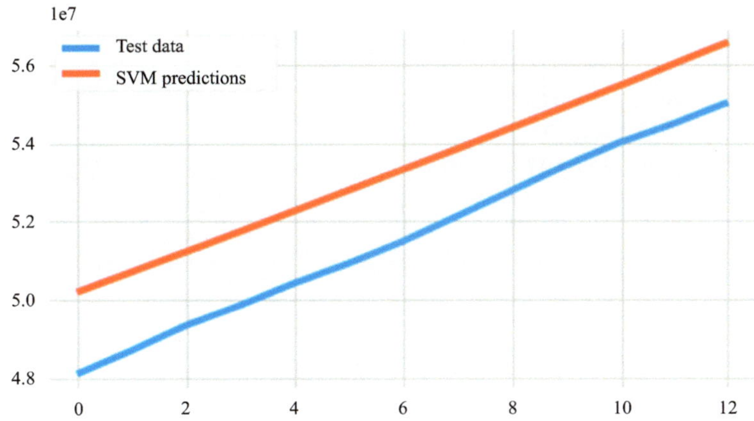

Figure 1.5 SVM prediction

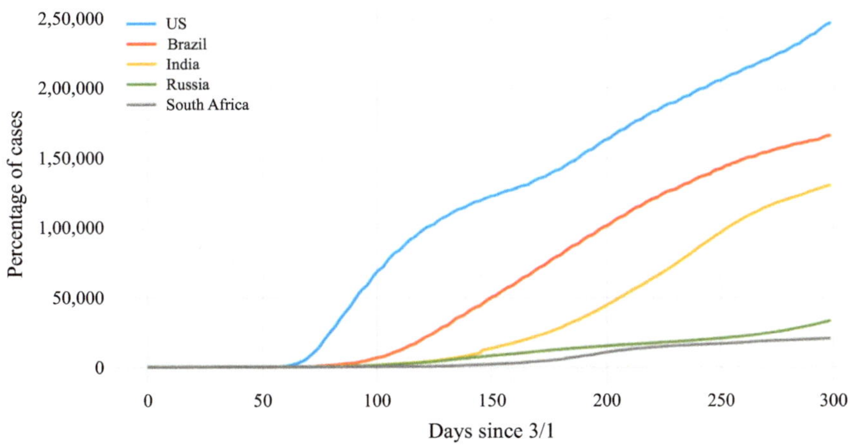

Figure 1.6 Coronavirus confirmed deaths cases

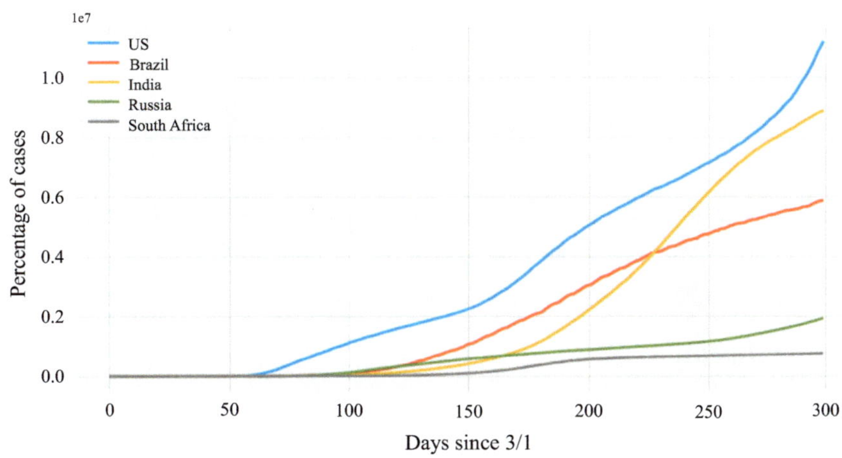

Figure 1.7 Coronavirus confirmed cases

Using the commands used above
MAE: 2519517.5968570937
MSE: 6857979171810.376

```
linear_model = LinearRegression(normalize=True, fit_intercept=False)
linear_model.fit(poly_X_train_confirmed, y_train_confirmed)
test_linear_pred = linear_model.predict(poly_X_test_confirmed)
linear_pred = linear_model.predict(poly_future_forcast)
print('MAE:', mean_absolute_error(test_linear_pred, y_test_confirmed))
print('MSE:',mean_squared_error(test_linear_pred, y_test_confirmed))
```

MAE: 2698714.792758974
MSE: 7865368274403.871

```
svm_test_pred = svm_confirmed.predict(X_test_confirmed)
plt.plot(y_test_confirmed)
plt.plot(svm_test_pred)
plt.legend(['Test Data', 'SVM Predictions'])
print('MAE:', mean_absolute_error(svm_test_pred, y_test_confirmed))
print('MSE:',mean_squared_error(svm_test_pred, y_test_confirmed))
```

Table 1.1 Comparison using different machine learning algorithms

Algorithm used	Bayesian search	Linear regression	SVM
R^2 confirmed	0.957443	0.96645	0.99599
R^2 expired	0.956738	0.96547	0.99429
R^2 active	0.957348	0.96666	0.97941

MAE: 1748047.8868652163
MSE: 3096060229804.693

Inference from Table 1.1

1. The values of mean absolute error and mean standard error are least in the support vector machine (SVM) algorithm which shows its efficiency in terms of speed and accuracy.
2. The value of the coefficient of regression is found to be closer to one in the case of SVM which indicates its accuracy and reliability over the other two algorithms used.

1.8 Conclusion

The planet is in the jaws of contamination with SARS-CoV2 (COVID-19). Early propagation estimation will help with the adoption of critical practices. Three types of algorithms have been compared and SVM produces better and more accurate results as compared to its two counterparts. This book chapter suggested using Johns Hopkins dashboard information to use AI and deep learning models for disease research. The analysis shows that one of the effective algorithms used for ML is the SVM help vector machine algorithm. In the case of the help vector machine algorithm, which reveals its precision, the value of mean absolute error is smaller. With a better and larger dataset, chances of a better accuracy increase. Researchers working in the same area are supported by this research study.

References

[1] R. Singh, R. Singh, and A. Bhatia "Sentiment analysis using machine learning technique to predict outbreaks and epidemics." *International Journal of Advanced Science and Research* (2018), 3(2), 19–24.

[2] D. S. Ting, L. Wei, V. D. Carin, and T. Y. Wong "Digital technology and COVID-19." *Nature Medicine* (2020), 1–3.

[3] D. Benvenuto, M. Giovanetti, L. Vassallo, S. Angeletti, and M. Ciccozzi "Application of the ARIMA model on the COVID-2019 epidemic dataset." *Data in Brief* (2020), 29, 105340.

[4] S. Deb and M. Majumdar "A time series method to analyze incidence pattern and estimate reproduction number of COVID-19." arXiv preprint arXiv:2003.10655 (2020).

[5] A. J. Kucharski, W. R. Timothy, C. Diamond *et al.* "Early dynamics of transmission and control of COVID-19: A mathematical modelling study." *The Lancet Infectious Diseases* (2020), 20, 553–558.

[6] S. K. Dey, Md. M. Rahman, U. R. Siddiqi, and A. Howlader "Analyzing the epidemiological outbreak of COVID-19: A visual exploratory data analysis (EDA) approach." *Journal of Medical Virology* (2020), 92, 632–638.

[7] R. Meredith, A. S. Azman, N. G. Reich, and J. Lessler "The incubation period of coronavirus disease 2019 (COVID-19) from publicly reported confirmed cases: Estimation and application." *Annals of Internal Medicine* (2020).

[8] H. M. Singer "Short-term predictions of country-specific Covid-19 infection rates based on power law scaling exponents." *International Conference on Electronic Devices, Systems, and Applications* arXiv preprint arXiv:2003.11997 (2020).

[9] Y. De Castro, F. Gamboa, D. Henrion, R. Hess, and J.-B. Lasserre "Approximate optimal designs for multivariate polynomial regression." *The Annals of Statistics* (2019), 47(1), 127–155.

[10] G. Klaus, R. K. Srivastava, J. Koutník, B. R. Steunebrink, and J. Schmidhuber "LSTM: A search space odyssey." *IEEE Transactions on Neural Networks and Learning Systems* (2016), 28(10), 2222–2232.

[11] U. Ojha and S. Goel "A study on prediction of breast cancer recurrence using data mining techniques." *Proceedings of the 7th International Conference Confluence 2017 on Cloud Computing, Data Science and Engineering*, pp. 527–530, 2017.

[12] S. Ghosh, S. Mondal, and B. Ghosh "A comparative study of breast cancer detection based on SVM and MLP BPN classifier," *1st International Conference on Automation, Control, Energy and Systems – 2014, ACES 2014*, pp. 1–4, 2014.
[13] A. Osareh and B. Shadgar "Machine learning techniques to diagnose breast cancer," *2010 5th International Symposium on Health Informatics and Bioinformatics, HIBIT 2010*, pp. 114–120, 2010.
[14] D. Bazazeh and R. Shubair "Comparative study of machine learning algorithms for breast cancer detection and diagnosis," *International Conference on Electronic Devices, Systems, and Applications*, pp. 2–5, 2017.
[15] M. S. B. M. Azmi and Z. C. Cob "Breast cancer prediction based on backpropagation algorithm," *Proceeding, 2010 IEEE Student Conference on Research and Development – Eng. Innov. Beyond, SCOReD 2010, no. SCOReD*, pp. 164–168, 2010.
[16] B. M. Gayathri and C. P. Sumathi "Comparative study of relevance vector machine with various machine learning techniques used for detecting breast cancer," *2016 IEEE International Conference on Computational Intelligence and Computing Research ICCIC 2016*, pp. 0–4, 2017.
[17] P. Boldog, T. Tekeli, Z. Vizi, A. Dénes, F. A. Bartha, and G. Röst "Risk assessment of novel coronavirus COVID-19 outbreaks outside China." *Journal of Clinical Medicine* (2020), 9(2), 571.
[18] R. Sujath, J. M. Chatterjee, and A. E. Hassanien "A machine learning forecasting model for COVID-19 pandemic in India." *Stochastic Environmental Research and Risk Assessment* (2020), 34, 959–972.
[19] A. Rupani, P. Whig, G. Sujediya, and P. Vyas "A robust technique for image processing based on interfacing of Raspberry-Pi and FPGA using IoT," *International Conference on Computer, Communications and Electronics (Comptelix)*, IEEE Xplore, 18 August 2017.
[20] P. Whig and A. Rupani "The development of big data science to the world." *Engineering Reports* (2019), 2(2), 1–7.
[21] P. Whig "Artificial intelligence and machine learning in business." *Engineering Reports* (2019), 2(2), 8–13.
[22] J. B. Chacko and P. Whig "Low delay based full adder/subtractor by MIG and COG reversible logic gate," *2016 8th International Conference on Computational Intelligence and Communication Networks (CICN)*, IEEE Xplore, 26 October 2017.
[23] C. Iwendi, A. K. Bashir, A. Peshkar *et al.* "COVID-19 patient health prediction using boosted random forest algorithm." *Frontiers in Public Health* (2020), 8, 357.
[24] S. Dhamodharavadhani, R. Rathipriya, and J. M. Chatterjee "COVID-19 mortality rate prediction for India using statistical neural network models." *Frontiers in Public Health* (2020), 8.
[25] P. Agarwal and P. Whig "Low delay based 4 bit QSD adder/subtraction number system by reversible logic gate," *2016 8th International Conference on Computational Intelligence and Communication Networks (CICN)*, IEEE Xplore, 26 October 2017.

[26] Covid19India.org (2020). India Covid-19 Tracker 2020. Available from www.covid19india.org/. Accessed on 7 April 2020.

[27] B. M. Weon "Doubling time tells how effective Covid-19 prevention works." medRxiv (2020). Available from www.medrxiv.org/content/10.1101/2020.03.26.20044644v1. Accessed on 4 April 2020.

[28] Google (2020). See how your community is moving around differently due to COVID-19. Available from www.gstatic.com/covid19/mobility/2020-03-29_IN_Mobility_Report_en.pdf. Accessed on 6 April 2020.

[29] Covid19India.org (2020). India Covid-19 Tracker 2020. Available from docs.google.com/spreadsheets/d/e/2PACX1vSc_2y5N0I67wDU38DjD h35IZSIS30 rQf7_NYZhtYYGU1jJYT6_kDx4YpFqw0LSlGsBYP8pqM_a1Pd/pubhtml. Accessed on 7 April 2020.

[30] S. P. Borgatti "Centrality and network flow." *Social Networks* (2005), 27(1), 55–71.

[31] T. Dwyer, S. H. Hong, D. Koschützki, F. Schreiber, and K. Xu "Visual analysis of network centralities," *Proceedings of the 2006 Asia-Pacific Symposium on Information Visualisation*–Volume 60, pp. 189–197, 2006, January.

[32] BBC News. "Coronavirus: Search for hundreds of people after Delhi prayer meeting." *BBC News* (2020). Available from www.bbc.com/news/world-asia-india-52104753. Accessed on 2 April 2020.

[33] S. Biswas "Will coronavirus lockdown cause food shortages in India?" *BBC News* (2020). Available from www.bbc.com/news/world-asia-india-52176564. Accessed on 7 April 2020.

[34] Y. Yadav "India lost more jobs due to coronavirus lockdown than US did during Depression." *The Print* (2020). Available from https://theprint.in/opinion/india-lost-more-jobsdue-to-coronavirus-lockdown-than-us-did-during-depression/397693/. Accessed on 8 April 2020.

[35] Press Trust of India. "Coronavirus: 1,445 cases liked to Tablighi Jamaat event, total crosses 4,000." *India Today News* (2020). Available from www.indiatoday.in/india/story/coronavirus-1-445-cases-liked-to-tablighi-jamaate-vent-total-crosses-4-000-1663962-2020-04-06. Accessed on 7 April 2020.

[36] P. L. Tu and J. Y. Chung "A new decision-tree classification algorithm for machine learning," *Proceedings Fourth International Conference on Tools with Artificial Intelligence TAI'92*, pp. 370–377. IEEE, 1992, November.

[37] C. M. Musil, C. B. Warner, P. K. Yobas, and S. L. Jones "A comparison of imputation techniques for handling missing data." *Western Journal of Nursing Research* (2002), 24(7), 815–829.

[38] M. Awad and R. Khanna "Support vector regression." In *Efficient Learning Machines*, pp. 67–80. Apress, Berkeley, CA, 2015.

[39] AlJazeera. "India: Coronavirus lockdown sees exodus from cities." *Aljazeera News Channel* (2020). Available from www.aljazeera.com/programmes/newsfeed/2020/04/india-coronavirus-lockdownsees-exodus-cities-200406104405477.html. Accessed on 6 April 2020.

[40] K. Garari "4.1 days doubling time for Coronavirus worrisome." *Deccan Chronicle* (2020). Available from www.deccanchronicle.com/nation/current-affairs/070420/41-daysdoubling-time-for-coronavirus-worrisome.html. Accessed on 7 April 2020.

Chapter 2

M-health: a revolution due to technology in healthcare sector

Mayuri Diwakar Kulkarni[1], *Ashish Suresh Awate*[1] *and Jyotir Moy Chatterje*[2]

Abstract

The term "lockdown" was introduced due to the COVID-19, and it drastically transformed the lifestyle of the human being. Before COVID-19 hit our society, we used to go to hospitals or clinics even for the same health issues, where doctors used to do clinical tests by physical examination. But this has drastically changed for COVID-19 norms; the physical examination is only applicable in critical care scenarios. Still in human life there are some diseases such as diabetes and blood pressure that are not critical but need regular consultation. Therefore, digitalization and communication revolution provide an effective solution, where basic consultation and patient monitoring can be performed easily through digital communication channels such as mobile phones, apps, or video-conferencing calls.

In this pandemic situation, it is necessary to maintain social distancing, and restriction has been imposed on traveling, which brings a greater restriction on how to do real-time monitoring of a patient from any location at any instant of time. This problem can easily be solved with the introduction of m-health technology in healthcare sector. It uses digital applications for remote monitoring, remote data collection, diagnosis, and treatment support. This revolutionary development has made diagnosis and prediction of diseases much convenient at early stages. Because of this, the human health problem is minimized.

This chapter will discuss how the m-health technology helps patients as well as healthcare workers. Due to this real-time monitoring, a patient can easily be diagnosed from his/her place. The chapter comprises what is m-health, working of m-health technology, impact of m-health technology on society. Also, this provides insight on all the aspects in m-health technology.

Keywords: M-health; IoT; COVID-19; Mobile technologies; Healthcare; WHO

[1]Department of Computer Engineering, SVKM's Institute of Technology, Dhule, DBATU Lonere, India
[2]Department of IT, LBEF, Asia Pacific University of Technology and Innovation, Kathmandu, Nepal

2.1 Introduction

Due to the outbreak of COVID-19 all over the world, transformation to a maximum extent to online service–based system has started. This transformation also took place in medical sector. This sector makes medical facilities available to patients on a digital platform. This digital platform provides support to patients either by making an appointment with a doctor or by online pharmaceutical ordering of medicines. This digital platform has enhanced the role in the sectors from booking, ordering to the online visiting to the clinics through video conferencing or through online meetings. Not only are these all, but also electronic health records are kept at doctors as well as patient's place. Due to this, the delays can be reduced. Hence, we can say that a digital platform has increased the reliability in healthcare sector too. But how has this transformation happened? It is not a change in a day.

Initially World Health Organization (WHO) introduced the information communication technology (ICT) in healthcare system. This concentrates on health education, record keeping, and data management [1]. From ICT, it is transformed toward e-health. This e-health is an electronic health system in which electronic processes and usage of Internet are more important. This e-health consists of ten e's in healthcare sector such as efficiency, enhancing quality, evidence based, empowerment, encouragement, education, enabling, extending, ethics, equality along with those additional features such as easy-to-use, entertaining, and exciting [2]. Later m-health introduced a system that focuses on various services to be offered, due to which mortality rate can be reduced. In addition, enhancement takes place due to the introduction of Internet of Things (IoT).

This online service system needs real-time data; hence the role of IoT introduced. The IoT comprises sensors, processors, and actuators connected to Internet. The use of IoT in the medical field provides real-time and accurate data to the medical practitioners. The adoption of IoT in the healthcare sector saves life by diagnosing and predication disease, followed by healing or counseling of patients and their beloved ones [3]. This provides more relief to patients in this pandemic situation where they need to always follow the guidelines of social distancing and lockdown regulations.

As per the WHO, m-health is defined as the "use of mobile and wireless technologies to support the achievement of health objectives." And as per the National Institutes of Health [4–6], m-health is "the use of mobile and wireless devices (cell phones, tablets, etc.) to improve health outcomes, health care services, and health research" [7].

2.1.1 History of m-health

The technology that generates, accumulates, and exchanges the medical information through wireless and mobile devices is known as m-health. Today we are using a wide variety of devices and applications such as diet apps, sleep monitoring, and fitness tracker. This all started way back in 1949 when AT&T introduced the first cell phone. But at times due to barriers of technology and lack of use, mobile devices had limited functionalities. As time went on the mobile industry grew rapidly with the introduction of smart phones, which opened the door for building and deploying mobile health applications. The mobile health industry grows rapidly and nowadays 50% of physicians use m-health applications to track their patients on a daily basis. But the mobile health application industry has been facing challenges due to lack of proper guidelines from government authority and legislation associated with it.

Today the mobile health industry is getting a big hand with wearable devices and associated applications. This wearable devices industry grows rapidly with an annual growth reported more than 20% each year [8]. Some common wearable technologies that had impact on the mobile health industry include smart watches, smart glasses, wristbands, footwear, and smart clothing. As the m-health industry continues to grow over the coming years, both wearable technologies and smartphone's capabilities likely positively impact the healthcare field and help to improve patient's care across the nation.

After the recommendation of the introduction of m-health in healthcare sector, a certain number of initiatives were taken by the various countries as follows:

- Inclusion of mobile technology to communicate various health-related issues.
- Testing and evaluating the use of m-health in a given situation.
- Conduction of ongoing programs using m-health.

2.1.2 What is m-health?

WHO categorizes the m-health services into 14 sectors (Figure 2.1). These services are health call centers, toll-free telephone services for the emergency, emergency management, disaster management, telemedicine, appointment booking, alert, community mobilization, health promotion, treatment compliance, data collection, decision support system, surveillance, and health awareness raising [9].

The roles of these services are explained briefly in the following:

Low-cost fastest communication is possible through the **messaging system**, transmitting messages through mobiles. This messaging system is available to users to offer information about testing and treatment method, availability of the health services. It is a very effective way to reach a wide spectrum of people in less time with lesser efforts. This one-way interactive tool is used for communication.

Data collection is used to gather the real-time data through the mobile phones, PDAs, or smart phones. This data gathering technique helps for engaging an effective use of information for various purposes such as analysis and diagnosis. By analyzing, data stakeholders can make some appropriate decisions.

Monitoring patients with the help of mobile technologies helps in an improvement of survival rate of patients. This is possible through **remote monitoring** for communicable diseases.

The shortage of healthcare workers in the developing countries may affect health services. Hence connecting to these healthcare workers with a source or mobile technology provides huge support. This will bridge the gap between patients and healthcare professionals.

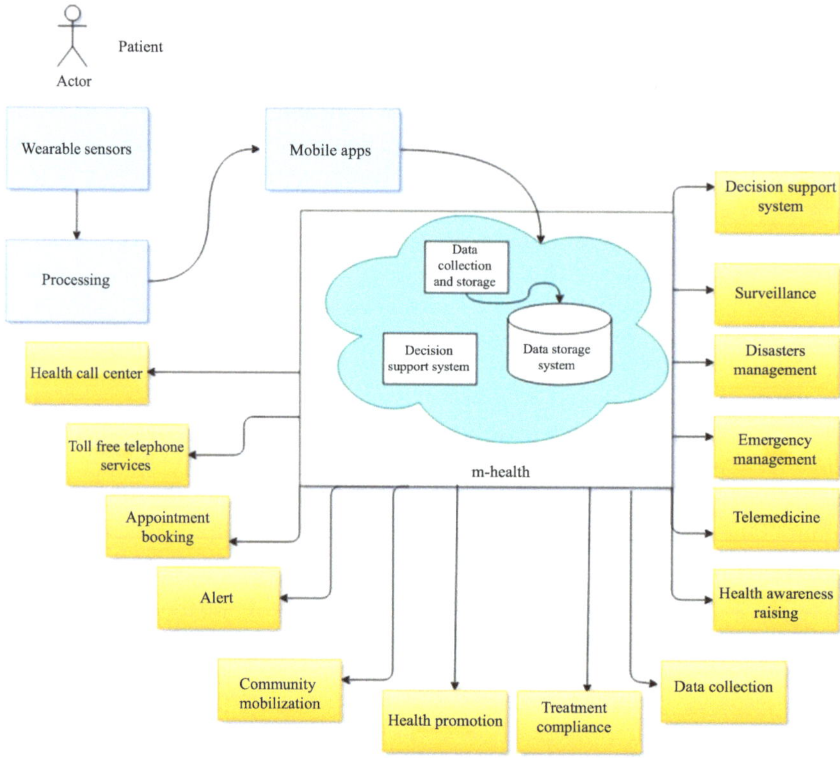

Figure 2.1 Overview of m-health

To **diagnose** the patient sitting at a remote place and providing the appropriate treatment is a very crucial task in the case of m-health. This would minimize the visits to hospitals and provide appropriate treatment to villages also. This facilitates providing appropriate symptoms and real-time monitored data of patients.

Through these calling and SMS services, arousing mass awareness is easily possible by connecting experts and patients who seek improvement. Patients get more benefits through this in comparison with visiting the clinics.

In the case of any disaster or pandemic-like situation, the use of SMS reaches each and every person who has mobile services. Due to this, the precautionary or primary relief to the needy people is easily available.

The probable date of vaccination, visit to experts' place, or **alert notifications** to the affected people will minimize the barrier in healthcare sector. This leads to appropriate medication facilities amongst the patients. This leads to fast cure for the diseases. This will help to improve the health status of a patient. Notifications alter the follow-ups process and improve treatment system that will be encountered.

Based upon all these assumptions and technological development along with the socioeconomic status of people, the m-health services are offered to the overall population. The prime concerns of m-health among these 14 services are [10] as follows:

Road traffic accidents, emergency obstetric care as emergency response system:

- Diseases like malaria, flu, diabetes, HIV/AIDS, TB surveillance, and control.
- Human resource management, supervision, and coordination.
- Telemedicine diagnostic and decision support for medical practitioners at a point of care, either synchronous or asynchronous mode.
- Clinical care and remote patient monitoring.
- Health monitoring and report collection.
- Health promotion, extension services, and community mobilization.
- M-learning related to healthcare among the public.
- Training for healthcare workers.

M-health is a part of e-health. The definition suggested by the WHO for m-health is medical and public health practice supported by mobile devices. This also includes the patient monitoring devices such as wearable sensors, personal digital assistants, and other wireless devices [9]. In a more precise way, Robert Istepanian in 2004 defines m-health as "mobile computing, medical sensor, and communications technologies for health care" [10] (Figure 2.2).

M-health is generally used in a field where it is determined, and treatment of diseases is dependent upon the reports of patients. This is feasible for patients to collect and share relevant data at any time without visiting a clinic. This also allows rapid convergence to optimal treatment.

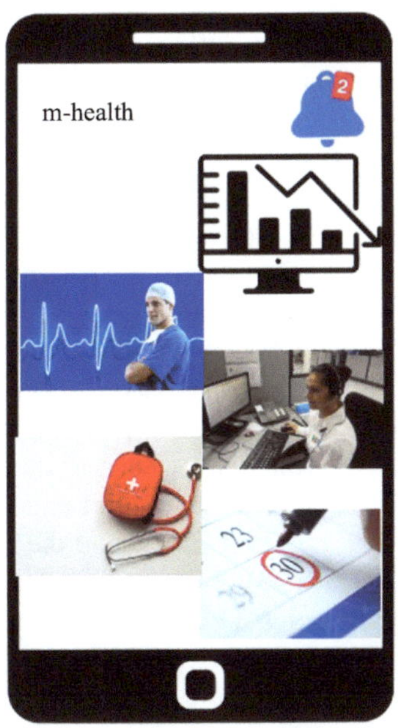

Figure 2.2 Services on mobiles

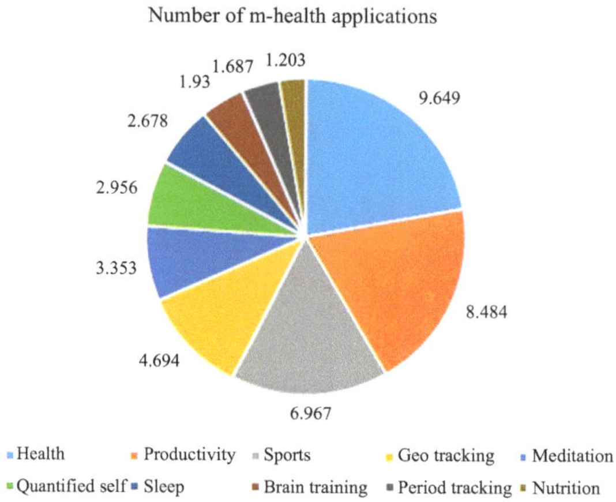

Figure 2.3 Use of different types of m-health apps globally used [12]

According to Statista, on the Google Play Store about 47,140 apps are available in the third quarter of 2020. This number rapidly grew in the last 5 years. In 2015, the numbers of apps present on the same platform were around 27,417 [11].

The use of different types of m-health apps is shown in Figure 2.3 [12]. These apps are for health monitoring such as productivity, sports, tracking, nutrition, sleep pattern, period tracking, and brains training.

2.1.3 Adoption of m-health by various countries

The use of m-health in **Australia** emphasizes diseases as cardiovascular and non-communicable that provide the services such as voice calling, text messaging, and mobile application support. In **China** m-health focuses on diseases such as cardiovascular diseases, diabetes, HIV, and hemophilia using text messaging and mobile applications. In **Malaysia**, the data is collected from the sensors, which depends upon inputs available from the sensors, addressed to the patient compliance. Countries like **New Zealand** adopted point-of-care devices and mobile videos to address issues of cardiovascular care, smoking, and adherence along with text messaging services. **Vietnam** focuses on education community–based physician's assistance for maternal and child health. **Cambodia** uses the service such as text messaging and follow-up of the patient using alert services for the disease such as diabetes and cleft palate issue. **South Korea** uses a disease diagnostic system and patient monitoring for skin diseases. **Singapore** uses text messaging for addressing the issue of asthma [13].

In **India**, there are a total of 73 mobile- or web-based applications developed and maintained by the Govt. of India. The developed apps are concentrating all the services to be offered by m-health as per the guidelines by the WHO.

The health app users in various countries are shown in Figure 2.4. The statistics shows, **China** is the leading country with 65% app users and India is the second most leading country with 63%.

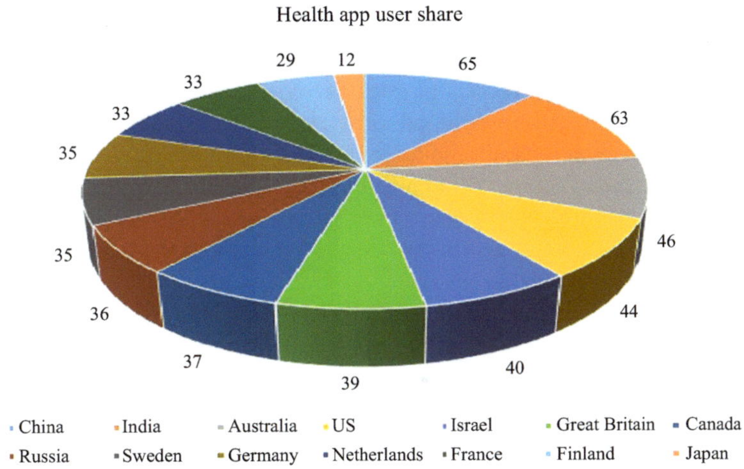

Figure 2.4 Usage of m-health applications all over world [14]

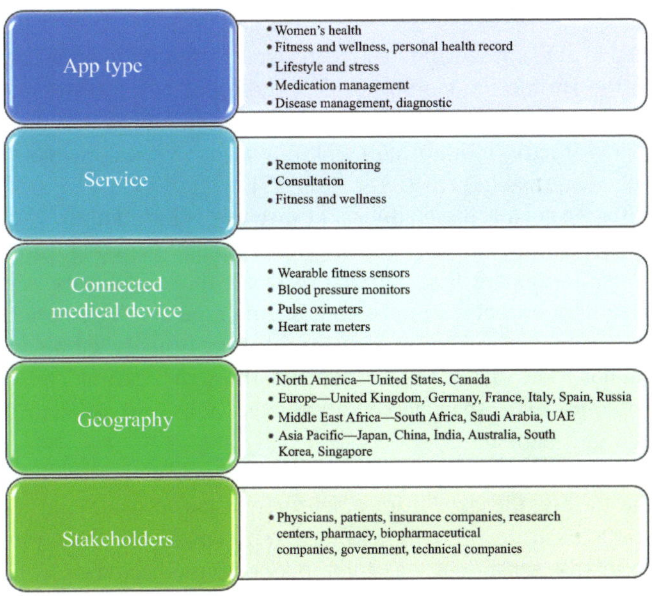

Figure 2.5 Segmentation of m-health app

M-health app has been segmented by types, services, connected medical devices, geography, and stakeholders [15,16]. This is explained in detail as shown in Figure 2.5.

App type segment contains fitness, wellness, and medication record keeping. This segment concentrates only on the day-to-day activities of patients, physician as well as the data maintained by the front-end health workers.

Service segment focuses on the aspects of remote monitoring, consultations with the wellness, and fitness issues.

Connected medical device segment uses wearable fitness sensors to monitor regular activities during exercise, physical activities, etc. The wearable sensors monitor blood pressure using a blood pressure sensor, monitor oxygen level of patients using an oximeter, monitor glucose in diabetic patients using a glucose-meter, monitor cardiovascular diseases using a heart rate (HR) sensor with wearable ECG.

Geography segment comprises various regions such as North America, Europe, Middle East Africa, and Asia Pacific. From these regions, various countries have adopted m-health services.

Stakeholder segment is nothing but physicians use this data from the m-health app and use that to diagnose disease, monitor health condition of patients. The biopharmaceuticals use this data to know the reactions of the medicines prescribed by a physician and depend upon that they can make the possible changes in the medicines. Government sector people use this data to manage the public health during critical conditions. Nowadays, data from the hospitals is used by the insurance providers to settle any claim.

2.1.4 Role of IoT in m-health

Sensors are used to sense real-time data. This data is used by medical practitioners. The data from the Biometric Monitoring Technologies can transform digital biomarkers for diagnosing and monitoring various diseases. Hence it is included in the m-health. These biometric monitoring technologies use various sensors to monitor HR, sleeping pattern, insulin sensitivity, etc. [17].

In the healthcare sector, the diagnosis of diseases is based upon various factors such as visual observation, touch sensing, or through listening problems from patients. All these things are incorporated in smart mobile phones. Visual observations of patients by a doctor are possible using cameras. A camera can capture images and takes videos of the patients. Later that data is analyzed by doctors using images and videos. The diagnosis of patients through hearing can be possible through microphones. The speech recognition technology is used to analyze the health condition of a patient.

The smart mobile phones consist of various sensors and wearable sensors connected. Due to this, the data from a sensor will be accessible at the m-health app. The sensors present in a mobile and wearable sensors are shown in Figure 2.6 that shows the inbuilt sensor such as microphone, camera, and externally we can connect required sensors such as glucose-meter, oximeter, and HR sensor.

Apart from mobile, various wearable devices are available from the companies like Apple, Sony, Samsung that manufacture products like smart watches, bracelets, headsets, and lenses. These devices monitor HR, sleep activity pattern, brain monitoring, glucose monitoring, and stroke monitoring, etc. [18].

Table 2.1 shows the externally connected sensors as well as inbuilt sensors present in a smart mobile phone to monitor real-time data to diagnose the medical condition of a patient [19].

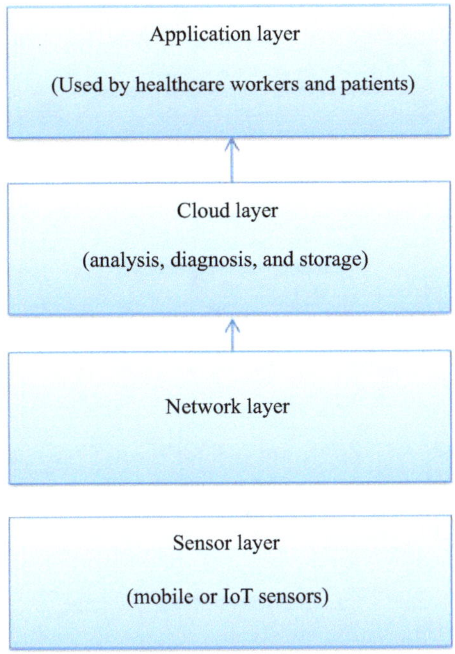

Figure 2.6 M-health with IoT devices

Table 2.1 Use of IoT in m-health

Sr. no	Monitoring disease	Sensors in mobiles	Additional sensors
1	Stress monitoring	Camera, fingerprint scanner, ambient light sensor, accelerometer/gyroscope, microphone, GPS, touch screen, Bluetooth [20]	Smart watch—heart rate sensor
2	Cardiovascular activity	Camera, microphone	Pulse sensor, ECG (wearable)
3	COVID-19	Microphone	Oximeter
4	Diabetes	–	Glucose sensor
5	Skin disease	Camera	–
6	Neurological disorders	–	EEG (wearable)
7	Eye health	Camera	–
8	Activity monitoring	Accelerometer, GPS, gyroscope, proximity sensor	–
9	Mental health and cognitive	Accelerometer, GPS, gyroscope, light sensor, camera, microphone	–
10	Respiratory and lung health	Microphone, camera	–

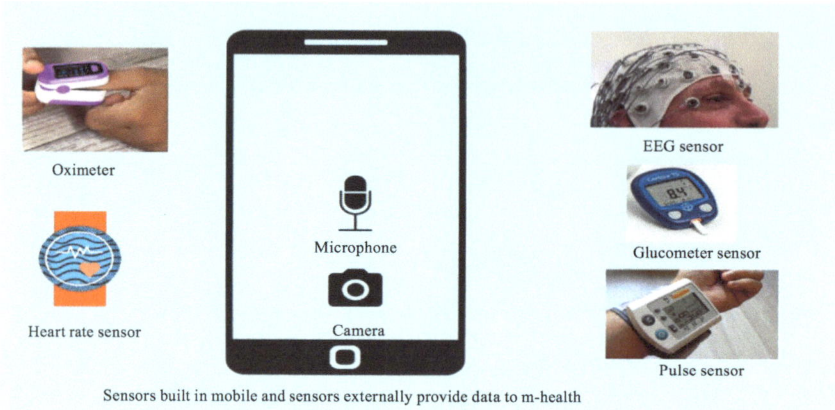

Figure 2.7 Layers in IoT for m-health systems

The IoT in an m-health uses the layered architecture. It consists of four layers such as sensor or physical layer, network layer, cloud layer, and application layer. The details of these layers are as follows:

Sensor layer: To a sensor layer various sensors are connected. These sensors receive real-time data that is given to the m-health application. Hence a sensor layer plays a very important role in the m-health application. Due to the availability of this real-time data, doctors can diagnose the level of a disease very accurately. This sensed data from the sensors is physical data that is then converted to digital form. This data later given to the network layer.

Network layer: Using various connectivity media such as Bluetooth, Wi-Fi, or Internet makes the data available in the network layer. The data is transferred from the network layer to cloud layer.

Cloud layer: This layer stores the data that can be used for analytics, diagnosis, or only for the storage. The analyzer system used the data for diagnosis purpose or for predictions and for preventive measures. The stored data at this cloud layer such as information of a patient and geographical details can be used at a time of disaster management. Data from the cloud is supplied to the application layer.

Application layer: This application layer provides data at an m-health app. These apps are used by patients, physicians, etc.

Figure 2.7 shows the layered architecture used in m-health sector [8].

2.1.4.1 Use of m-health during COVID-19

In China, NTCC established an Emergency Telemedicine Consultation (ETC) System that alerts and responds to the network. This ETC is built upon a doctor-to-doctor approach. This uses three-layered architecture such as telemedicine service platform, telemedicine cloud layer, and telemedicine service application layer [21]. A telemedicine service platform is used by specialists and health workers in regional hospitals to provide immediate diagnosis and consultation. This is used for consulting with patients, for education and training, patient monitoring, etc. This could reduce the spread of COVID-19. The middle layer is a telemedicine cloud layer that allows capture, store, and processing of patient records. Due to this, appropriate treatment can be possible. The telemedicine service application layer features consultation from experts' treatment team to municipal hospitals, country level hospitals to fight against COVID-19 [21].

M-health plays a crucial role in monitoring the COVID-19 infected people who are in home quarantine or self-quarantine using various mobile apps. This also analyzes the patient's symptoms using wearable devices and through which it monitors whether it is required to admit a patient in a hospital. These wearable devices monitor pulse rate and sleep patterns [22].

2.1.5 M-health to maintain social distancing

The main motto of introducing m-health by the WHO in the healthcare sector is to reach out to each patient or to the healthcare expert so that they either will be relieved or to monitor, consult, or to educate using mobile apps. In the pandemic COVID-19 where until the introduction of vaccines for COVID-19, only the preventive major stated by the WHO are social distancing and wearing mask with sanitization. In such scenarios, m-health played a very important role such as guiding people through the apps, monitoring home quarantine people using these apps, medical record sharing, and bringing pharmaceutical support to patients through home delivery of drugs. Not only this, but also contact tracing, maintaining social distancing using proximity sensors or using wireless networks, etc. are the other ways [23].

2.2 Discussion

2.2.1 M-health to maintain social distancing

Cardiovascular health monitoring is monitored by the physicians using ECG as well as embedded sensors such as camera and microphone. Skin diseases are monitored using videos: videos of bare skin of fingertip as inputs. The video is monitored by the doctors, and depending on videos, skin diseases are diagnosed. Front and back camera used to monitor the heart as well as respiration rate. Wearable ECG is used to check cardiovascular diseases. By using images of eye fundus diagnosis of diabetic macular edema, diabetic retinopathy (DR) is made possible. This can be done through a smartphone camera. Similarly, skin diseases can be diagnosed using images. This helps experts to identify skin cancer cell carcinoma, squamous cell carcinoma, and melanoma. Mental health monitoring can be possible through sensors such as accelerometers, GPS, microphones, and cameras present in smartphones. This determines the daily stress, sleep patterns, geospatial activities, and kinesthetic activity to monitor health conditions [19].

2.2.2 Impact of m-health during COVID-19

During COVID-19, 79.5% showed their interest to adopt m-health in China [24]. WHO launched a dedicated messaging service with the WhatsApp and Facebook to keep people safe during the pandemic. WHO used the messaging languages as Arabic, English, French, Hindi, Italian, Spanish, and Portuguese, and due to this, it is possible to reach out up to 2 billion people by providing latest information regarding COVID-19. WHO also provided the latest COVID-19 reports, because of this, decision-making becomes easier [25].

To combat COVID-19, the m-health app plays a very essential role. These 115 health apps help people to combat COVID-19 by providing various features. The app development is mostly done by governments or by the Ministry of Health. The 99% apps were free and developed by the governments, for their citizens to combat COVID-19 [26]. Table 2.2 indicates the apps designed by various countries.

Maximum applications are developed and maintained by the Govt. of United States, which are 28, to fight against COVID-19. India is at second position with five apps. The counties like Italy, Kingdom of Saudi Arabia, Mexico, Spain, Vietnam, and Global developed four apps.

These apps are developed and designed by the various governments as the data or the information of the people is sensitive.

Table 2.3 shows m-health apps introduced by various countries during pandemic COVID-19. The table also shows that the usage in a form of downloads in the table itself also explains the usage of the m-health app for various purposes such as contact tracing [27], geo-location identification of the users, notification as well as consultation.

From Table 2.3, it is clear that m-health in COVID-19 is used for data collection. This collected data is used by a person to know the contacts and approximate contact time whenever he/she is infected due to COVID-19. From that it is easily possible to know the count of people who may have chances of being infected. This collected data is used to avoid disasters. Due to this, the health force receives an alert and they can prepare accordingly. On the other hand, it helps a general user by a timely notification system.

Table 2.2 COVID-19 m-health app developed by various countries

Sr. no.	Number of apps [26]	Country [26]
1	28	United States
2	5	India
3	4	Italy, Kingdom of Saudi Arabia, Mexico, Spain, Vietnam, Global
4	3	Canada, Australia, France, Netherlands, UAE
5	2	Malaysia, Ireland, South Korea, United Kingdom
6	1	Armenia, Austria, Bahrain, Bolivia, Brazil, Columbia, Czechia, Denmark, Egypt, Georgia, Hungary, Indonesia, Iceland, Jamaica, Jordan, Kuwait, Latvia, Mali, Morocco, New Zealand, North Macedonia, Pakistan, Poland, Portugal, Qatar, Republic of Cyprus, Republic of Fiji, Romania, Singapore, Sri Lanka, Switzerland, Thailand, Tunisia, Turkey, and Uruguay

Table 2.3 Features of various m-health apps designed by various counties with the number of downloads/users

Sr. no	Country	App	Features	Language	Downloads
1	India	Aarogya Setu App [28]	Contact Tracing app, Geo-location-based COVID-19 statistics ICMR-approved labs information, risk status users	English, Hindi, Marathi, Gujarati, Bengali, Punjabi, Odia, Telugu, Tamil, Malayalam, Assamese	1,569,600 [29]
2	Canada	COVID alert [30]	Notification app that alerts before the symptom of COVID-19, Contact tracing	–	6,557,294
3	Canada	ABTrace Together	Contact tracing app	–	
4	United Kingdom	NHS COVID-19 app	Trace, Alert, Check-In, Symptoms, Test, and Isolate [31]	English, Welsh, Bengali, Urdu, Gujarati, Punjabi, Chinese, Romanian, Turkish, Arabic, Polish, Somali [32]	
5	United Kingdom	COVID-19 NI mobile app [33]	COVID-19 Symptom Checker, Advice, and guidance "chatbot" [33]	–	–
6	Australia	Coronavirus Australia app [34]	Updates of COVID-19 and symptoms checker	–	1 million
7	Australia	COVID-SAFE [35]	Contract tracing and official assistance to understand and contain spread of COVID-19	–	7 million

In the case of home isolation conditions by calling the affected patient, health workers can advise on the safety precautions as well as counseling to the patients. This m-health record keeping software avoids the visits of patients to clinics.

2.2.3 Global government initiatives on e-health and m-health

The policy reforms in healthcare play an important role in the adoption of m-health. These policies need to be consumer-friendly and must have win–win situations for both service user and provider. Globally, various countries' governments are already taking positive initiatives in this sector, for example:

- Indian government introduces mHelp—is an initiative of the m-health-collaborative environment that aims at building the pool of expertise and a good number of global health stakeholders using mobile technology. These technologies are expected to be interconnected and provide the direct consultations, tools, and network of expertise in this field [36].
- The new legislation has been introduced by South Korea for removing barriers in remote monitoring and consultation in healthcare as a part of "ubiquitous health."
- To enhance collaboration and ultimately for improving the effectiveness and efficiency of regulatory processes applicable to Internet-based medical applications and wireless-enabled medical devices in the United States. Recently the Memorandum of Understanding has been signed between Food and Drug Administration and Federal Communications Commission.
- The European Union have provided support for various pilot projects related in the area of personal healthcare system, including m-health, which consist of technology development and market development for it and have provided proper guidelines to demonstrate the benefits of these systems. Also they introduced blazing trail initiatives that provided a prospect to gather and share related works in m-health.
- The appointment of a national coordinator for e-health is one of the major steps taken by the Pakistan government to promote health in the country. The Pakistan government also released an action plan for e-health that includes the use of telemedicine services.

2.2.4 *Applications of m-health in monitoring health*

As we know, today's smartphones have a bundle of sensors. We can use these sensors to sense various health parameters to extract a person's health condition in both active and passive ways. To understand individual's mental and physical health, we can club the data measured by a mobile sensor with other information in devices such as SMS, call logs, and apps use to get a pattern that helps to track it for long duration. So we can say that m-health is an efficient and cheap way to monitor individual's health. Following are some ways we can monitor individuals in different diseases with the help of mobile sensors and wearable devices.

2.2.4.1 Monitoring cardiovascular health

To monitor cardiovascular health the vital signs measured by physicians are HR or pulse rate. HR measurement of patients will help practitioners to diagnose heart-related diseases. Conventionally, ECG is used to extract the HR and HR variabilities (HRV). But for ECG you need expertise to extract HR and HRV and patients need to be stationed at some place. Now in the advancement of wearable devices, HR and HRV can be obtained by a fitness tracker. But these wearable and portable ECG required additional sensors that can be saved by exploring the mobile phone camera and microphone.

By deriving photoplethysmogram (PPG) signals from videos of bare skin by using mobile phone camera sensors, we can find HR and HRV of patients. The light absorption characteristics of hemoglobin in blood differ from the surrounding body tissues such as flesh and bone. PPG estimates the volumetric changes in blood by detecting the fluctuation of transmissivity and/or reflectivity of light with arterial pulsation through the tissue. So HR and HRV parameters are extracted by PPG signals either by measuring pulse-to-pulse time difference in time-domain [37] or by finding the dominant frequency in the frequency domain from the fingertip using the flashlight and the camera of a smartphone.

2.2.4.2 Monitoring pulmonary health

The pulmonary diseases such as cough, asthma, chronic obstructive pulmonary disease, and lung cancer are caused due to air pollution and smoking tobacco. Therefore, the early detection of these lung diseases and continuous monitoring of pulmonary health are paramount for timely and effective medical intervention. Many researchers used the microphone of a smartphone to detect the sound of a cough and breathing and analyzed the recorded audio signals in efforts to develop a cost-effective and portable tool for a faster assessment of pulmonary health. The smartphone can be used for lung rehabilitation exercise [37].

2.2.4.3 Monitoring ophthalmic health

DR is one of the common complications of diabetes, which, if diagnosed late and left untreated, can lead to blindness. Current medical diagnosis of DR is very expensive, needs an expert and skilled photographer, requires special processing and storage of films. A low cost and effective solution is proposed by using a modern day smartphone camera with the cloud-based storage, and processing can be an efficient way to remote screening and diagnosis of ophthalmic diseases.

2.2.4.4 Mental health assessment

The today's generation smartphones have a number of embedded sensors such as accelerometer, GPS, light sensor, and microphone. The data from these sensors can be collected passively with the smartphone, which aggregate with the individual's phone usage information such as call logs, SMS pattern, and apps usage that may be used to extract the individual's behavior and understand one's mental health. For example, an individual's stress level or emotional state can be deduced from their voice while talking over the phone and recording the conversation with the smartphone's microphone. In addition, the accelerometer can provide information about physical activity and movement during sleep. The GPS can provide information about the location and thus the context and variety of activity. Therefore, the smartphone enables a less intrusive and more precise alternative to the traditional self-reporting approach, and it may be very useful in assessing the mental well-being of an individual.

2.2.5 Benefits of m-health technology [38]

- The mobile devices nowadays are low cost and able to provide real-time access to related data about social interactions, behavior, diseases, disorders, and a host of other physical and physiological variables.
- The sensors in smartphones discussed earlier provide great support to monitor patient health remotely with respect to chronic diseases such as diabetes, hypertension in which continuous monitoring is needed.
- The m-health can be a great weapon to monitor the health of senior citizens.
- The wearable devices such as smart watches are used to display critical information with respect to monitor your mental and physical health without direct intervention of mobile phone application.

2.2.6 Barriers to m-health [38]

To adopt the m-health, the following are the major barriers as follows:

- aversion to innovation,
- less proper infrastructure,
- technology procurement cost,
- proprietorship,
- lack of legislation and a regulating body.

With these barriers the m-health devices are mobile and remote, and they are worked on wireless technology that comprises more concern such as security threat than that of wired technology. The most common mobile device security threats include the following:

- Loss, theft, and replacement: Due to small size, mobile devices have majority of chances that they can be stolen, lost, or slid from pocket or exchanged due to advancement in technology.
- Off-site data storage: Nowadays the storage capacity of mobile devices has increased enormously, which enables the devices to expose corporate-sensitive data.
- Always accessing particular network on a mobile device is beyond the control of anyone.

2.2.7 Challenges for m-health technology [38]

As mobile technology touches the healthcare arena that has sensitive data, the IT administrators are faced with several unique challenges as follows:

- How to release trust and certificates for m-devices so that users can access health information effectively?
- What are the ways to grant access to the server?
- How to define data storage policy on the m-devices?
- How to implement a data recovery policy for the misplaced, formatted, or lost devices?

- What is the data-erasing policy for lost or misplaced devices? And how can it be implemented efficiently?
- Which security protocols are best suited for medical application?
- How should data privacy policies be implemented?

2.2.8 Future of m-health [39, 40]

The future of the m-health system in terms of technology is as follows:

1. Due to continuous upgrading in m-health, the applications will be more user-centric. In user-centric applications the engagement of the user will be increased because of enabling the gamification in the apps. Hence it will motivate users to continue their treatment plans.
2. Due to the introduction of the cloud, an interoperability feature can be available. This will encourage the use of API as well as the development of new protocols collecting electronic health records and to maintain that record in the cloud.
3. AI-driven diagnostics and care management are also possible.
4. Data analytics and precision medicine will transform the approach of patient care [41].

2.3 Conclusion and future work

M-health is the extension to e-health. Due to advancements in m-health, the livelihood of the people improved. The services and online support from m-health is a ray of hope in the medical field as well as in disaster management systems. Diagnosis of disease and remedy on the same are possible due to usage of wearable IoT as well as sensors in a mobile. M-health plays a very essential role during COVID-19 such as online counseling, consultation, and many more services. By introducing various technologies such as AI, the diagnostics availability can increase. This could help in critical situation such as pandemics or where the proficient professionals are not available. In the near future, the robotics will provide assistance to medical professionals. Hence we can say that continuous updating in the m-health can come up with a new paradigm in the healthcare sector. This will enhance the way of medical facility to the patient without reaching to clinic, without delaying for the treatment and without waiting for the expert's opinion. Due to this, people will be more specific toward their health issues. This could help to remote place people where still medical facilities have not reached yet but smartphones or mobile phones reached.

References

[1] www.frontenders.in/blog/information-communication-technology-health-care.html [Accessed: 27-May-2021].

[2] G. Eysenbach, "What is e-health?" *Journal of Medical Internet Research*, vol. 3, no. 2, p. E20, 2001. https://doi.org/10.2196/jmir.3.2.e20.

[3] https://evisit.com/resources/what-is-mhealth/ [Accessed: 25-May-2021].

[4] R. Sujath, J. M. Chatterjee, and A. E. Hassanien, "A machine learning forecasting model for COVID-19 pandemic in India," *Stochastic Environmental Research and Risk Assessment*, vol. 34, pp. 959–972, 2020.

[5] C. Iwendi, A. K. Bashir, A. Peshkar, *et al.*, "COVID-19 patient health prediction using boosted random forest algorithm," *Frontiers in Public Health*, vol. 8, p. 357, 2020.

[6] S. Dhamodharavadhani, R. Rathipriya, and J. M. Chatterjee, "COVID-19 mortality rate prediction for India using statistical neural network models," *Frontiers in Public Health*, vol. 8, 2020.

[7] https://news.careinnovations.com/blog/what-is-mhealth-how-is-it-different-from-telehealth [Accessed: 25-May-2021].

[8] A. Behmanesh, N. Sayfouri, and F. Sadoughi, "Technological features of internet of things in medicine: A systematic mapping study," *Wireless Communications and Mobile Computing*, vol. 2020, pp. 1–27, 2020.

[9] www.who.int/goe/publications/goe_mhealth_web.pdf [Accessed: 25-May-2021].

[10] www.who.int/goe/mobile_health/mHealthReview_Aug09.pdf [Accessed: 27-May-2021].

[11] mHealth Apps Market Size, Share & Trends Analysis Report By Type (Fitness, Medical), By Region (North America, APAC, Europe, MEA, Latin America), And Segment Forecasts, 2021–2028, Published Date: Feb, 2021, Base Year for Estimate: 2020, Report ID: GVR-1-68038-555-7, Format: Electronic (PDF), Historical Data: 2016–2019.

[12] www.statista.com/statistics/1180843/health-related-mobile-apps-worldwide-number-by-focus/ [Accessed: 25-May-2021].

[13] M. Anthony, J. Jonnagaddala, N. Gudi, R. Islam, P. Narasimhan, and S. Liaw, "mHealth for integrated people-centred health services in the western pacific: A systematic review," *International Journal of Medical Informatics*, vol. 142, p. 104259, 2020.

[14] www.statista.com/forecasts/1181436/share-of-health-app-users-by-country [Accessed: 25-May-2021].

[15] Mordorintelligence.com, "Mobile Health (mHealth) Market Size, Share, Industry Trends | Growth Analysis Report 2021 to 2026 – Mordor Intelligence", *Mordorintelligence.com*, 2021. [Online]. Available: www.mordorintelligence.com/industry-reports/mobile-health-market [Accessed: 07-Jun-2021].

[16] Grandviewresearch.com, "mHealth Apps Market Size Worth $149.3 Billion By 2028", *Grandviewresearch.com*, 2021. [Online]. Available: www.grandviewresearch.com/press-release/global-mhealth-app-market [Accessed: 07-Jun-2021].

[17] B. Bent, K. Wang, E. Grzesiak, *et al.*, "The digital biomarker discovery pipeline: An open-source software platform for the development of digital

biomarkers using mHealth and wearables data," *Journal of Clinical and Translational Science*, vol. 5, no. 1, p. e19, 2021.

[18] https://aabme.asme.org/posts/medical-sensors-laying-the-foundation-for-continuous-patient-monitoring [Accessed: 27-May-2021].

[19] S. Majumder and M. J. Deen, "Smartphone sensors for health monitoring and diagnosis," *Sensors*, vol. 19, no. 9, p. 2164, 2019.

[20] K. Woodward, E. Kanjo, D. Brown, *et al.*, "Beyond mobile apps: a survey of technologies for mental well-being," *IEEE Transactions on Affective Computing*, 2020. Early access: https://doi.org/10.1109/TAFFC.2020.3015018.

[21] Y. Zhai, Y. Wang, M. Zhang, *et al.*, "From isolation to coordination: How can telemedicine help combat the COVID-19 outbreak?" *medRxiv*, 2020, doi: https://doi.org/10.1101/2020.02.20.20025957.

[22] C. P. Adans-Dester, S. Bamberg, F. P. Bertacchi, *et al.*, "Can mHealth technology help mitigate the effects of the COVID-19 pandemic?" *IEEE Open Journal of Engineering in Medicine and Biology*, vol. 1, pp. 243–248, 2020.

[23] D. Giansanti, "The role of the mHealth in the fight against the Covid-19: Successes and failures," *Healthcare*, vol. 9, no. 1, p. 58, 2021.

[24] S. Yang, Y. Chen, L. Zhou, Y. Huang, and J. Dai, "Willingness to adopt mHealth among Chinese parents during the COVID-19 outbreak: Cross-sectional questionnaire study," *JMIR mHealth and uHealth*, vol. 9, no. 1, p. e23155, 2021.

[25] Who.int, "WHO Health Alert Brings COVID-19 Facts to Billions via WhatsApp", *Who.int*, 2021. [Online]. Available: www.who.int/news-room/feature-stories/detail/who-health-alert-brings-covid-19-facts-to-billions-via-whatsapp [Accessed: 02-Jun-2021].

[26] M. Almalki and A. Giannicchi, "Health apps for combating COVID-19: Descriptive review and taxonomy," *JMIR mHealth and uHealth*, vol. 9, no. 3, p. e24322, 2021.

[27] A. S. R. Srinivasa Rao and J. A. Vazquez, "Identification of COVID-19 can be quicker through artificial intelligence framework using a mobile phone–based survey when cities and towns are under quarantine," *Infection Control & Hospital Epidemiology*, vol. 41, no. 7, pp. 826–830, 2020.

[28] MyGov.in, "Aarogya Setu Mobile App", *MyGov.in*, 2021. [Online]. Available: www.mygov.in/aarogya-setu-app/ [Accessed: 04-Jun-2021].

[29] Play.google.com, 2021. [Online]. Available: https://play.google.com/store/apps/details?id=nic.goi.aarogyasetu [Accessed: 04-Jun-2021].

[30] H. Canada, "Download COVID alert: Canada's exposure notification app", *Canada.ca*, 2021. [Online]. Available: www.canada.ca/en/public-health/services/diseases/coronavirus-disease-covid-19/covid-alert.html [Accessed: 04-Jun-2021].

[31] nhs.uk, "What the app does – NHS COVID-19 app support – NHS.UK", *nhs.uk*, 2021. [Online]. Available: www.covid19.nhs.uk/what-the-app-does.html [Accessed: 02-Jun-2021].

[32] nhs.uk, "Translations – NHS COVID-19 app support – NHS.UK", *nhs.uk*, 2021. [Online]. Available: www.covid19.nhs.uk/translations.html [Accessed: 02-Jun-2021].

[33] NI, "European mhealth hub | Covid-19 NI", *Mhealth-hub.org*, 2021. [Online]. Available: https://mhealth-hub.org/covid-19-ni [Accessed: 02-Jun-2021].

[34] 2021. [Online]. Available: www.health.gov.au/resources/apps-and-tools/coronavirus-australia-app [Accessed: 04-Jun-2021].

[35] Covidsafe.gov.au, "COVIDSafe app", *Covidsafe.gov.au*, 2021. [Online]. Available: www.covidsafe.gov.au/ [Accessed: 04-Jun-2021].

[36] www.nhp.gov.in/miscellaneous/m-health [Accessed: 25-May-2021].

[37] https://mhealthintelligence.com/news/the-history-of-mobile-health-from-cell-phones-to-wearables [Accessed: 19-Jun-2021].

[38] www.ncbi.nlm.nih.gov/pmc/articles/PMC4121723/ [Accessed: 19-Jun-2021].

[39] www.pgs-soft.com/blog/mhealth-top-5-trends-for-2021-and-beyond/ [Accessed: 27-May-2021].

[40] www.mckinsey.com/industries/healthcare-systems-and-services/our-insights/finding-the-future-of-care-provision-the-role-of-smart-hospitals# [Accessed: 16-Jun-2021].

[41] https://mhealthintelligence.com/news/the-future-of-mhealth-may-be-health-industry-collaboration [Accessed: 27-May-2021].

Chapter 3

Analysis of Big Data in electroencephalography (EEG)

Sagar Motdhare[1], Garima Mathur[1] and Ravi Kant[2]

Abstract

Human beings have expansive tendencies and coherent thinking abilities. A few of these are grown hereditarily, while a few are displayed in the course of knowledge. These progressions may be seen in various scales along with elements of neurons. Subsequently, it is fundamental to examine the neuronal conduct in tremendous information sizes above various human networks. "Big Data analytics" is arising quickly as an examination zone in the research area. It goes about as an apparatus to aggregate, examine, and oversee enormous amount of disparate, organized and unstructured information, especially in the current clinical frameworks. Big Data idea is unfathomably useful in the sickness discovery region like identification of epileptic seizure. In any case, the conversion pace and exploration openings are deferred by several essential matters in the Big Data model. The fundamental target of this section is to numerically display the information created by an electro-encephalography (EEG) acquisition method. Utilization of Big Data in dealing with an immense measure of information is proposed to investigate. Furthermore, we explore the utilization of Big Data in epileptic EEG assessment.

Keywords: Artifacts; Big Data; Compression standard; Electroencephalography (EEG); EEG activity; EEG application; EEG channels; EEG framework; EEG recording system; EEG data storage; EEG video; Electrode placement system; Epilepsy; Human mind; Mathematical model; Medicine; Neurology; Sampling rate; Sample size; Seizure

3.1 Introduction

Previous methods applied in the area of medication were focused on the discovery of illnesses and their seriousness. These locations were subject to a few specific medical

[1]ECE Department, Poornima University, Jaipur, India
[2]Ericsson, Plano, USA

methodologies in addition to techniques. Thus, there persists a need of creative technique to comprehend as well as dissect the degree of sicknesses. Inferable from the current progressions in innovation, the information delivered is well-off in substance like pictures, sounds and videos when contrasted with the information utilized from different sources, which is restricted. This prompts more trouble in creating and inferring the most significant important data. Also, in long electroencephalography (EEG) data, essential data was not removed. Subsequently, the definite assessment of the EEG information created can be utilized as an improved way to deal with separate huge information, accordingly, permitting precise illness discovery/expectations [1,2].

An EEG-seizure-distinguishing framework has numerous troubles. In the first place, since EEG is a non-stationary signal, so epileptic in addition to non-epileptic examples can modify all through the signal on behalf of dissimilar patients. Secondly, an EEG signal that is acquired by means of intracranial terminals would make a tremendous amount of consistent information that leads to the colossal data issue. This huge measure of information delivered accordingly requires a protected stockpiling framework that can be utilized for the ongoing information calculation [3].

Gen Li surveyed about deep learning for examining EEG information in order to interpret the action of human mind and diagnose the illness and clarified insights regarding different models for knowing the subtleties of recurrent neural network as well as convolution neural network [4,5]. Luo *et al.* inspected the new advancement and achievements in the field of Big Data implementations in the healthcare area and summed up the difficulties, gaps as well as chances to get better and progress Big Data implementations in the area of healthcare [6]. Golmohammadi *et al.* introduced a three-pass framework that can accomplish superior arranging EEG occasions of clinical pertinence [7]. Sendi *et al.* introduced a Spark-based AI approach to deal with the seizure discovery issue utilizing direct dimensionality decrease and order. Utilizing this methodology, they accomplished a normal exactness, affectability, particularity across all patients [8]. Golmohammadi *et al.* examined a superiorly performing EEG examination framework dependent on the standards of machine learning calculations as well as Big Data is projected [9]. Doma and Pirouz analyzed the epoch information from the sensor channels of EEG as well as performed a similar examination of various AI procedures that were tried with and without principal component analysis for decrease in dimensionality. Network investigation was likewise used for hyper-boundary tuning for every one of the tried AI models above Spark cluster for bringing down implementation period [10]. Gutierrez and Husain examined the plan and advancement of EEG workbench: a prototyping system for building EEG information investigation structure for the Android stage. EEG information depicts the action of neuron populaces in the cerebrum and is obtained through terminals set on explicit situations in the skull. EEG signals have been demonstrated to be adequately extraordinary among people and along these lines appropriate for use in the confirmation cycle [11]. De Dea *et al.* researched the exceptional part of rest through EEG otherworldly investigation of three diverse spindle epochs (ante, spindle, and post) to give extra and nitty-gritty data on rest cerebrum working in attention deficit hyperactivity disorder. These highlights can be investigated through notable large information examination strategies [12]. Nahmias *et al.* surveyed feature-based approaches as well as deep learning put together methodologies with respect to their capacity to recognize the expected presence of Dilantin, Keppra or none. The creators recognized sufferers consuming either anticonvulsant or individuals taking no meds; just as linking the two anticonvulsants. Furthermore, they discovered various ways to deal with be best for various gatherings of groupings [13]. Mansoor *et al.* investigated the abilities of brain computer interface (BCI) frameworks and led a review to expand and upgrade the unwavering quality and precision of the BCI frameworks. An organized outline was given, which comprises the information obtained, highlight extraction and arrangement calculation techniques utilized by various scientists in the previous some years. Several arrangement calculations for BCI based on EEG frameworks are tensor classifiers, versatile classifiers, move learning loom and profound knowledge, just as a few different methods [14].

3.2 Methodology

Analysis of Big Data is a computational strategy that executes exemplary part in understanding the patterns of EEG and connections among the signals in enormous datasets. Discovery of epilepsy from the EEG signal is a genuine guide to illustrate the utilization of 3Vs of information. The 3Vs of Big Data analytics are variety, velocity and volume. These 3Vs can portray various EEG functionalities information accordingly delivered. The subtleties of 3Vs in Big Data are shown in Figure 3.1. Despite the fact that the EEG signal with epileptic seizure is intricate, it very well may be altogether dissected by Big Data that helps subsequently removing commendable data [1].

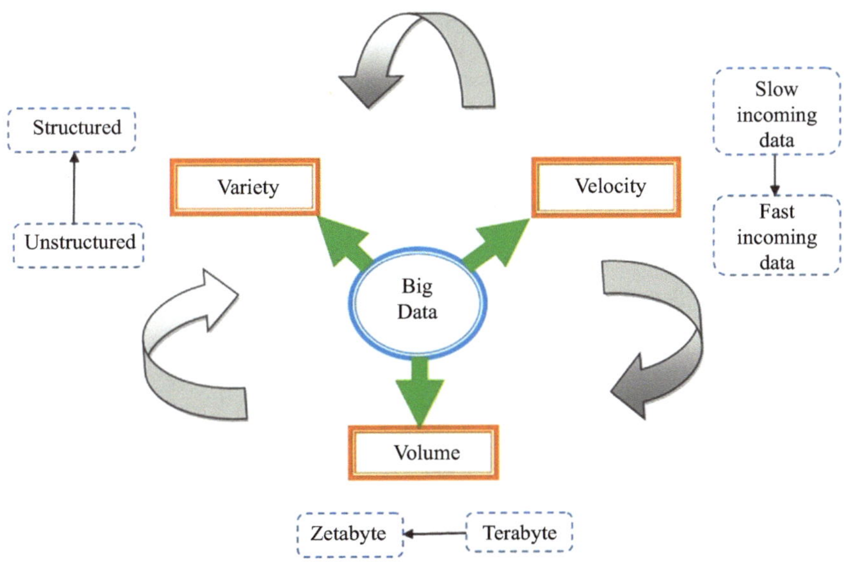

Figure 3.1 Three Vs of Big Data [1] (adapted from Big Data Analytics in Healthcare (Studies in Big Data, Vol. 66))

The biological information that are unpredictable and huge in size need top to bottom assessment. So one can adjust these information boundaries and can think of new technologically enhanced firm products. With the help of such progressions, the information may be put away and examined by scientists effectively. Every one of these impromptu creations is conceivable through Big Data analytics [1].

The information of the EEG with epileptic conditions would be classified as structured or unstructured, which is produced on or after tremendous clinical or potentially nonclinical guides. Such information are further used to decide different classes available in an EEG signal with epileptic information. In this interval, the epileptogenic movement examination is completed by means of Big Data. This agreement will give a comprehensive look to conceivable examination zone in epileptic sickness discovery and might be forecast too [2].

EEG is a viable apparatus to dissect the usefulness of the mind of human. An electrical movement of the cerebrum on millisecond timescale and at a lesser rate than erstwhile mind imaging innovations is given by an EEG signal. The chronicle of the human mind in indigenous habitat erstwhile than inside a research facility setup is permitted by EEG. A viable investigation of the arising strategies is encouraged in order to dissect the neuronal conduct and provide further bits of knowledge [15].

It is vital to work on the complex and reliant conduct of the EEG information alongside the information investigation. Likewise, the safe information stockpiling, getting to and utilizing the information are fundamental. The investigation of consistent EEG needs time-area subtleties. Static information will not give the genuine time data of the persistent information. Likewise, at some stage in the information transformation from consistent to computerized, the transient data of the information must be taken into consideration. Despite the fact that the information storage is accessible, the EEG information procured were infrequently put away in the precedent since the capacity and loading are responsible to restrictive software. Likewise, the speed of information assortment is confined by setup transmission capacity, outlay as well as adaptability of the information [15,16].

3.3 EEG signal recording

A digital EEG framework changes over the waveform keen on a progression of mathematical qualities. This cycle is acknowledged as analog-to-digital conversion. The qualities can be put away in the processor memory, controlled and afterward redisplayed as waveforms on the screen. Mathematically, the pace at which the waveform information is examined to change over it is called the "sampling rate."

The "sampling rate" is typically communicated in Hertz, for instance 200 Hz is 200 times each moment. The least tolerable rate of sampling is 2.5 times more prominent than the most noteworthy rate of recurrence of premium, yet largely advanced EEG frameworks will test at 240 Hz. A few accounts that include recording movement straightforwardly from the mind facade might boast action of an elevated recurrence, for instance 200 Hz. Thusly, various computerized EEG frameworks will have discretionary inspecting paces of 480 Hz accessible.

Inspecting at pace lesser than this will imply that, when the signal is changed over rear-to-analog type, it will not take after the real waveform.

The next factor that influences the precision of the waveform is known as "sampling skew." Sampling skew happens whilst all channels are not examined at the same time. Numerous advanced EEG frameworks test channel 1 first, then, at that point test channel 2, then, at that point channel 3 and so on. "Sampling skew" is defined as the delay between testing of every channel. In order to decrease the sampling skew, several computerized frameworks utilize burst mode sampling. This speeds up amid progressive directs inspecting to lessen the measure of sampling skew. "Display" is the last factor that influences the exactness of advanced EEG waveforms. Its exactness relies upon the quantity of focuses or pels (pixels) that are accessible. "Screen resolution" is defined as the quantity of pel accessible. Screen resolution is portrayed in figures that address the pel accessible in the even and perpendicular alliance.

Modification of the montage "online" at the instance of recording or "offline" subsequent to the recording is finished can control digitized EEG signals. The "remontaging" is cultivated with the help of recording all the channels of EEG by means of a typical location terminal. Notwithstanding the montage utilized to show the information whilst its recording is being done, the information is put away in the PC memory in like manner reference style. This permits the information to be shown utilizing various montages sometime in the not-too-distant future. Since computerized frameworks store the simple sign as mathematical qualities, remontaging is a basic deduction measure that brings about dropping of the normal reference (Figure 3.2).

EEG is a viable instrument to analyze the usefulness of the human cerebrum. An electrical activity of the mind is given by an EEG signal on millisecond timescale at a lesser cost than erstwhile brain imaging technologies. The account of the human mind is permitted by EEG in common habitat apart from inside a research center setup. It works with the successful examination of the arising strategies to break down the neuronal conduct and offer further bits of knowledge. This clears way for a wide scope of chances by empowering the commitment of huge number of scientists and extending the conceivable outcomes of various experimentations.

It is vital to work on the perplexing and reliant conduct of the EEG information alongside the information investigation. Likewise, the protected information stockpiling, getting to and utilizing the information are fundamental. The investigation of nonstop EEG needs time-domain subtleties. Static information will not

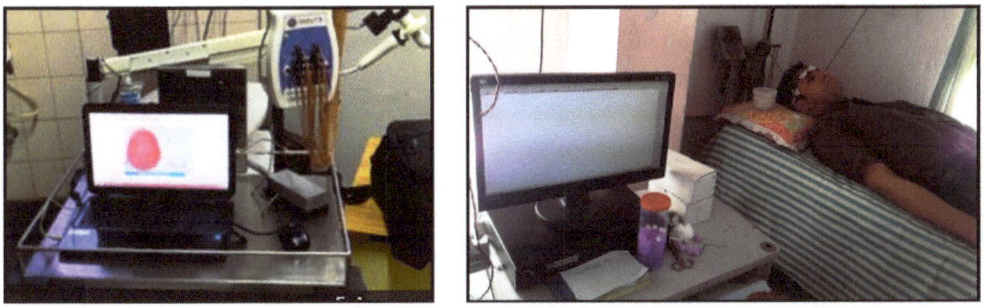

Figure 3.2 EEG signal recording

offer the genuine time data of such constant information. Likewise, for the period of the information change commencing constant to digital, the temporal data of the information must be considered. Despite the fact that the information storage space is accessible, the EEG information gained were seldom put away in the past since the capacity and downloading is at risk to restrictive programming. Moreover, the speed of information assortment is limited.

3.4 Activity/action of EEG

The activities/actions of EEG can be classified into four different frequency bands:

- Beta action: more than 13 Hz
- Alpha action lies between 8 and 13 Hz
- Theta action lies between 4 and 7 Hz
- Delta action: less than 4 Hz

"Beta movement" is a typical action that can be observed when the eyes are shut or open. It will in general be found at channels recorded from the middle or frontage of the skull. A few medications may expand the measure of beta movement in the EEG. "Alpha movement" is likewise an ordinary action that can be observed in waking grown-ups. Mostly, it is found at channels that are recorded from the rear of the scalp. It is genuinely balanced; moreover, it has voltage ranging from 40 to 100 μV. It is possibly observed whilst the eyes are shut and ought to vanish otherwise diminish in voltage when the eyes are open. "Theta-action" can be classified as together usual in addition to unusual movement that relies on the condition and age of the patient. It is typical in grown-ups, if the patient is sluggish. Anyway, it can likewise demonstrate brain disorder on the off chance that it is found in a patient who is ready as well as alert. In more youthful patients, theta movement might be the primary action found at channels recorded at the rear and focal spaces of the skull. "Delta-action" is just ordinary in a grown-up, quiet in the event that is in moderate to profound rest. On the off chance that it is observed at some previous time, it will demonstrate brain disorder. Unusual activity might be found taking all things together or a few channels relying upon the essential brain setback.

Aforesaid are simply short depictions of a portion of the more straightforward waveforms that might be found in some single recording of EEG. Blends of above-mentioned designs are conceivable that can make understanding of the record troublesome. Unusual action is not generally explicit to any situation and could propose a couple of various findings.

3.5 EEG applications

The significant jobs of EEG are as a guide to analyze epilepsy. Nonstandard patterns such as sharp waves, spikes and complex waves can be observed. The sort of commotion and the space of the brain that it is recorded from will help the doctor in endorsing the right medicine for that kind of epilepsy.

Epileptic patients that cannot be constrained by medicine will frequently go through a medical procedure to eliminate the harmed tissue. EEG assumes a significant part in restricting this tissue. Unique terminals can be embedded through the cortex or on the other hand a matrix of anodes put straightforwardly on the outside of the cortex. These accounts, frequently called long-term monitoring for epilepsy, can be concluded for periods going from 1 day to many weeks. Which spaces of the cerebrum ought to be carefully taken out is shown by the recorded EEG.

Sufferers who are profoundly insentient, to recognize brain dead and conceivable reversible situations, can take help of EEG research. Electro-cerebral inactivity or electro-cerebral silence is characterized as non-EEG action for more than 2 μV in voltage while recording from electrode on the head, which is 10 cm or additionally separated.

Utilizing the 1020 global scheme of position of electrodes, the normal space amid electrodes in a grown-up is 6–6.5 cm. Nonetheless if a similar movement was recorded utilizing larger interelectrode distance, a few action may be observed. Accordingly, some 2-fold distance terminal linkages are suggested, for instance FP1-C3, F3-P3, C3-O1.

Display sensitivities of at least 2 μV/mm are mandatory. Anyway, advanced EEG frameworks have the additional benefit of having sensitivity standards of 1.5 and 1 μV/mm. This 50%–100% expansion in sensitivity would permit a further sure appraisal of the existence or nonappearance of a 2-μV signal.

The EEG is additionally utilized to examine different situations that might influence cerebrum capacity like strokes, mind wounds, liver and kidney infection and dementia.

3.6 Mathematical model

The principle purpose of this part is to numerically show the information produced by an EEG recording framework. The utilization of Big Data is proposed to investigate in dealing with a tremendous measure of information. This part gives the numerical model to figure the measure of information created by EEG recordings. It is shown that with a boost in the sampling rate, bigger information is delivered, which perpetually builds the intricacy of recording. Consequently, it is seen that the tremendous measure of information should be dealt with for EEG examination.

Let us assume that if EEG data is recorded for V hours, then for P minutes it is agreed by

$$P = V \times 60 \tag{3.1}$$

Thus, entire amount of samples for each second of EEG recordings are

$$Q = \frac{\{(P)(60)(s)\}}{y} \tag{3.2}$$

where Q is the amount of samples present each second, s stands for seconds, y is the duration of EEG data containing sample (s).

Also, the entire number of bits B_N needed to encode Q samples is agreed by

$$B_N = Q \times B \text{ bits} \tag{3.3}$$

Subsequently for every patient on the off chance that we regard as information for a day by means of distinct channel, B_N bits of information is created. On the off chance that we demand paradigm of 10–20-electrode framework for recording of EEG (Figure 3.3),

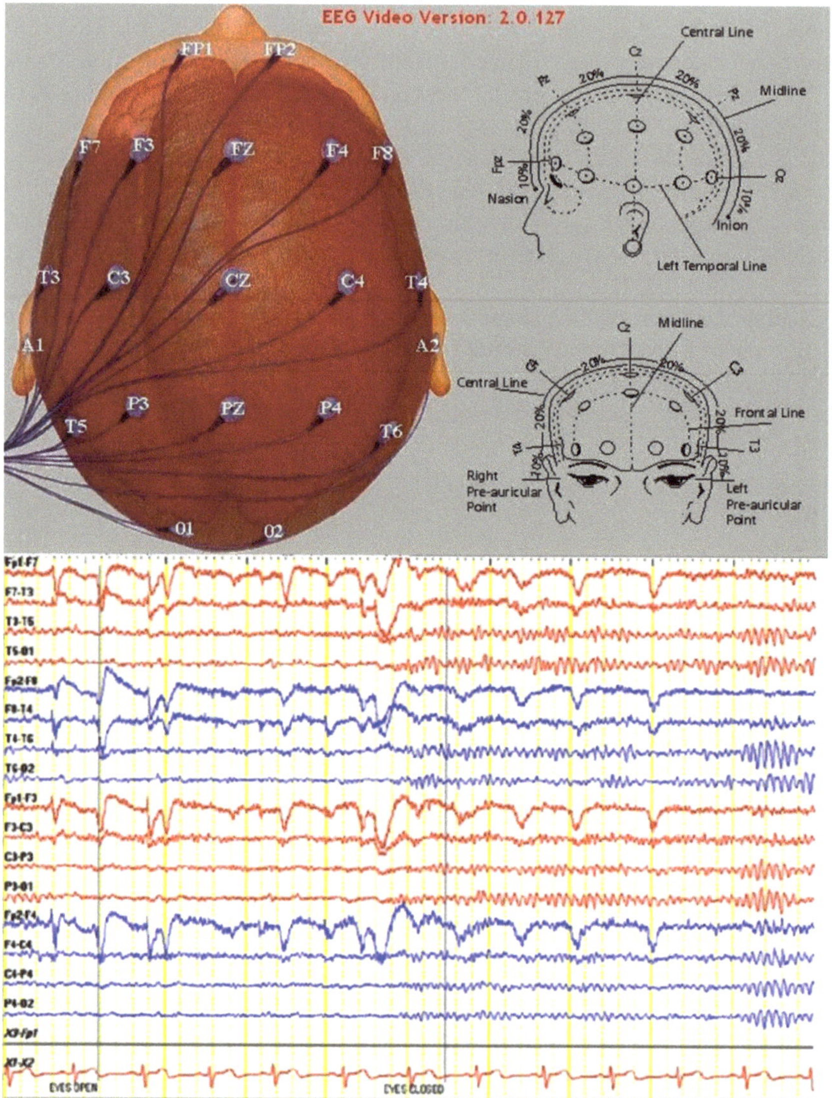

Figure 3.3 10–20 Placement of electrodes on scalp and EEG signals from different locations of brain

Table 3.1 Data generated by EEG recording system

Duration (h)	Data generated for single-channel EEG	Data generated for 24-channel EEG
1	55 MB	165.02 MB
24	1.2 GB	4 GB
72	4.1 GB	12 GB

aggregate sum of EEG information produced with H channel recording is specified by

$$Z = B_N \times H \tag{3.4}$$

where H is the channel recording, Z is the sum of EEG data created with H channel recording.

The hard and fast data delivered by an EEG recording framework for a variety of range at sampling frequency of 256 Hz is shown in Table 3.1. Information delivered will increment since the quantity of channels utilized on behalf of recording expanded can be seen very well. By means of an increment in the sampling pace, bigger information is delivered, which perpetually builds the intricacy of recording. Consequently it is seen that the tremendous measure of information should be dealt with in the support of EEG examination [1].

3.7 Across the boundaries of small sample sizes

Huge data sets empower an enhanced practical run of intra-individual variety; furthermore, the utilization of the huge information investigation can be better utilized for epileptogenic movement recognition utilizing AI and profound learning for more precise outcomes all through various applications. Powerful information presents the executives are fundamental for an assortment of information scales to guarantee the quality boundaries like information norms and information approval for a fruitful examination. Huge information presents a powerful information of the board framework to analysts for better overseeing and sharing the information proficiently with no significant endeavors in information cleaning and information course of action. For instance, in epilepsy recognition, huge EEG information are accessible for the examination, location and perhaps the expectation of epileptic seizures. Quite possibly the main objectives in seizure location is to discover improved biomarker meant for the recognizable proof of illness movement. Huge scope examination of EEG empowers to attain understanding of epileptic cycles and accordingly working with before time seizure identification.

3.8 EEG signal analytics and seizure analysis

Enormous amount of information obtained from EEG signal monitoring devices cannot be stored after a specific purpose of time. This prompts the absence of assessment of the information. Since the specificity of the EEG signal massively relies upon the sickness style, different EEG handling procedures are accessible to find essential highlights commencing the EEG information. These highlights would then be able to be pre-prepared by an AI calculation that gives subtleties of the sickness.

Streaming information investigation in medication alludes to a methodical utilization of ceaseless information and its connected clinical data created through applied examination, specifically prescient examination. These investigations can be either diagnostic or predictive. These grouping subtleties can be demonstrated further to give different instruments like ready frameworks and offering notice to clinicians [15].

Epilepsy, quite possibly the most well-known neurological conditions described by epileptic seizures, is the second most basic neurological problem behind stroke, as indicated by the World Health Organization. Seizures may happen, paying little heed to the conditions or host ascribes. Patients with epilepsy experience the ill effects of abrupt and unanticipated seizures, for the period of which they cannot secure selves and are powerless alongside suffocation, passing or hurt due to blacking out in addition to auto collisions. Until now, this infection is primarily treated with drugs and medical procedure; no fix exists, and therapies with anticonvulsants are not totally solid for all of sorts of epilepsy.

EEG undertakes a noteworthy part in distinguishing epilepsy, as it approximates contrasts in voltage swaps involving anodes alongside the subject's scalp by sensing ionic flows streaming within cerebrum neurons and gives fleeting and spatial information with reference to the mind. Location with EEG requires an immediate assessment by a doctor just as a significant measure of time and exertion. Moreover, specialists with varying degrees of demonstrative experience in some cases report discrepant suppositions on the indicative outcomes. Thusly, the advancement of a computerized, PC-helped technique for the analysis of epilepsy is desperately required. While EEG assumes significant parts in observing the cerebrum action of patients with epilepsy and diagnosing epilepsy, a specialist is expected to examine all EEG chronicles to recognize epileptic action. This strategy is clearly tedious and dreary, and an ideal and exact analysis of epilepsy is vital for start antiepileptic drug treatment and consequently decreases the danger of future seizures and seizure-related inconveniences.

In epilepsy finding, tremendous EEG information are accessible in favor of the investigation, discovery and perhaps the expectation of epileptic seizures. Perhaps, the main objectives within seizure recognition are to discover enhanced biomarker for the recognizable proof of ailment succession. Huge scope examination of EEG empowers to acquire knowledge of epileptic cycles also in this manner encouraging early seizure recognition [16].

As of now, perfect-seizure-investigation frameworks are not accessible. In this way, there is a necessity to advance execution of the seizure examination frameworks. To distinguish "interictal and ictal" occasions in the EEG is the fundamental point of an epileptic seizure identification framework (Figure 3.4). The remembrance of a system is consolidated as a globular buffer. The capacity of the buffer is

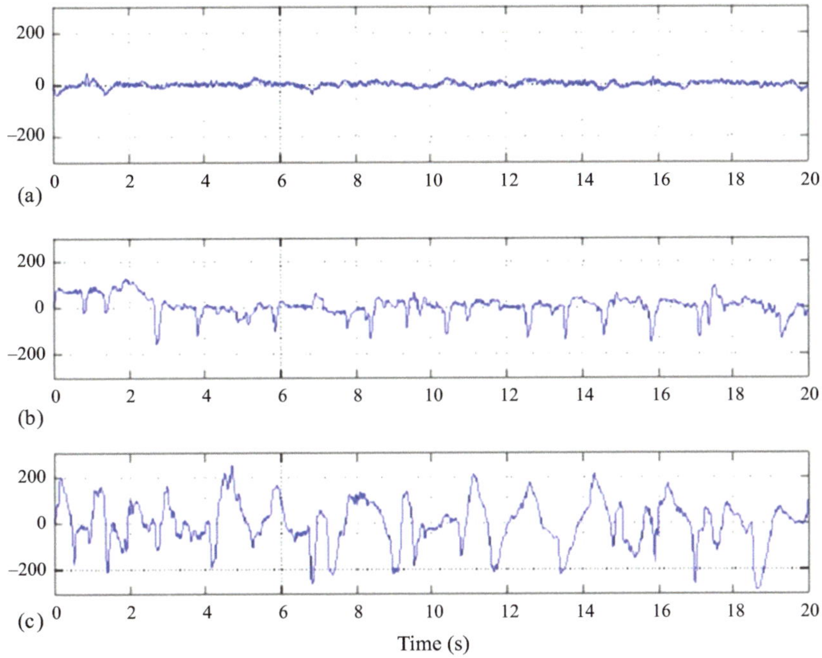

Figure 3.4 Typical EEG waveforms corresponding to epilepsy ((a) interictal, (b) preictal and (c) ictal stage)

to accumulate the epileptic information with the end goal that the hour of event of the epileptic structure action can be identified and explored. The put away information in the PC can be gotten to by a staff part in the facilities. In the event that the epileptic action does not happen, the memory is overwritten by the new information. To accumulate epileptic information, commencement by the master is of significance, given that PC-based identification might offer mistaken outcomes. This is on the grounds that bogus epileptic action might be caught by the framework and accordingly investigated [17].

3.9 EEG digital video

A video EEG accounts what a patient is performing or encountering on video tape whilst an EEG assessment records your brainwaves. The reason for existing is to have the option to perceive what is going on when a patient contains a seizure or occasion and contrast the image with what the EEG records simultaneously. Blares that happen during the test are likewise recorded. This may get if an individual discussion generates sounds during an occasion. By performing this, specialists perusing the EEG can notify if the seizure or occasion was identified with the electrical movement in the cerebrum. Assuming this is the case, we would describe this epilepsy seizure. Video EEG is generally useful to decide whether seizures with uncommon highlights are really epilepsy to recognize the kind of seizures, and to identify the locale of the cerebrum anywhere, seizures start. Finding the locale unequivocally is fundamental if epilepsy medical procedure is being thought of. Different calls for video EEG tests incorporate: EEG telemetry, EEG monitoring or video EEG monitoring. Normally, these expressions indicate exactly the identical mania. The objective of testing is ordinarily to record commonplace seizures or occasions and to maintain patient safe. Now and again bringing meds possibly will show the way down to additional seizures than expected or one might have a greater seizure or else one that keeps going longer than ordinary. Specialists and attendants may have to offer seizure meds that take steps rapidly to discontinue stretched or rehashed seizures on the off chance that they happen during the testing.

Owing to the headway in the know-how, VCR recording devices were put back by computerized recordings in lengthy haul video EEG recording frameworks. As a whole the computerized video EEG recording frameworks, right now the prominently utilized video design paradigm, are Moving Picture Experts Group (MPEG). It is utilized as the touchstone video design on the grounds that it can oblige well-built outline sizes. The circle gap is stored by utilizing the compression factors of 8:1 and 30:1. A 100:1 extra compression factor might corrupt the video eminence. Likewise, when the quality just as the movement of the video increments, less compression can be acquired. The series of pressure can be altered by a factor of at least 2. The compression reach will be in the reach somewhere in the assortment of 3.4 and 4.5 Mbps, in MPEG-2. Excluding MPEG-2, other standard MPEG designs are MPEG-4, MPEG-7 and MPEG-21 [18].

Table 3.2 depicts the aggregate sum of video EEG information put away in a DVD circle. In favor of model, on the off chance that 128 channels of EEG are utilized in the midst of an examining pace of 1 000, which will create an information of 256 kbps. In order to accumulate the video EEG information caught at the rate of 256 kbps, one DVD of standard size 4.7 Gbps is needed [19].

The amount of information produced by continuous EEG recording can be critical. Verifiably, the investigation and capacity of this information have been trying because of moderately restricted computational assets. These difficulties persevere today, regardless of the pervasiveness of modest gigaflop workers and terabyte stockpiling frameworks, for an alternate explanation: the setup clinical work stream for EEG examination separates for current informational collections.

Table 3.2 Data generated and stored in DVDs

No. of channels	Compression standard	Sampling rate	Kilo bytes per second (kbps)	Per day data generation (GB)	Storage capacity in DVDs (GB)
128	–	200	51	5	1.0
128	MPEG-1	1 000	256	25	4.5
128	MPEG-2	1 000	812	75	15

The present status of the workmanship recording frameworks currently obtains many channels of EEG information at high examining rates. These huge scope informational indexes can be a huge number of times bigger than customarily gained clinical EEG, which is ostensibly gathered at 200–500 Hz. Albeit the equipment part of gathering, examining and putting away this information is practical, the "best quality level" of investigation by human master visual audit of whole records is not. The sheer expansion in information for present day chronicles puts a critical strain on epilepsy monitoring unit staff and assets for everything except the least complex of investigations. In addition, the chase for multiscale occasions going in term from milliseconds to minutes requires more itemized and rehashed audit of EEG. The requirement for solid computerized examination apparatuses in clinical and research electrophysiology is obviously perceived, and there is a developing local area of scientists seeking after these objectives. The field ought to positively profit with equal endeavors in other clinical fields, like genomics, that are driving endeavors in database management, data mining and pattern recognition.

3.10 EEG data storage and its management

A subject with epilepsy might catch different seizures in a daytime. Notwithstanding the ictal and postictal actions, bury ictal information ought to likewise be saved with the normal EEG tests. Consequently, it is fundamental for an exceptionally arranged and oversaw record framework. The EEG record framework comprises a home observance document that will be in an ASCII format. This document is the sole wellspring of record for gear's settings and data that incorporates the name of patient, montages, setting information of equipment (PC as well as intensifier), account of every EEG records of sufferer explicit and clinic unit numeral. This record style additionally incorporates instance and date data with respect to all the progressions completed.

Interpreting the recorded EEG document assists in the investigation plus improvement of the epileptic seizure location frameworks. Annotations give data regarding the areas and epochs of the seizure spikes within EEG information.

Patient's EEG records are likewise the piece of the PC frameworks that carries the benchmark EEG information together with ictal and interictal data recorded and distinguished by specialists or by PC programs. These record frameworks are displayed to give different significant capacities, for example (i) quick exploring of usual signals of EEG, (ii) to give quick admittance to signals of EEG number of channels, (iii) following the advancement of additional precise seizure location or forecast frameworks and (iv) to lay up together "continuous" in addition to "non-continuous EEG information" [20].

EEG information demonstrating is helpful for creating applications in the area of medical services, just as in the design of BCI. A framework can be developed that incorporates web-server that can be utilized to transfer and store EEG information. A proficient self-changing brain signal demonstrating framework can flawlessly catch and break down EEG brainwave information. The stage gives easy to understand interface secure information stockpiling and examination abilities for wave investigation, factual examination and unmitigated grouping utilizing various machine learning algorithms. An orderly technique to see how the variety of crude informational indexes utilized in preparing models influences the exactness of machine learning algorithms, which can investigate the exhibition of AI calculations under different computational executions [21].

Brain research is presently a quickly developing scientific field. Large amount of data, different information formats and nonstandardized domain portrayals lead to contrary outcomes and translations of neuroscientific data and to troublesome correspondence among research centers and scientific teams. Neuroinformatics, a recently settled scientific field, gives coordination across all levels and sizes of neuroscience. The research group has added to the structure of a neuroinformatics framework by creating and incorporating data management for EEG/ERP (EEG, event related potential) research [22].

3.11 Big Data in epileptic EEG analysis

Consistent EEG signals that have high resolution have deterrents like its amount also, pace of the dataset and information created on or after different screens for each patient. EEG signals additionally deal with issues identified with the intricacy of spatiotransient nature. Because of this, guaranteeing adequacy of seizure recognition or prediction frameworks would be troublesome also, consequently the strength of the ceaseless observing frameworks [16].

As of now, various epilepsy detection frameworks are accessible that use the adjustment in arrangement commencing any one wellspring of biological discrepancy. These frameworks go about as a ready gadget particularly in crisis circumstances. Figure 3.5 depicts the nonexclusive epileptic seizure discovery/

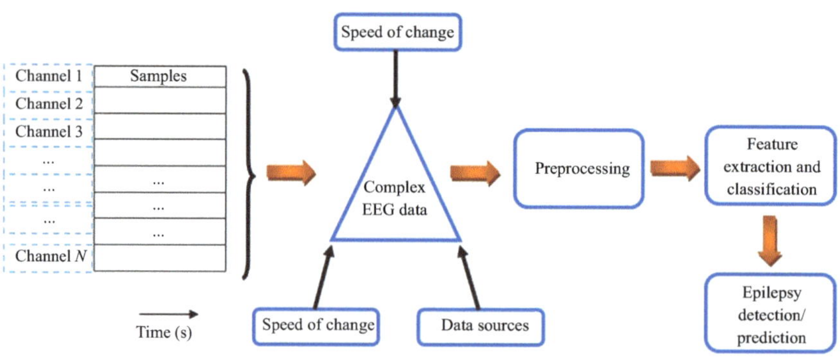

Figure 3.5 Epileptic seizure recognition/prediction structure using Big Data analytics [1] (adapted from Big Data Analytics in Healthcare (Studies in Big Data, Vol. 66))

expectation framework utilizing huge information investigation. Be that as it may, these frameworks will in general be problematic, explicitly in instantaneous epileptic observing frameworks. They might still lean to offer bogus alerts and this might be the reason for immense uneasiness for patients as well as overseers. These frameworks possibly will not work precisely, because of the absence of earlier clinical information also, examination is finished by utilizing solitary biological varieties of signal. There is an interest meant for flexible methodology that can associate these biological variations incredibly fine in the multichannel time series EEG information [23,24].

As large quantity of uninterrupted information alongside the erstwhile patient's data is brought about in hospitals, progressed capacity frameworks are critical. By means of the capacity to stockpile the information, recovering it is tedious as well as costly. Big Data employability encourages a quick recovery of enormous volumes of such information furthermore conveys by means of logical demonstrating. In the exploration field, frameworks like Hadoop, MapReduce and MongoDB are generally utilized [2].

EEG handling based on Big Data intended for the improvement of assessment support scheme in hospitals is getting boundless [25]. This empowers the neurologist by means of the information of data with reference to the patient along with artifact eliminated signals. These signals are conveyed at instance with the upgrades in patient consideration frameworks. The essential explanations behind the advancement of aforesaid frameworks are because of the creation of immense measure of EEG information in hospitals for each patient. Along these lines, decision support systems in hospitals are profoundly valued by the scientist's society [26].

3.12 Conclusion

EEG information grandstands a gigantic variation in data, including information produced by development of muscles, video data, instruments impedances; the extensive scope of this process and the amount of information alongside its different kinds have prepared the epileptic seizure recognition or expectation a Big Data issue. As of now, enhancements in data storage present a substitute arrangement while taking care of colossal measure of information in assorted storage medium. Yet, several storage frameworks are restricted via the variety of the information kinds. Undesirable reprocessing of the information is restricted by the expanded utilization of "metadata along with recording time-stamps" on different instances, despite the fact that the previous outcomes are stored in the framework stage. Henceforth, the information representation utilized ought to have the option to bring about Big Data by empowering analysts to carry out elucidative examination exclusive of letting completely go over information. Such investigation would assist with getting new knowledge as of them. Additionally, the presentation metrics must be taken into consideration alongside its time and convey ability, while consolidating Big Data in the observing clinical gadgets. For dealing with

EEG Big Data, real-time epileptic recognition frameworks may be thought in prospect [27,28].

Quite possibly the main objectives in epilepsy research is to distinguish better biomarkers, both of intense changes and disease progression. Utilizing neural designing strategies, a significant objective of the lab is to describe new biomarkers that demonstrate the circumstance and area of seizures, particularly those found in EEG signals. The most encouraging biomarker is at present high frequency oscillations (HFOs). HFOs have a reasonable relationship with epileptic networks, yet it is muddled how to carry out them in a clinically significant and safe design [29]. The essential objective is to create and decipher apparatuses that will permit clinicians to use HFOs and improve clinical consideration. The main impediment of HFO research is distinguishing them. Most clinical examinations have depended upon manual survey that requires numerous hours and is certifiably not a suitable clinical arrangement. Mechanized calculations can be valuable; however, they are inclined to recognizing relics [30].

Practically all past R&D endeavors, including EEG, and seizure recognition, have been led on little data sets. Frequently, these data sets are bad portrayals of the sort of information found in medical conditions. Transient artifacts, not normal in data sets gathered underneath study conditions, can essentially debase execution. Of course, in spite of high correctness introduced in the exploration writing, the exhibition of monetarily accessible frameworks has been deficient in clinical settings. There is as yet extraordinary interest for an automated structure that accomplishes a stumpy bogus caution rate in scientific implementations [31].

EEG (electroencephalograms) is a test used to discover issues identified with electrical movement of the cerebrum and utilized for the analysis of conditions like epilepsy and so on. EEGs can be long contingent upon a patient's condition. Previously, the data created from different sources is used to be restricted in a short-sighted structure. With the headway of innovation, we are assaulted with rich substance like images, videos, audios. This has put a strain on our ability to beat this information and infer data. Comparable is the situation with the information created from long EEG records. The investigation of the information produced by EEGs can cause significant damage and can utilize a superior methodology. With the headway of our clinical capacities, we need to ensure that we advance the innovation to make up for lost time and have the option to see such humongous information, yet in addition identified with as of now analyzed examples and perform authentic information match-ups [32,33].

3.13 Future scope

Big Data analytics is coming to help on this front. Big Data analytics is a computational strategy that is playing out a quintessential job in understanding the examples, relations in a huge dataset from any sort of source. The information could be in any structure. The progressions in the Big Data analytics field are making it simpler, quicker and more exact to investigate the information produced from long EEG accounts. This is the future and an incredible illustration of the assembly of all parts of science.

References

[1] Yedurkar, D.P., and Metkar, S.P.: Big data in electroencephalography analysis. In: Kulkarni, A., Siarry, P., Singh, P., Abraham, A., Zhang, M., Zomaya, A., and Baki, F. (eds) *Big Data Analytics in Healthcare. Studies in Big Data*, vol 66. Springer, Cham.

[2] Kaur, K., and Rani, R.: Managing data in healthcare information systems: many models, one solution. *Computer* 48(3), 52–59 (2015).

[3] Yu, W.D., Kollipara, M., Penmetsa, R., and Elliadka, S.: A distributed storage solution for cloud based e-healthcare information system. In: *Proceedings of the IEEE 15th International Conference on e-Health Networking, Applications and Services (Healthcom'13)*, pp. 476–480, Lisbon, Portugal (2013).

[4] Li, G., Lee, C., Jung, J., Youn, Y.C., and Camacho, D.: Deep learning for EEG data analytics: a survey. *Concurrency and Computation: Practice and Experience* 32. 10.1002/cpe.5199. (2019).

[5] Khairandish, M.O., Sharma, M., Jain, V., Chatterjee, J.M., and Jhanjhi, N.Z.: A hybrid CNN-SVM threshold segmentation approach for tumor detection and classification of MRI brain images. *IRBM* (2021).

[6] Luo, J., Wu, M., Gopukumar, D., and Zhao, Y.: Big data application in biomedical research and health care: a literature review. *Biomedical Informatics Insights* 8, 1–10. (2016).

[7] Golmohammadi, M., Torbati, A., Diego, S., Obeid, I., and Picone, J.: Automatic analysis of EEGs using big data and hybrid deep learning architectures. *Frontiers in Human Neuroscience* 13, 76. (2019).

[8] Sendi, M.S.E., Heydarzadeh, M., and Mahmoudi, B.: A spark-based analytic pipeline for seizure detection in EEG big data streams. In: *Annual International Conference of the IEEE Engineering in Medicine and Biology Society*, Jul 2018, pp. 4003–4006.

[9] Golmohammadi, M., Harati Nejad Torbati, A.H., Lopez de Diego, S., Obeid, I., and Picone, J.: Automatic analysis of EEGs using big data and hybrid deep learning architectures. *Frontiers in Human Neuroscience* 13, 76. (2019).

[10] Doma, V., and Pirouz, M.: A comparative analysis of machine learning methods for emotion recognition using EEG and peripheral physiological signals. *Journal of Big Data* 7, 18. (2020).

[11] Gutierrez, L. and Husain, M.: Design and development of a mobile EEG data analytics framework. In: *2019 IEEE Fifth International Conference on Big Data Computing Service and Applications (Big Data Service)*, 2019, pp. 333–339.

[12] De Dea, F., Ajcevic, M., Stecca, M., *et al.*: A big-data-analytics framework for supporting classification of ADHD and healthy children via principal component analysis of EEG sleep spindles power spectra. *Procedia Computer Science* 159, 1584–90. (2019).

[13] Nahmias, D.O., Civillico, E.F., and Kontson, K.L.: Deep learning and feature based medication classifications from EEG in a large clinical data set. *Scientific Reports* 10, 14206. (2020).

[14] Mansoor, A., Usman, M.W., Jamil, N., and Naeem, M.A.: Deep learning algorithm for brain-computer interface. *Scientific Programming* 2020, 12 p (2020).

[15] McCullough, J.S., Casey, M., Moscovice, I., and Prasad, S.: The effect of health information technology on quality in U.S. hospitals. *Health Affairs* 29(4), 647–654 (2010).

[16] Drew, B.J., Harris, P., Zègre-Hemsey, J.K., *et al.*: Insights in to the problem of alarm fatigue with physiologic monitor devices: a comprehensive observational study of consecutive intensive care unit patients. *PLoS One* 9(10), (2014).

[17] Chen, J., Dougherty, E., Demir, S.S., Friedman, C.P., Li, C.S., and Wong, S.: Grand challenges for multimodal bio-medical systems. *IEEE Circuits and Systems Magazine* 5(2), 46–52 (2005).

[18] Fogg, C., Mitchell, J., Pennebaker, W., and LeGall, D.: *MPEG Video Compression Standard*, 1st edn. Springer, New York, ISBN: 978-0-412-08771-4. (1996).

[19] Niedermeyer, E., and Lopes, F.: *Electroencephalography: Basic Principles, Clinical Applications and Related Fields*, 5th edn. Lippincott Williams & Wilkins Publishers, Philadelphia (2005).

[20] Lesser, M.P., Stochaj, W., Tapley, D., and Shick, J.M.: Bleaching in coral reef anthozoans: effects of irradiance, ultraviolet radiation and temperature on the activities of protective enzymes against active oxygen. *Coral Reefs* 8(4), 225–232 (1990).

[21] Golmohammadi, M., Torbati, A.H., Diego, S.L., Obeid, I., and Picone, J.: Automatic analysis of EEGs using big data and hybrid deep learning architectures. *Frontiers in Human Neuroscience* 13, 76. (2019).

[22] Borckardt, J.J., Nash, M.R., Murphy, M.D., Moore, M., Shaw, D., and O'Neil, P.: Clinical practice as natural laboratory for psychotherapy research: a guide to case-based time-series analysis. *American Psychologist* 63(2), 77–95 (2008).

[23] Kaisler, S., Armour, F., Espinosa, J.A., and Money, W.: Big data: issues and challenges moving forward. In: *46th Hawaii International Conference on System Sciences*, pp. 995–1004. (2013).

[24] Gotman, J.: Automatic recognition of epileptic seizures in the EEG. Electroencephalography. *Clinical Neurophysiology* 54(5), 530–540 (1982).

[25] Belle, A., Kon, M.A., and Najarian, K.: Biomedical informatics for computer-aided decision support systems: a survey. *Scientific World Journal* 2013, 8 pp (2013).

[26] Thuraisingham, R.A., and Gottwald, G.A.: On multiscale entropy analysis for physiological data. *Physica A: Statistical Mechanics and its Applications* 366, 323–332 (2006).

[27] Cuzzocrea, A., Song, I.-Y., and Davis, K.C.: Analytics over large-scale multidimensional data: the big data revolution. In: *Proceedings of the ACM 14th International Workshop on Data Warehousing and OLAP*, pp. 101–104 (2011).

[28] Puce, A., and Hämäläinen, M.: A review of issues related to data acquisition and analysis in EEG/MEG studies. *Brain Sciences* 7(12), 58. (2017).

[29] Rashid, A., and Qureshi, I.M.: Eliminating electroencephalogram artefacts using independent component analysis. *International Journal of Applied Mathematics, Electronics and Computers* 3(1), 48. (2015).

[30] Achanccaray, D., and Meggiolaro, M.: Detection of artifacts from EEG data using wavelet transform, high-order statistics and neural networks. In: *XVII Brazilian Conference on Automatica* (2008).

[31] Devuyst, S., Dutoit, T., Stenuit, P., Kerkhots, M., and Stanus, E.: Removal of ECG artifacts from EEG using a modified independent component analysis approach. In: *2008 30th Annual International Conference of the IEEE Engineering in Medicine and Biology Society*, 2008, 5204–5207. (2008).

[32] Marino, M., Liu, Q., Vlastimil, K., *et al.*: Adaptive optimal basis set for BCG artifact removal in simultaneous EEG-FMRI. *Scientific Reports* 8(1). (2018).

[33] Dora, C., and Pradyut Kumar, B.: Robust ECG artifact removal from EEG using continuous wavelet transformation and linear regression. In: *2016 International Conference on Signal Processing and Communications (SPCOM)*, 2016. (2016).

Chapter 4
An analytical study of COVID-19 outbreak

Shipra Gupta[1], Vijay Kumar[2], P. Patil[3] and Lajwanti Kishnani[4]

Abstract

Today, the effect of COVID-19 has become a worldwide problem. The transmission of this virus from one human being to another is a serious concern. This virus can spread from one person to another due to contact of a contaminated surface. The virus can survive on the surface of metal, wood, plastic, glass, disposal goods, etc. The survival time of the virus depends upon the nature of surface. To destroy the virus from the contaminated surface, some specific concentrations of alcoholic chemicals such as ethanol, propanol and sodium hypochlorite are required. The uses of exposure time of these chemicals depend upon the percentage of concentration. One successful method to control the transmission of virus is to make people stay at their home as virus needs human body for transmission from one place to another. The spreading rate of virus through human being is very high. However, this virus has spread across the whole world and the survival of human beings is very difficult in the present scenario, but also there are some positive aspects that have been observed. Due to low movements of vehicles, air pollution, and due to industrial lockdown, air and water pollution have decreased.

Keywords: Analytical study; COVID-19; Effects on world; Effects on life of people; Effect on environment; Hydrogen peroxide; HCoV-22pE; HCoV-NL63; HCoV-OC43; HCoV-HKU1; HCoV-22Pe; Leprosy; MERS-CoV; MRSA; Measles; MHV; Propanol; SARS-CoV; TGEV; TGEV; Variant of virus; Zika

[1]School of Management, Graphic Era Hill University, Dehradun, India
[2]Department of Physics, Renewable Energy by Recycling of Waste Papers, Graphic Era Hill University, Dehradun, India
[3]Department of Mechanical Engineering, Graphic Era Deemed to be University, Dehradun, India
[4]Professional Communication, American College of Dubai, Dubai, UAE

4.1 Introduction

Many types of viruses are available in the world like smallpox, diarrhea, Marburg, plague, infectious malaria, HIV/AIDS, influenza, cholera, Ebola, rabies, pneumonia, Middle-East respiratory syndrome (MERS), dengue, hantaviruses, anthrax, MRSA "superbug," pertussis, tetanus, meningitis, syphilis, SARS, leprosy, measles and Zika. Except these, some new viruses are infecting the people from last two decades. One dangerous virus at this time is related to the coronavirus family. The coronaviruses that can affect human beings have a large group. When these viruses become in touch with the human beings, they show the symptoms of pneumonia in beginning [1,2]. HCoV-229E (HCoV-229E, HCoV-NL63, HCoV-OC43 and HCoV-HKU1), HCoV-NL63, HCoV-OC43, HCoV-HKU1, SARS-CoV and MERS-CoV are the only six CoVs that had been known till 2007 [3]. In 2002–03, first time, the citizens of Guangdong, China suffered from SARS-CoV. Symptoms of this virus observed were high fever, headache and cough [4]. Due to its high transmission nature among human beings, it was spread across 29 countries, which infected more than 8,000 persons with about 800 deaths [5,6]. The citizens of Saudi Arabia in 2012 were suffered from MERS-CoV, and symptoms at that time are again just like pneumonia. At that time, 35% was the death rate [7]. The transmission of this virus was limited with geography boundaries [8] and the transmission was break down in the Middle-East countries [9,10]. At present, transmissible gastroenteritis virus (TGEV) and mouse hepatitis viruses (MHV) are also included in the family of SARS-CoV.

In December 2019, the citizens of Wuhan city, China suffered from a new member of this family, coronavirus. In the capital of Hubei, China, this disease was first identified in 2019 and now has spread globally. At present, this virus has created the pandemic of 2019–20 [11,12]. Common symptoms of this disease are high fever, breathing problem, cough, muscles pain and throat infection [13,14]. As per one report of March 23, 2020, the death rate of infected patients was about 4.4%; however, it might vary from 0.2% to 15% depending upon the age and health of the patients [15,16].

The possibility of spreading of this virus through respiratory droplets during cough is lower than transmission through the human body [17]. The possibility of transmission through the contact of a contaminated surface is very high. This virus can survive on surfaces of many materials like metal, plastic up to 5 days. The time of diagnosing this disease is generally 2–14 days [13,18]. For suspected persons of virus, using masks (N-95) is suggested. However, the normal healthy person can use the masks made by simple clothes [19,20]. Right now, we have no vaccines or injections for the treatment of this virus.

The total infected cases from COVID-19 [21–23] were 184,247,550, total deaths due to this virus were 3,987,466 and recovered cases were 168,626,075 (as on July 4, 2021) [24–26]. A total of 196 countries around the world are affected by this problem. Maximum countries impose lockdown to prevent further spreading in people and healthcare settings. In different virus infections, the time required for cure is 1–4 days in seasonal flu, 1–7 days for swine flu, 2–14 days for MERS, 2–10 days for SARS and 2–14 days or 2–24 days for novel coronavirus COVID-19 [24,27]. The persons who are infected by COVID-19 experience the following symptoms: 98% cases showed only fever; 76% suffered from cough; 44%, muscle pain; 8%, headache; and only 3% suffered from diarrhea [28,29]. The aim of this review was to brief the data available about this dangerous virus so that the society will take it seriously and also aim at being aware of the positive and negative aspects.

4.2 Review of literature

This study is very useful at this time when the whole world is facing this problem of infectious COVID-19. As per many experts and WHO, it is a very crucial problem that is spreading continuously across the globe. The limitation to break this virus chain is imposing lockdown in cities, states and all countries so that human body is not available to carry this virus. As per one study of China, coronavirus may be available in human beings manure and toilet after cure and even his/her COVID-19 report becomes negative. The flies present near the manure and toilet can spread this virus. One member of this family, MERS-CoV, can survive on the surface of steel for 24 h, at the surface of plastic till for 4 days at 20 °C [30]. It can be removed from the surfaces of steel and plastic by the use of ethanol of 80% concentration, by 2-propanol of 75% concentration within 30 s [31], by povidone-iodine of 7.5% within 15 s [32]. SARS-CoV can survive on the surfaces of metals, wood, papers, plastic and disposable gown up to 2–5 days at room temperature [19,33]. It can be removed from these surfaces by use of ethanol of concentration (95%, 85%, 80% and 78%) within 30 s [20,31]. A chemical 2-propanol with 100% and 75% concentration can also be used, which can remove the virus only in 30 s [31,34]. 1-Propanol of 30% concentration can remove the virus only in 30 s [34], formaldehyde with hydrogen-peroxide with 1% concentration only in 2 min [34], glutardialdehyde of 2.5% concentration from 2 to 5 min [21,35], povidone-iodine of 0.23%–0.47% concentration can remove the virus only in 15 s to 1 min, [35,36]. TGEV and MHV survive on the surface of steel up to 28 days at a temperature of 4 °C–20 °C. MHV takes about 10 min to remove it from the surface of steel. The chemicals that are used to remove this virus are ethanol of 70% concentration, 2-propanol of 50% concentration, benzalkonium chloride and chlorhexidine digluconate of 0.05% concentration, sodium hypochlorite of 0.001% concentration, formaldehyde of 0.7% concentration [27,37]. HCoV survives on the surface of steel (up to 5 days), aluminum (up to 2–8 h), glass (up to 5 days), PVC (up to 5 days), silicon rubber (up to 5 days) ceramic and Teflon (up to 5 days), and it can bear the temperature up to 21 °C [38,39]. HCoV can only be removed from the surfaces by benzalkonium chloride with a concentration of 0.2% [27,40].

4.2.1 The history of identification and spreading in the world

On December 31, 2019, some people in Wuhan city in China reported about the symptoms that were found in the sell market of beavers and snakes. Till today, it is still not been clear that which animal is responsible for inventing the coronavirus COVID-19. After 1 week, Chinese health authorities had announced that this virus belongs to the family of SARS and MERS coronaviruses [41–43]. After 2 days, in Wuhan, the first death was declared due to COVID-19. In January 13–15, 2020, health officials of Thailand and Japan announced that they found coronavirus COVID-19-infected confirmed cases in their respective countries. It means that this virus could spread outside of China. Japan and Thailand began to screen everyone coming from Wuhan city. From January 17, 2020, the United States began doing health checkup at airports for all people coming from Wuhan and, later checking started for all people coming from China. One confirmed case was also found in Washington State on January 21, 2020. China suspended its in-and-out traveling from January 23, 2020. Soon the movement became banned from the other cities in Hubei. On January 24, 2020, the number of infected persons increased very rapidly in Wuhan city. Temporary hospitals and nursing homes were arranged for taking care of the infected patients. On January 30, the United State Centers for Disease Control and Prevention announced that this virus could transmit from one human body to another, and that was why confirmed cases continued to rise rapidly. Scientists, doctors and researchers of the whole world started working to find effective treatment and/or invent vaccines [44–47].

4.3 Method

As the number of cases of COVID-19 has been increasing continuously in across the whole world, and it seems that a study should be done about this virus. It will make the people to be aware of the seriousness of this problem as in many countries, citizens are not taking it seriously. This manuscript will brief the people about its spreading rate so people may become aware of the prevailing danger worldwide due to this disease. To review, a bibliographic database of life sciences and biomedical information has been prepared. Medical Literature Analysis and Retrieval System has also been studied. All the current information is taken from the website of worldometer.info that continuously updates the data about the novel COVID-19. About 44 published manuscript/reports have been studied for this study and data is given in a review of literature section and some is in a tabular form.

4.4 Results

Most of the data describe the pandemic situation of novel COVID-19. In this study, it was also seen that survival timing and temperature of various viruses are different. Survival timing of MERS-CoV, TGEV, MHV and HCoV vary on steel, PVC, silicon rubber and ceramic surface from 2 days to 28 days at 20 °C–30 °C. SARS-CoV viruses can survive on the surface of all metals, wood, paper, glass, plastic and disposable gown from 1 day to 5 days at room temperature. The nature of present virus is different from the other viruses of their family. It can transmit from one human being to another. It is also seen that one virus can infect

406 people. Its growth rate of transmission is so fast that first 1 lakh persons were infected in 67 days while the next 1 lakh were infected only in 10 days and the third 1 lakh person were infected only in 4 days worldwide. It means the people of all countries should be aware of the prevailing dreadful situation. This chain of infection can be broken by the use of alcoholic chemicals like ethanol, propanol, benzalkonium chloride, hydrogen peroxide and povidone-iodine. This manuscript can play an important role for this purpose.

Figure 4.1 shows the top most 20 countries having maximum numbers of infected and death cases. Table 4.1 represents the percentage of death rates from confirmed cases and all cases with respect to ages of people. How the percentages are changed with respect to sex is given in Table 4.2. The percentages of death rates of prehistoric case are given in Table 4.3. The growth rates of death with respect to dates, ages and countries are also given by three graphs (Figures 4.2 and 4.3).

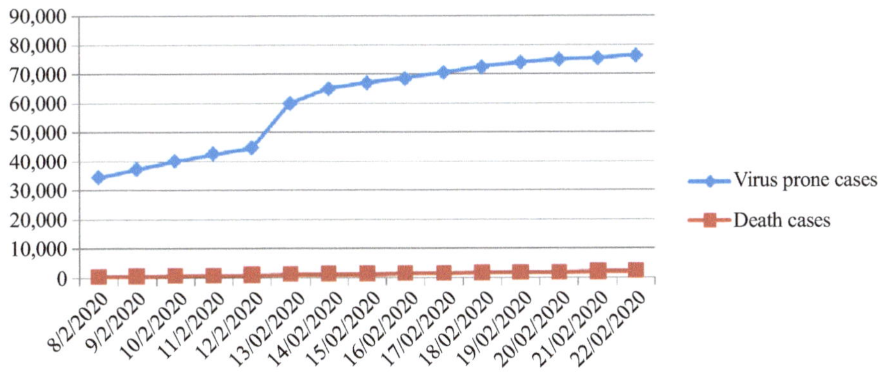

Figure 4.1 Graph between virus prone and death cases with respect to dates in month of February, 2020 [1]

Table 4.1 The fatality rates with respect to age of employees [24]

Age (years)	Percentage of rate of death (only in virus confirmed patients)	Percentage of rate of death (in all cases)
More than 80	21.9	14.8
70–79		8.0
60–69		3.6
50–59		1.3
40–49		0.4
30–39		0.2
20–29		0.2
10–19		0.2
0–9		No fatalities

Table 4.2 Rate of death in confirmed cases of infection by virus and all cases with respect to sex [24]

Sex	Percentage of rate of death (for confirmed cases)	Percentage of rate of death (for all cases)
Male	4.7	2.8
Female	2.8	1.7

Table 4.3 Rate of death in preexisting medical conditions [24]

Preexisting condition	Percentage of rate of death (for confirmed cases)	Percentage of rate of death (for all cases)
Cardiovascular disease	13.2	10.5
Diabetes	9.2	7.3
Chronic respiratory disease	8.0	6.3
Hypertension	8.4	6.0
Cancer	7.6	5.6
No preexisting conditions	–	0.9

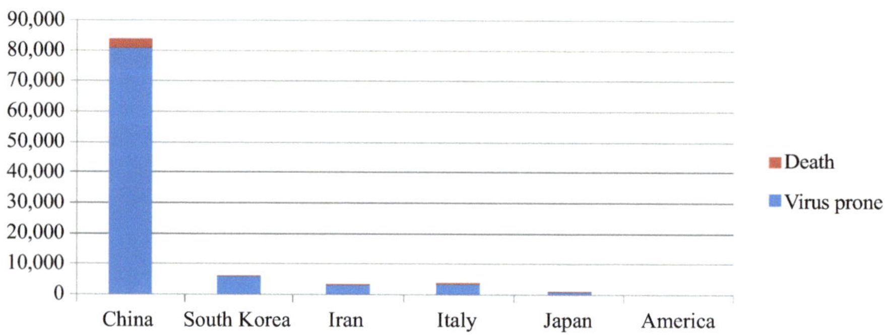

Figure 4.2 Number of infected and death cases with respect to countries (as on starting of end on February, 2020) [1]

4.5 Discussions

Novel coronavirus COVID-19 affects the people and society in many ways. The effects of this pandemic situation are not good for the universe. Some direct and indirect effects of this pandemic situation on human beings and nature are as follows:

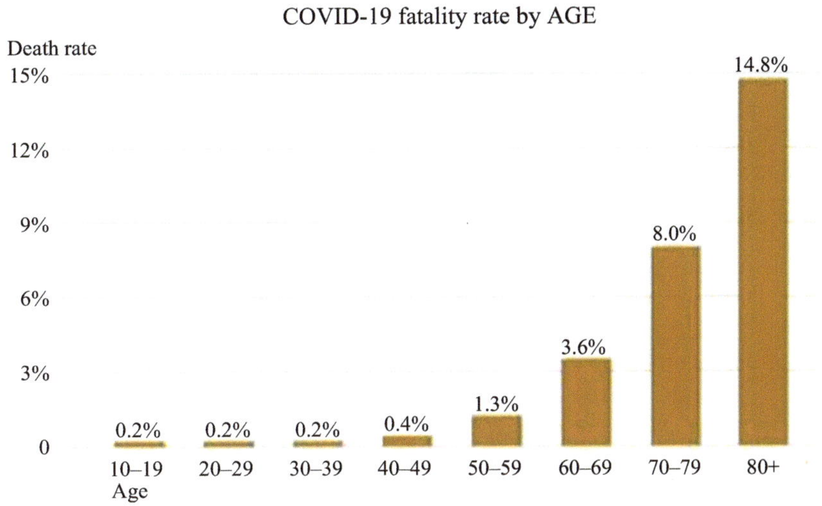

Figure 4.3 Death rate with respect to age of infected persons [1]

1. **Effect on food habits:** It is seen that the infection of the virus had started from the places where only the consumption of nonvegetarian food is practiced. A lot of amount of harmful germs are available inside the bats and snakes. When human beings use these as food, sometimes the germs present in bodies do not die and enter into the body of human beings. No study is available, which can establish that it can start from a person of vegetarian habit, but this virus can transmit from a nonvegetarian to a vegetarian person. Another aspect of this pandemic situation is that we are forgetting the real food habits. Right now, we are using fast food that is not healthy for our health. Perhaps this situation can give a lesson to improve our food habits.
2. **Effect on climate:** It was understood from the previous study, the transmission of viruses like SARS-CoV and MERS-CoV of coronavirus family depends upon the climate, that is why the spreading of these viruses is limited and easy to be controlled. But the nature of novel coronavirus COVID-19 is not controlled by climate change. It has been spread in all countries of different climates. To control it or break the chain, governments of many countries declared a lockdown or temporary curfews in their countries. However, it is not favorable for our economy, but during this period, manufacturing in industries is stopped, which may help to improve the climate.
3. **Temperature:** As per the previous reports, the novel coronavirus COVID-19 cannot survive beyond 25 °C. But no academic or experimental theory is available to prove it. It is also seen that the places where temperature is greater than 25 °C, infection cases are available. It means that virus cannot die by only raising temperature, rather it also depends upon exposure time. To break the chain of this virus, the movements of two, three and four wheelers

have been decreased on roads. It will also help to decrease the risk of global warming.

4. **Air pressure:** No study is available that relates the air pressure to the coronavirus. Air pressure affects human health, but whether it does affect COVID-19 is not known.
5. **Pollution:**
   (i) **Air pollution:** There is no report available that says that COVID-19 is affected by air pollution. But due to lockdown, the target to decrease the air pollution to a certain level by 2030 can be achieved only in 1 year, because the movements of trains, buses, cars and airplanes have considerably decreased. All domestic and international flights are stopped by a number of countries.
   (ii) **Sound pollution:** Factories, industries, buses, trucks, trains and airplanes that are responsible for sound pollution are stopped due to lockdown situation. Therefore, the level of sound pollution has decreased unexpectedly.
   (iii) **Water pollution:** This virus cannot be removed by only plain water. The bleached soap water can break the shape of virus and can remove it from the surface. There is no direct relation between COVID-19 and water pollution, although nowadays, people are not present at beaches and ships are not moving in sea. Factories that emit polluted water are temporary closed; most of the hotels that emit polluted water and pass it to river are closed. These aspects of COVID-19 show that it may become the reason to decrease water pollution. However, it also creates a huge loss on economy of a country.

6. **Average income per person:** Due to the lockdown situation in a country, the incomes of labors, shopkeepers, industrialists and common persons have been affected. The total income of the people has decreased. Thus, average income per person has decreased due to this pandemic situation.
7. **Gross domestic product (GDP):** As per person, average income has decreased in the present scenario, which may affect GDP. Every country requires a lot of expansion to fight against this virus, but the manufacturing of all products has come to a standstill. This will affect the GDP of every country.
8. **Education:** Education is the most essential part of students in country. Due to the lockdown situation, students cannot go to schools, colleges and universities. The conduct of examinations of students is also affected. Some universities and colleges are trying to teach students online, but it could not be arranged by every university or college. It seems that this period has become a great curse on students.
9. **Age group:** The virus COVID-19 affects each and every person and it has been spreading only by contacts of infected persons. If a member is infected due to this virus, it is a possibility that every member of family gets infected by this virus. The probability of recovery of young persons is more than old-aged persons.

10. **Currency factors:** The exchange of currency is much responsible for spreading this virus. The purchase and sell are made by currency in country. If money is handed over by an infected person, it can affect all persons who will handle it directly. Online payments play an important role in this situation.
11. **Body weight:** To stop the chain of virus spreading, a policy, work-from-home, is declared by governments and private offices. In this policy, employees have to work from home by the help of Internet. Due to a less movement of people, the weight of the employee may increase. It is suggested that employees should do something to get rid of this problem.
12. **Blood pressure:** When employees work in office, they remain well accustomed with its homogeneous atmosphere. In the work-from-home policy, working in a new environment without any supporting staff is challenging. At home, the frequency of taking food also increases, which may be the reason to increase the blood pressure of a person.
13. **Waste papers:** In the garbage of a city, 35% waste papers are available. In general, the waste papers can emerge due to written examinations of students, class teaching and the manual working of offices and hotels. In the present scenario, hotels, offices are closed. Teaching and examination are being done online, which may decrease the amount of waste papers. As we know that paper-mill industries are responsible for greenhouse gas emission, dirty and polluted water release and land pollution. Electricity and fuel oil are also considerably consumed by the paper-mill industry. The present scenario will help to decrease the amount of waste papers.

4.6 Precautions

From the previous analysis, it is suggested that people should follow the following instructions:

1. People should keep their surroundings clean.
2. When any person enters home, he/she should wash his hands properly by a beach soap or an alcoholic sanitizer.
3. During this period, the use of flight should be minimized as passengers in flight may come from different countries.
4. The use of public transports such as buses, trains and any other conveyances should be reduced.
5. The proper arrangement of sanitization at every transport station should be made.
6. Proper and suitable masks should be used.
7. As the transmission of this virus is highly possible from one human being to another, in Guangzhou and southern Guangdong province, robots are used for many purposes. A similar method should be adopted by us.
8. Vegetarian and nonvegetarian foods should be cooked separately, and, especially, nonvegetarian foods should be consumed after proper cooking.

4.7 Conclusions and future scope

From the previous analysis, it is concluded that the most dangerous part of coronavirus COVID-19 is human-to-human transmission. It can also transmit from the contaminated surfaces of steel, aluminum, metal, wood, plastic, PVC, papers and disposable gowns of human beings. This chain is continuously increasing. Borders of countries, climate, temperature and distances cannot stop this virus from spreading. It can even survive on these surfaces from some hours to many days. Some specific types of alcoholic chemicals like sodium hypochlorite, propanol and ethanol with different concentrations can break the chain of this virus. If human beings are not coming in contact with this, its transmission and spreading can break. Many countries are decided to follow the lockdown situation for their citizens. Perhaps, China uses this technology to stop this virus and now, the numbers of infected cases are very low. Every person should understand the present situation of the world and should cooperate to control this virus.

Acknowledgment

The authors are grateful to the management of Graphic Era Hill University Dehradun for providing all necessary facilities.

References

[1] Yvonne X. L., Yan L. N., James P. T., and Ding X. L. 'Human corona viruses: A review of virus–host interactions'. *Diseases* 2016, vol. 4, pp. 1–28.

[2] Pene F., Merlat A., Vabret A., *et al.* 'Coronavirus 229E-related pneumonia in immunocompromised patients'. *Clin. Infect. Dis.* 2003, vol. 37, pp. 929–32.

[3] Vander H. L. 'Human coronaviruses: What do they cause'. *Antivir. Ther.* 2007, vol. 12, pp. 651–58.

[4] Walsh E. E., Shin J. H., and Falsey A. R. 'Clinical impact of human coronaviruses 229E and OC43 infection in diverse adult populations'. *J. Infect. Dis.* 2013, vol. 208, pp. 1634–42.

[5] Frieman M., and Baric R. 'Mechanisms of severe acute respiratory syndrome pathogenesis and innate immunomodulation'. *Microbiol. Mol. Biol. Rev.* 2008, vol. 72, pp. 672–85.

[6] Peiris J. S. M., Guan Y., and Yuen K. Y. 'Severe acute respiratory syndrome'. *Nat. Med.* 2004, vol. 10, pp. 88–97.

[7] Kim Y., Cheon S., Min C., *et al.* 'Spread of mutant middle east respiratory syndrome coronavirus with reduced affinity to human CD26 during the South Korean outbreak'. *mBio* 2016, vol. 7, pp. 236–41.

[8] Graham R. L., Donaldson E. F., and Baric R. S. 'A decade after SARS: Strategies for controlling emerging coronaviruses'. *Nat. Rev. Microbiol.* 2013, vol. 11, pp. 836–48.

[9] Oboho I. K., Tomczyk S. M., Al-Asmari A. M., *et al.* 'MERS-CoV outbreak in Jeddah—A link to health care facilities'. *N. Engl. J. Med.* 2015, vol. 372, pp. 846–54.

[10] The Korean Society of Infectious Diseases; Korean Society for Healthcare-associated Infection Control and Prevention. 'An unexpected outbreak of middle east respiratory syndrome coronavirus infection in the Republic of Korea'. *Infect. Chemother.* 2015, vol. 47, Korea, pp. 120–2.

[11] Velavan T. P., and Meyer C. G. 'The COVID-19 epidemic'. *Trop. Med. Int. Health* 2020, vol. 7, pp. 278–80.

[12] Jin Y. H., Cai L., Cheng Z. S., Cheng H., Deng T., and Fan Y. P. 'A rapid advice guideline for the diagnosis and treatment of 2019 novel coronavirus (2019-nCoV) infected pneumonia'. *Mil. Med. Res.* 2020, vol. 7(1), pp. 4–13.

[13] Mahtani S., Berger M., O'Grady S., and Iati M. 'Hundreds of evacuees to be held on bases in California; Hong Kong and Taiwan restrict travel from mainland China'. *The Washington Post* 2020, p. 7.

[14] World Health Organization. Coronavirus disease 2019 (COVID-19): Situation report, 47. WHO; March, 2020.

[15] Wei X. S., Wang X., Niu Y., *et al.* 'Clinical characteristics of SARS-CoV-2 infected pneumonia with diarrhea'. *Rochester NY.* 2020, vol. 35, pp. 46–62.

[16] Chen N., Zhou M., Dong X., Qu J., Gong F., and Han Y. 'Epidemiological and clinical characteristics of 99 cases of 2019 novel coronavirus pneumonia in Wuhan, China: A descriptive study'. *Lancet* 2020, vol. 395, pp. 507–13.

[17] Hessen M. T. Novel Coronavirus Information Center: Expert guidance and commentary. Elsevier Connect. Archived from the original on 30 January 2020, Retrieved 31 January 2020.

[18] Lai C. C., Shih T. P., Ko W. C., Tang H. J., and Hsueh P. R. 'Severe acute respiratory syndrome coronavirus 2 (SARS-CoV-2) and coronavirus disease-2019 (COVID-19): The epidemic and the challenges'. *Int. J. Antimicrob. Agents.* 2020, vol. 55(3), pp. 105924–30.

[19] Lai M., Cheng P. K., and Lim W. W. 'Survival of severe acute respiratory syndrome coronavirus'. *Clin. Infect. Dis.* 2005, vol. 41, pp. 67–71.

[20] Rabenau H. F., Kampf G., Cinatl J., and Doerr H. W. 'Efficacy of various disinfectants against SARS coronavirus'. *J. Hosp. Infect.* 2005, vol. 61, pp. 107–11.

[21] Nagaraju R., Subhash Chandra Bose P., Ravi G., Damineni S., and Valluru R. 'A review on current status of buccal drug delivery system'. *Res. J. Pharm. Tech.* 2020, vol. 13(6), pp. 2954–62.

[22] Sujath R., Chatterjee J. M., and Hassanien A. E. 'A machine learning forecasting model for COVID-19 pandemic in India'. *Stochastic Environ. Res. Risk Assess.* 2020, vol. 34, pp. 959–72.

[23] Iwendi C., Bashir A. K., Peshkar A., *et al.* 'COVID-19 patient health prediction using boosted random forest algorithm'. *Front. Public Health* 2020, vol. 8, p. 357.

[24] www.worldometers.info/coronavirus/coronavirus-symptoms [Accessed: 23-Feb-2021].

[25] Zheng Y. Y., Ma Y. T., Zhang J. Y., and Xie X. 'COVID-19 and the cardiovascular system'. *Nat. Rev. Cardiol.* 2020, vol. 17(5), pp. 259–60.
[26] Al-Tawfiq J. A., Abdrabalnabi R., Taher A., Mathew S., and Rahman K. A. 'Infection control influence of Middle East respiratory syndrome coronavirus: A hospital-based analysis'. *Am. J. Infect. Control.* 2019, vol. 47, pp. 431–4.
[27] WHO. Infection prevention and control during health care when novel coronavirus (nCoV) infection is suspected. WHO; 2020. Interim guidance. 25 January 2020.
[28] Yen M. Y., Lu Y. C., Huang P. H., Chen C. M., Chen Y. C., and Lin Y. E. 'Quantitative evaluation of infection control models in the prevention of nosocomial transmission of SARS virus to healthcare workers; implication to nosocomial viral infection control for healthcare workers'. *Scand. J. Infect. Dis.* 2010, vol. 42, pp. 510–15.
[29] Alshammari M., Reynolds K. A., Verhougstraete M., and O'Rourke M. K. 'Comparison of perceived and observed hand hygiene compliance in healthcare workers in MERS-CoV endemic regions'. *Healthcare (Basel, Switzerland)* 2018, vol. 6, pp. 6–122.
[30] Vandoremalen N., Bushmaker T., and Munster V. J. 'Stability of Middle East respiratory syndrome coronavirus (MERS-CoV) under different environmental conditions'. *Euro Surveill.* 2013, vol. 18, pp. 32–45.
[31] Sidharta A., Pfaender S., Vielle N. J., Dijkman R., Friesland M., and Becker B. 'Virucidal activity of WHO-recommended formulations against enveloped viruses, including Zika, Ebola, and emerging coronaviruses'. *J. Infect. Dis.* 2017, vol. 215, pp. 902–6.
[32] Eggers M., Eickman M., and Zorn J. 'Rapid and effective virucidal activity of povidone-iodine products against Middle East respiratory syndrome CORONAVIRUS (MERS-CoV) and modified vaccinia virus ankara (MVA)'. *Infect. Dis. Ther.* 2015, vol. 4, pp. 491–501.
[33] Shu-Ming D., Xin-Sheng Z., Rui-Fu W., *et al.*, SARS Research Team, 'Stability of SARS coronavirus in human specimens and environment and its sensitivity to heating and UV irradiation'. *Biomed. Environ. Sci.* 2003, vol. 16, pp. 246–55.
[34] Rabenau H. F., Cinatl J., Morgenstern B., Bauer G., Preiser W., and Doerr H. W. 'Stability and inactivation of SARS coronavirus'. *Med. Microbiol. Immunol.* 2005, vol. 194, pp. 1–6.
[35] Kariwa H., Fujii N., and Takashima I. 'Inactivation of SARS coronavirus by means of povidone-iodine, physical conditions and chemical reagents'. *Dermatology* 2006, vol. 212, pp. 119–23.
[36] Eggers M., Koburger-Janssen T., Eickman M., and Zorn J. 'In vitro bactericidal and virucidal efficacy of povidone-iodine gargle/mouthwash against respiratory and oral tract pathogens'. *Infect. Dis. Ther.* 2018, vol. 7, pp. 249–59.
[37] Saknimit M., Inatsuki I., Sugiyama Y., and Yagami K. 'Virucidal efficacy of physico-chemical treatments against coronavirus and parvoviruses of laboratory animals'. *Jikken Dobutsu Exp. Anim.* 1988, vol. 37, pp. 341–5.

[38] Warnes S. L., and Little Z. R. K. 'Human coronavirus 229e remains infectious on common touch surface materials'. *mBio* 2015, vol. 6, pp. 1697–15.

[39] Sizun J., Yu M. W., and Talbot P. J. 'Survival of human coronavirus 229e and OC43 in suspension and after drying on surfaces: A possible source of hospital-acquired infections'. *J. Hosp. Infect.* 2000, vol. 46, pp. 55–60.

[40] Wood A., and Payne D. 'The action of three antiseptics/disinfectants against enveloped and non-enveloped viruses'. *J. Hosp. Infect.* 1998, vol. 38, pp. 283–95.

[41] Kampf G., Todt D., Pfaender S., and Steinmann E. 'Persistence of coronaviruses on inanimate surfaces and their inactivation with biocidal agents'. *J. Hosp. Infect.* 2020, vol. 104, pp. 246–51.

[42] Yen M. Y., Lu Y. C., Huang P. H., Chen C. M., Chen Y. C., and Lin Y. E. 'Quantitative evaluation of infection control models in the prevention of nosocomial transmission of SARS virus to health care workers: Implication to nosocomial viral infection control for health care workers'. *Scand. J. Infect. Dis.* 2010, vol. 42, pp. 510–15.

[43] Alshammari M., Reynold K. A., Verhougstraete M., and O'Rourke M. K. 'Comparison of perceived and observed and hygiene compliance in health care workers in MERS-CoV endemic reasons'. *Health Care* 2018, vol. 6, pp. 122–9.

[44] Huang C., Wang Y., Li X., *et al.* 'Clinical features of patients infected with 2019 novel coronavirus in Wuhan, China'. *Lancet* 2020, vol. 395, pp. 497–506.

[45] Wang D., Hu B., Hu C., *et al.* 'Clinical characteristics of 138 hospitalized patients with 2019 novel coronavirus-infected Pneumonia in Wuhan China'. *JAMA* 2020, vol. 323, pp. 1061–9.

[46] WHO. Coronavirus disease 2019 (COVID-19). Situation report 23. WHO; 2020.

[47] Dhamodharavadhani S., Rathipriya R., and Chatterjee J. M. 'COVID-19 mortality rate prediction for India using statistical neural network models'. *Front. Public Health* 2020, vol. 8, pp. 441.

Chapter 5

IoT-based smart healthcare monitoring system

Hakan Yüksel[1]

Abstract

The Internet of Things (IoT) has enormous potential to provide patients with better medical facilities in healthcare. At the same time, it facilitates the work of healthcare workers. In this work, the proposed system is to develop a web- and mobile-based application through sensors that communicate through networked devices and help monitor and record patients' medical information and health data. The proposed output of the system is to establish a system that will provide medical assistance in general standards to patients by grasping the information about their health conditions through the wearable device provided on the Internet, even in the most remote areas where there are no hospitals. In the developed device, a micro-controller that can record the patient's body temperature, oxygen saturation and heart rate was used. In the case of any medical emergency, the system can provide the necessary information to inform the doctors of the patient and family about the current health status of the patient and complete medical information. In addition, the collected information will provide an advantageous approach in decision-making and will provide the necessary information when the general health values are exceeded.

The main purpose of the study can be summarized as follows:

- Obtaining patient's health information via IoT.
- Collection and evaluation of information.
- Providing IoT-based health solutions.

Keywords: Arduino; Body temperature; Development boards; ESP-8266; Healthcare; Health information; Health monitoring; Heart rate; Internet of Things; IoT in healthcare; Microcontroller; Mobile-based software; Oxygen saturation; Smart healthcare service; Sensors; Software; ThingSpeak; Wearable technology; Web-based software; Web services

[1]Department of Computer Technologies, Technical Science Vocational School, Applied Science University of Isparta, Isparta, Turkey

5.1 Introduction

The Internet of Things (IoT) architecture can be roughly summarized as consisting of a lower sensor layer, an intermediate network layer and an upper application layer. Labels, one of the main methods of obtaining information at the bottom, are increasingly used in various business areas. The use of RFID tags is expected to replace existing barcodes in various business areas over time.

From past to present, Internet technologies continue with noticeable growth, and different needs and technologies are developed every day. IoT is one of the leading technologies developed in-line with these needs [1].

The IoT aims to connect physical objects such as machines, sensors and smart devices to the Internet, collect and process data from connected network devices and automatically execute certain business processes based on the data processed. In short, the IoT aims to create a dynamic global network infrastructure by connecting various virtual and physical objects [2]. It can also be defined as a system of devices that connect and share information through various communication protocols to communicate with each other and create an intelligent network. The IoT has started to be implemented rapidly in the fields of energy, environment, tourism, security, transportation and health.

Today, smart wearable technology product applications in the field of health are frequently encountered due to factors such as the expensiveness of health services, the development of microcontroller technology, sensor sizes, shrinkage in relation to the development of technology and significant developments in the world of wearable technology [3,4]. These systems allow the activities of people (sick or healthy individual) to be monitored all day and enable complex health practices to be performed at low costs. IoT-based healthcare applications can potentially provide comprehensive patient care in a variety of settings, such as outside the healthcare field (at home, etc.), acute (requiring short-term care) and long-term (requiring patient care). The data are collected and processed on a server with the help of communication technologies. In this way, healthcare professionals can quickly access more valuable information in the diagnosis and treatment of the disease [5].

Studies such as smart sensors, remote monitoring and medical device integration took place in the applications of the IoT in the field of health [6–8]. The fact that it has the potential to not only keep patients healthy and safe but also improve the service delivery practices of healthcare personnel is a potential factor in the use of the IoT in the field of health. Through the developed devices, patients and their doctors can communicate more, and more information flow is provided. Therefore, increasing patient–doctor interaction increases solution-oriented satisfaction [9].

Smart patient monitoring systems are systems that enable vital signals received from patients to reach servers in health centers and specialist personnel such as doctors and nurses through servers. All information from the sensors is collected by the network and processed and sent to the receiving unit for transmission to the server. In today's applications, the sensor can be connected directly to the Internet.

The data can be viewed on a smart device or any computer connected to the Internet, if desired. The server processes the data from the sensors and can share it over the Internet using a wired or wireless connection. Finally, the transferred data should be transmitted to the server computer in a regular and sequential manner. The data saved on the server are shared with other units when requested [10]. The general scheme of the smart patient monitoring system is shown in Figure 5.1.

Smart patient monitoring systems can be configured in various ways. A smart system designed to monitor health status can contain many sensors, triggers, smart fabrics and electronic textiles, power supplies, wireless devices, microcontroller units and processors, as well as software. These systems can process vital signals such as body temperature, heartbeat, blood pressure, oxygen ratio in the blood and respiratory rate. The data obtained through the sensors can be transmitted to the relevant specialists in the health center via the IoT. By making use of the data coming from the sensors, the specialist can follow the patient's condition without the need to meet face to face. Today, intelligent systems can process instantaneous data and send notifications to specialists, and patients are gaining increasing importance. The patient can easily use these systems in his daily life, so that the patients' health information is monitored instantly without going to the health center or hospital, and as a result, patients are prevented from wasting time going to the hospital or health center frequently [11,12]. Moreover, these systems can also make an emergency call to the relevant health centers in possible emergencies.

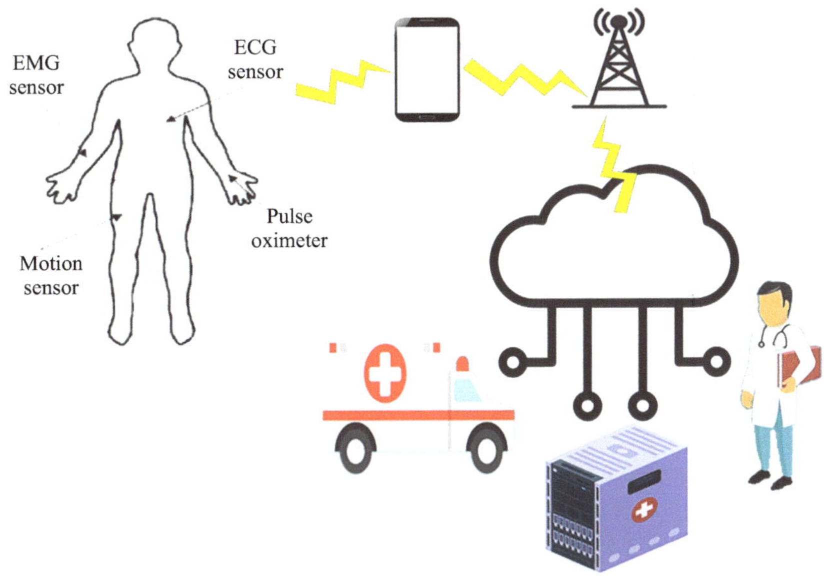

Figure 5.1 Smart patient monitoring system

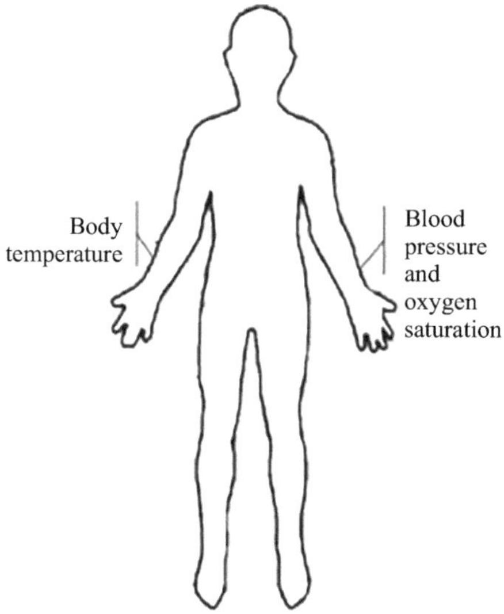

Figure 5.2 Receiving positions of health data in the human body

Various health data on the patients' bodies are obtained with the help of the sensors shown in Figure 5.2. Through these measurements, steps such as identifying the disease, treating the disease and monitoring the disease are carried out.

Although body temperature is not the same in all people, it is generally around 36.5°C in healthy people. Body temperature is not a disease, but one of the symptoms of possible disease. Average body temperature may vary due to factors such as the person's age, gender, muscle activity and external temperature. A body temperature that is higher than normal (hyperthermia) or lower than normal (hypothermia) can be a sign of any disease. However, other symptoms should be carefully monitored in order to definitively identify the disease [13].

The pulse is the pressure on the veins of the blood pumped by the heart with each beat. It is the feeling of how many times the heart contracts in a minute with different techniques. With each contraction, the blood is first sent to the aorta and then to the other vessels with pressure. Their elastic structure, the vessels constantly expand and then narrow. This enlargement can be felt by groping in places close to the surface, such as the wrist, temple and groin. While the heart rate may differ from person to person due to different factors such as age, gender and physical structure, it is normal to observe pulse changes due to different reasons such as body temperature, physiological changes, physical activity and emotional changes, drug use, illness and stress [14].

The pulse is the pressure on the veins of the blood pumped by the heart with each beat. It is also expressed as the number of heart contractions per minute. The pressure created by the contraction of the heart is transmitted to other vessels, especially the aorta. The elastic structures of the vessels constantly expand and contract. This change is felt by gripping near the skin, such as the temple and wrist.

The number of heartbeats may differ from person to person due to parameters such as age and physical structure, especially gender. In addition to these, heart rate changes can be observed due to different reasons such as body temperature, physiological changes, physical exertion, emotional changes, stress and illness [14].

Blood pressure, the pressure force exerted by the heart on the blood continues through the veins in the body. This pressure force is also felt on the vessel walls. The pressure exerted by the blood on the vessel wall is called blood pressure. Blood pressure decreases when the heart relaxes and increases when the heart contracts. The blood pressure that occurs when the heart relaxes is called the small blood pressure, and the blood pressure that occurs when the heart contracts is called the high blood pressure. The systolic blood pressure value in a normal person should not exceed 140 mmHg. The diastolic pressure should not be more than 80 mmHg. High or low blood pressure can harm the body. High blood pressure can strain blood vessels and cause bleeding. On the other hand, low blood pressure causes organs not to receive enough oxygen [15].

The oxygen rate in the blood is carried to the cells in our body by means of the hemoglobin cells in the arterial blood. Since the number of hemoglobin cells in the blood is limited, there is a certain amount of oxygen that the blood can carry. The ratio of the amount of oxygen carried by the blood to the maximum amount of oxygen it can carry gives the oxygen saturation value of the blood. This value is known in medical language as SpO_2. The SpO_2 method can be defined as a method that sends 960-nm red and 660-nm infrared light waves to the blood and determines the oxygen rate in the blood according to the amount of light reflected back. The functional SpO_2 value in a normal person is around 95% [16]. The SpO_2 method can be easily measured from external organs such as earlobe, fingertip or nose.

Respiration rate is the process of expelling carbon dioxide gas from the blood through the lungs and providing oxygen to the cells in the body. The respiratory rate in a normal adult person is 10–15 breaths/min.

Problems that can be seen in the body when breathing stops are as follows:

- cardiac tenderness per minute,
- 1–4 minute: tendency to damage per minute,
- 4–6 minute: onset of brain damage per minute,
- Brain damage in the 6th to 10th minute,
- +10 minute: irreversible brain damage can occur within minutes.

As can be seen, a person whose breathing stops can be damaged in a very short time in the brain and nerve tissues [17].

Body temperature, respiratory rate and blood pressure along with pulse are the most basic vital signs that show the instant situation of the person. Changes in findings in this group, including heart rate, provide useful information about the general condition of the person.

Intelligent, low-cost and low-energy sensors used in smart monitoring technologies are designed to receive and assist patients with a wealth of health information. These systems provide fast and secure data retrieval. As the IoT technology develops, wireless sensors, mobile devices, smart wearable technology products will make a great contribution to health services by providing a smart environmental structure.

In this study, a functional remote device that reduces the cost of potentially long-term (requiring patient care), acute (requiring hospital care) and out-of-hospital patient care saves time and cost by eliminating the need for the patient to go to the health center and works by minimizing patient life. It is aimed to design a smart patient monitoring system. The developed device can measure the patient's body temperature, oxygen saturation and heart rate.

In this part of the study, first of all, studies in the field of smart health services will be examined in order to draw attention to the developments in the IoT technology in the literature. Afterward, the evaluation of the smart health services model developed based on IoT within the scope of hardware and software and the presentation of necessary information about the system structure were transferred section by section.

5.2 Related work

Smart wearable systems (SWS) were the first examples used in the field of health within the scope of the IoT. SWS, which are systems designed to monitor the patient 7/24 and to warn them when necessary, have been included in our daily lives as factors that have increased their prevalence and made life easier in the last 10 years, and their number is increasing rapidly [18]. According to the research conducted by PwC (Price Waterhouse Coopers) in the USA in 2014, 56% of the participants stated that the average life expectancy will increase within 10 years due to the use of AGSs, and 46% of them prevent obesity by controlling their nutrition and exercise activities [19]. Researcher thinks that it can be passed when the applications of IoT related to health services are examined: tracking of objects and people (patient or staff), identification and verification, automatic data collection and remote sensing.

When the literature is examined, it is seen that there are more system designs that receive information from the individual and transfer it to a central server, thus enabling health providers to obtain information about the individual's health status. Khan has designed a wireless IoT and RFID-based patient-tracking system that detects body temperature, blood pressure, electroencephalography (EEG) signs and the amount of glucose in the blood, especially electrocardiogram (ECG), for the regular follow-up of the patient by the healthcare providers. The sensor data obtained from the patient are transferred to the smart phone and computer with RFID technology. These devices were sent to the structures in health systems via the Internet using network services [20].

A multibody sensor network structure was developed by Lebepe *et al.* to learn the stress situation in real time. With this sensor network, body temperature, galvanic skin response and heart rate are detected, and it is desired to make some estimation about the stress state of the person. The received information was transferred to the phone via Bluetooth connected to a microcontroller. The information on the phone was recorded and analyzed in a database on a server [21].

Alexander and Arun performed ECG measurement with a lightweight, portable and contactless armband that can be connected to android-based smart devices. The real-time signals from the data were converted under microprocessor control in an ECG sensor for amplification and filtering purposes. The processed data were sent to mobile phones for viewing via Bluetooth technology. The test results showed that the long-term measurements of the system are stable, easily portable and easy to use. In addition, it has been shown that the system can have information about whether there is any abnormality in cardiac activities by checking the records of the patient or health server in detail [22].

Kaplan *et al.* developed the family physician monitoring system. Physiological signs such as nonelectrical blood pressure, pulse, body temperature and SpO_2 were transmitted in accordance with health standards. Graphical signals (ECG, electromyography (EMG), etc.) were also displayed graphically and transmitted to a smart device. However, it has been stated that these obtained signals do not have a medical value due to the common signal suppression rate and low sampling frequency of the measurement system. An e-health sensor platform (Arduino Health Kit), which works together with the programming platform of the widely used Arduino Uno development board, was used to measure these signals. The obtained information was transferred wirelessly to a mobile application with the 2.4-GHz HC-05 Bluetooth 2.0 module [23,24].

Delrobaei *et al.* focused on the design of an IoT-based wearable device for the monitoring of body tremor, which is one of the symptoms of Parkinson's disease, in the home environment of the patient. Many sensor systems have been tried to objectively measure the tremor status of Parkinson's patients. These systems include gyroscope, accelerometer, goniometer (joint range of motion measurer), EMG and optical motion capture systems [25]. It has been stated that inertial measurement units combining these sensors offer a new approach.

MercuryLive, a structure that allows home monitoring of people with Parkinson's disease using wearable sensors, has been developed. MercuryLive is built from a web-based graphical user interface client with three layers on the basis of wearable sensors, data acquisition engine, live data streaming and web services used for storing sensor data, as well as video conferencing capability to increase communication efficiency. It has been stated that the main computers of the server in the system provide the opportunity to collect, store and securely provide patient data, and provide both visual and graphical patient follow-up with its graphical user interface [26].

In mobile patient monitoring applications, various network technologies are used to transfer data between sending and receiving centers. Otto *et al.* designed wireless body sensor network architecture for monitoring the health status of patients. The system consists of multiple sensor nodes and a network coordinator that monitors the user's body movement and heart activity. It consists of a server and a digital assistant working on the computer within the system [27].

A smart health monitoring system has been developed that uses mobile devices to collect real-time health data from errors and store this information on network servers connected to the Internet. These data were used to determine medical diagnosis using a network of sensors after being acquired by a wearable device [28].

For the rehabilitation of the patient in daily life, the LiveNet system, a flexible wearable platform, has been developed for real-time dataflow and condition classification. Data received with sensor networks were classified and analyzed on Linux-based Zaurus PDA. It has been stated that LiveNet can be used for classification in many areas such as ECG, EEG, emotion perception, stress perception, follow-up of Parkinson's patients and perception of critical health conditions of soldiers. It is stated that the system also has Bluetooth, GPRS, GSM, GPS, cameras and RTT modem technologies for communication. HMM (hidden Markov model) and FFT techniques have been applied with LiveNet for critical situations of soldiers [29].

For risky patients, the wearable wrist band called AMON has been carried out as a different study that detects the pulse, blood oxygen amount and body temperature of the patients and transmits wireless data to the healthcare providers over the network [30].

Wristbands, which have become more popular in recent years, have been designed for athletes, an IoT-based wearable device that measures the pulse (heart rate) and the amount of oxygen in the blood. In the designed device, STM32-based microcontroller series was used to detect these parameters from the athlete. The use of the wireless transmission module provides data transmission to the smart devices of athletes, trainers and healthcare professionals for processing and analyzing the athlete's blood oxygen amount and heart rate information according to the needs of different users [31].

Many different applications have been developed that detect and monitor biological signals. Using a smart chair, a system has been developed that can continuously monitor the ballistocardiogram and physiological signals of ECG in sitting position for scale [32].

Using the Intel Galileo development board, the system was developed that collects various health data and uploads them to the database server used by healthcare professionals. One of the main goals of the developed system is to reduce the effort caused by patients going to the hospital each time to control their health parameters [33]. A similar study by Sahoo *et al.* examined the healthcare management system and the large amount of patient records obtained from various reports. They analyzed health parameters to predict the patient's future health conditions. They developed a cloud-based big data analytics platform to predict health conditions using probabilistic tools [34].

Smart wearables have much more efficient power management than traditional devices. At the same time, they have devices that can communicate with health servers 24/7 as they can connect to a network server. In addition to these, they should be able to correct their mistakes by training themselves with continuous measurements. Nagavelli and Guru Rao [35] proposed a new method for estimating disease severity from patient medical records using a statistical approach based on data mining, which expressed as the degree of disease probability threshold.

A data model has also been developed to use and record IoT data. Researchers have developed a source-based ubiquitous data accessing method to globally collect and publish data from IoT devices. They also offered an emergency medical service based on how IoT data are collected and used across different platforms [36].

When the studies in the literature were examined, it was determined that the majority of the researchers followed the health system of the patients and went to develop a new model and system with the study they focused on (stress control, abnormal heart activities, hypoglycemia, acute, etc.). In addition, body area network technology has started to be used actively with the widespread use of smart patient monitoring systems. Considering the patient's health history and qualifications (region of residence, gender, race, etc.), diseases that are at risk are identified, and it has been observed that the most appropriate portable device that the person can use according to a proactive approach continues actively.

5.3 Proposed method

The smart healthcare monitoring system designed in this study consists of two main parts: hardware and software. In the hardware part of the system, it has been realized as a structure that enables the measurement of the data in the body of the person using sensors and the transfer of the data to the Internet environment (web services). In the software part, there are software that perform the wireless transmission of the data received from the sensors, web services, database applications and mobile applications. In addition, there is an embedded software system in order to extract meaningful information from the data obtained. The general structure and working principle of the designed system is shown in Figure 5.3.

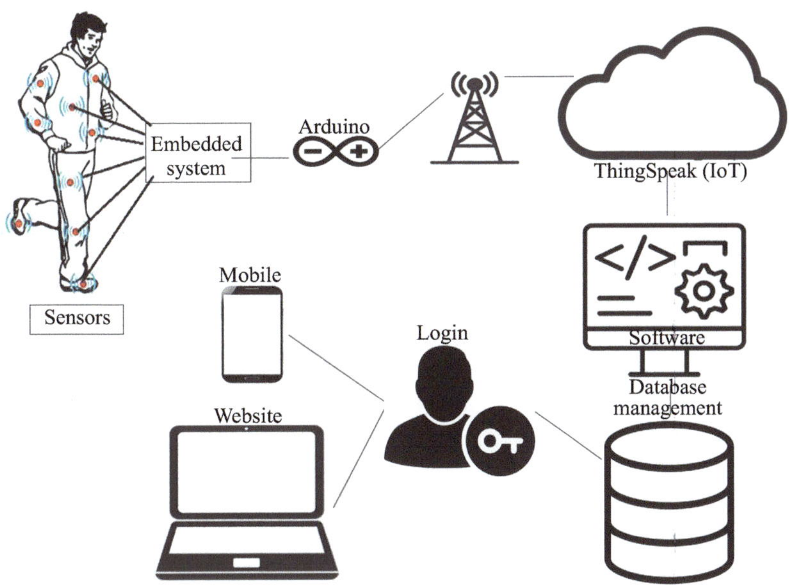

Figure 5.3 Proposed system model

Various health parameters (body temperature, oxygen saturation and heart rate) are obtained by the sensors on the practitioners using the system, and this information is transmitted to a network unit determined as an access point (AP) by using the Arduino Wi-Fi module in the IoT standard. Since this information transmitted to web services comes as a collective data structure, first of all, these data are distinguished. Health data measured from sensors are transferred to the Internet environment via web technology services. In addition, this information on the web is saved on a database server for permanent recording. Users or healthcare professionals can view this information saved on the server via the web page or mobile application.

5.3.1 Hardware

In this hardware unit, there are sensors (pulse, blood oxygen saturation and body temperature) to obtain the health data of the person and a development board to which these sensors are connected.

5.3.1.1 Development board

As a microcontroller technology in the system, Arduino Uno development board, which has become very common in recent years and is very practical to implement and contains an Atmel ATmega328-based microcontroller, is used. Features such as supporting the open source software philosophy, having numerous hardware and sensor support, and being cost-effective, were effective in the selection of this platform [37].

The Arduino platform consists of an Atmel microcontroller combination that includes program memory, data memory and input and output channels integrated into the system. The hardware units required for the operation of the system are already available on the integrated card. Due to this advantage, many electronic applications can be made quickly with Arduino-based circuit boards. Special software is available for Arduino programming. C/C++ language is used in the program [38].

Arduino can receive the data around it through the many sensors it supports and can understand its environment the modules that can be added to it. In addition, many technologies such as Wi-Fi, RJ45 Ethernet port, Bluetooth, biological sensors as well as memory cards can be used easily peripheral hardware units called modules that can be mounted on Arduino products [39,40].

There are many types of Arduino boards. In the realized project, Arduino Uno R3 board was used in the circuit adapted to the body of the person. The transfer of the data coming from the person's body to the Internet is provided with the ESP-8266 Wi-Fi module. Biological sensors were used to detect health data.

5.3.1.2 Arduino Uno R3

The Arduino Uno is connected to the computer with a USB and provides power to the sensor with an operating voltage of 5 V. Atmel ATmega328 IC, the Arduino is controlled with the desired programming. The recommended supply voltage is in the range of 7–12 V. It runs at 16 MHz and has 2 kB of memory. The

Table 5.1 The basic features of Arduino boards [43]

Microcontroller	ATmega328
Digital I/O	14 (6 of them support PWM)
Analog input	6
Operating voltage	+5 V DC
Supply voltage	7–12 V DC
Limits of supply voltage	6–20 V
DC current per I/O	40 mA
Current for 3.3 V	50 mA
Flash memory	32 kB
SRAM	2 kB
EEPROM	1 kB
Clock	16 MHz
Other specifications	4 LEDs (TX, RX, Pin 13, power indicator), reset switch

Arduino is connected to the computer to control the pins on the Arduino. Arduino has 14 digital input/output pins. Six of them are used as PWM outputs. There is also a reset button and ICSP header on the board [41,42]. The basic features of Arduino Uno are given in Table 5.1.

5.3.1.3 ESP-8266: Wi-Fi module

Wi-Fi modules are the ones used to upload or receive data by connecting to the Internet via any Wi-Fi. These modules allow data transfer from Arduino to web servers using the standard HTTP protocol [44]. ESP-8266 Wi-Fi module was used for the developed system. One of the most capable modules used to connect to the Internet via Wi-Fi is the ESP-8266. ESP-8266 can also work independently without the need for any microcontroller. There are also different versions of this module.

ESP-8266 module includes a 32-bit Tensilica L106 microcontroller that can operate at 80–160 MHz. The module directly supports TCP/IP, 802.11.b/g/n communication protocol and WPA/WPA2 use. The module has two serial communication channels in order to communicate with peripheral units and supports SPI, UART, I2C and I2S protocols over these channels. It has a 10-bit ADC input for measuring from the external environment, 17 GPIO inputs and 4 PWM channels for analog output. A PCB antenna can be used for communication, as well as an external antenna can be attached to increase the communication distance. With two MIMO (multiple inputs and multiple output) support, there can be more than one antenna on the receiver and transmitter. This feature, a single wireless network, can be established within 1 km [45–48].

ESP-8266 modules usually need to be updated before they can be used. For this reason, the ESP-8266 was updated before the electronic circuit was installed. The ESP-8266 connects to the Wi-Fi network specified in the microcontroller using the username and password specified in the microcontroller. After the connection process is successful, the information from the sensors is sent to the IoT platform through this module.

5.3.1.4 MAX30102: pulse and oxygen saturation sensor

The MAX30102 sensor in Figure 5.4 can measure vital signs of a person's oxygen saturation and heart rate.

Pulse oximetry is a noninvasive procedure used to measure the peripheral capillary oxygen saturation level in the blood. It is calculated as the amount of oxygen dissolved in the blood (hemoglobin and deoxyhemoglobin). The sensor measures the absorption spectra of oxygenated hemoglobin (HbO_2) and deoxygenated hemoglobin (Hb). It is evaluated using two different wavelengths of light, namely, red light (660 nm) and infrared light (940 nm). Oxygenated hemoglobin (HbO_2) has high absorption at 940 nm, and deoxygenated hemoglobin (Hb) at 660 nm.

The probe used for pulse oximeter measurement is placed in areas such as earlobe or fingertip. These are the places where the tissue layer in our body is the thinnest. Pulse oximeter generally contains two different working techniques. These are known as reflectance (where the transmitter and receiver are placed opposite each other) and transmittance (where the transmitter and receiver are placed on the same side) [49].

The MAX30102 uses two different wavelengths for SpO_2 measurements. In the MAX30102, infrared and red LEDs are used to identify individual PPG signals. Infrared and red LEDs have different AC and DC amplitudes, so these signals need to be filtered. For this process, an *R* ratio is determined along with SpO_2. The expression *R* is known as an "ratio of the odds." The following equation shows the calculation of the *R* value:

$$R = \frac{AC_{red}/DC_{red}}{AC_{IR}/DC_{IR}}$$

Once the *R* expression is determined, a curvilinear approach or a lookup table is used to estimate SpO_2. These data are typically collected through empirical methods. The patient's age, gender, medical and general health conditions may affect the accuracy of SpO_2 measurement. In this study, SpO_2 values in the 0.4–3.4

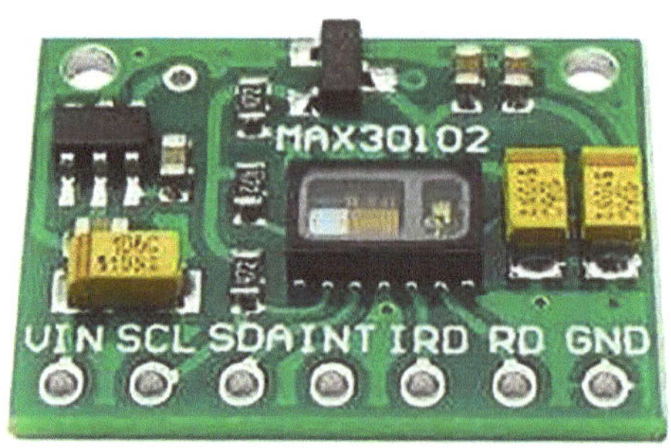

Figure 5.4 MAX30102 sensor

R value range were calculated using data equation derived from the Prahl [50] best fit straight-line approach:

$$SpO_2 = 104 - 17R$$

Heart rate information can also be obtained with the MAX30102 sensor. In this application, the heart rate information is again obtained by the MAX30102 sensor. The DS18B20 sensor was used to measure body temperature via an SpO_2 module.

5.3.1.5 DS18B20: body temperature sensor

Body temperature gives important clues in the diagnosis of some diseases and in determining the general condition of the patient. DS18B20 temperature sensor is a module on which resistor connections are made, and it has been brought in for easy supply and signal output. The pin configuration of a DS18B20 temperature sensor board is shown in Figure 5.5. There is a DS18B20 1-line digital temperature sensor. This sensor gives values in the range of 9–12-bit with values in the range of −55°C to 125°C (±0.5°C). The most important feature of the sensor is its high sensitivity and it is a digital sensor, not an analog one. In this way, a more stable temperature measurement is realized. The DS18B20 has a unique 64-bit serial number engraved in it. This sensor, which can be easily used for heat measuring devices, in projects that measure temperature, can be used with many microcontroller systems, especially Arduino.

Features of the heat sensor

- Temperature −10°C to 80°C (accuracy of ±0.5°C)
- Operating voltage: 3.0–5.0 V
- 9- or 12-bit selectable resolution
- A single digital pin can be used for communication with the 1-wire interface

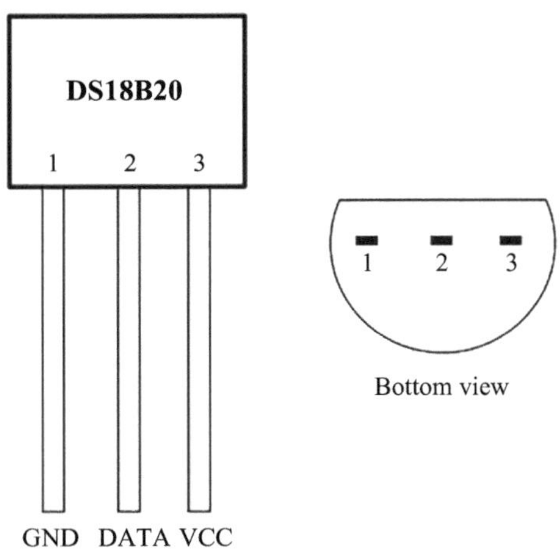

Figure 5.5 Pin configuration of a DS18B20 sensor

- There is a temperature limit warning system
- Response time of less than 750 ms
- Three wire (red wire—VCC, black cable—GND, white cable—DATA)
- 6-mm diameter, 30-mm long stainless steel sheath
- 1-m-long cable

5.3.1.6 DHT11: temperature sensor

DHT11 is used to measure humidity and temperature values of indoor and outdoor environments. An 8-bit microcontroller is integrated in its internal structure. The DHT11 sensor measures the temperature value with the NTC temperature measurement unit and measures the humidity value with the resistive humidity measurement unit. The configurations between the sensor and the controller card must be properly calibrated in order to make the measurements correctly [51].

DHT11 is a humidity and temperature sensor unit that can output digital signals. It is efficient and reliable in long-term work. Thanks to its high-performance 8-bit microprocessor, it provides fast and quality response. The unit measures temperature between 0°C and 50°C with a margin of error of 2°C, and a humidity meter with an error margin of 5% RH between 20% and 90% RH. In Table 5.2, the operating range values of the relevant sensor are given.

5.3.2 Software

The coordinated operation of the designed system with the hardware architecture is carried out by using various software technologies. The software used in the system can be examined in two parts as embedded system software and web and mobile technologies software. With the embedded system software, the data received from the patient's body via sensors are arranged and transferred to the unit to be used over the network. The data are transferred to the Arduino Wi-Fi module, which is used as a gateway, as a 1-byte data string. First of all, the start bit of the data coming to the Wi-Fi module is extracted, then successively incoming data packets are assigned to predefined values in order. Thus, the data coming from the microcontroller circuit is separated and ready to be transferred to web services.

The platform and programming technologies used in the implementation of the web application in this study are briefly mentioned in the following:

- *Visual Studio.NET*: It is an application development platform developed for the .NET platform. One of its biggest features is that it offers a common application development platform called IDE (integrated development environment).

Table 5.2 DHT11 sensor measuring ranges

Features	Measure
Operating temperature	0°C–50°C
Temperature tolerance	±1°C
Humidity range	20%–90%
Humidity tolerance	±4%

- *SQL Server*: It is a comprehensive database platform that can provide data management. An SQL Server provides reliable storage for structured and relational data that allow building and managing data applications with high performance and availability.
- *Asp.NET:* It is a web application developed by Microsoft. It also includes technologies that allow the development of XML-based web services. Asp.Net codes work based on common language runtime. In other words, it is possible to develop Asp.NET-based applications with all software languages under the .NET framework. In other words, as in java technology, the code written by the programmer is translated into a common language by a virtual script layer before it is run.
- *Android Studio*: It is an environment developed for programmers. In this environment, software developers can create applications suitable for devices with Android operating system. The testing process of these applications can also be carried out in Android Studio. Java is used as the programming language. Also, Android Studio's operating system is Cross-platform. This means multiplatform software. In this way, software distribution can be realized for more than one operating system.

The developed web service: It provides an access base to different interface tools that can be used by specialists or patients to access the data recorded on the server at any time. The data can be viewed by both the web page and the mobile application by entering the user name and password by the expert or the relevant person who wants to view the data received from the person. The website used was developed using Microsoft Visual Studio, and the mobile application was developed using Android Studio interface programs.

5.3.3 ThingSpeak: an IoT web service

ThingSpeak is a free data platform designed for the IoT. It collects and stores data in real time. ThingSpeak is a web-based open API IoT-based information platform that converts external components used for IoT into their own data and is used to store sensor data [23]. ThingSpeak communicates as a "data packet" carrier between the Internet connection and the cloud and receives, records, analyzes, observes and operates the detected graph from the connected sensor to the main microcontroller [46].

Its applications and API keys: It can simply communicate with other platforms. A ThingSpeak platform is used to collect and analyze data from devices and present these analysis and values to the user. At the same time, working information of the device can be shared over social media platforms (Twitter, etc.) with the applications offered on the ThingSpeak platform, and critical values can be sent to the mobile device as a notification.

In this study, instantaneous measurements were made from the sensors on the system. The received data were sent to ThingSpeak IoT interface with an ESP-8266 microcontroller–based Wi-Fi module.

5.3.4 Structure and working principle of the system

Vital data received through the sensors in the patient's body will be sent to the Arduino Wi-Fi module via the embedded system, and from there it will be transferred to the Internet environment via an AP. The data transferred to the Internet will be saved in the database on the server by means of web services. The data recorded in the database will be presented to authorized persons (identified persons within the system) via the website and mobile application designed to be used and queried when necessary. The flowchart of the created software is shown in Figure 5.6.

The designed microcontroller system measures a total of five data, three vital data and two ambient data, in the patient's body, and transmits them simultaneously to the Wi-Fi module. After these transmitted data are saved in the database via web services, they are presented to the relevant experts and people in the form of a

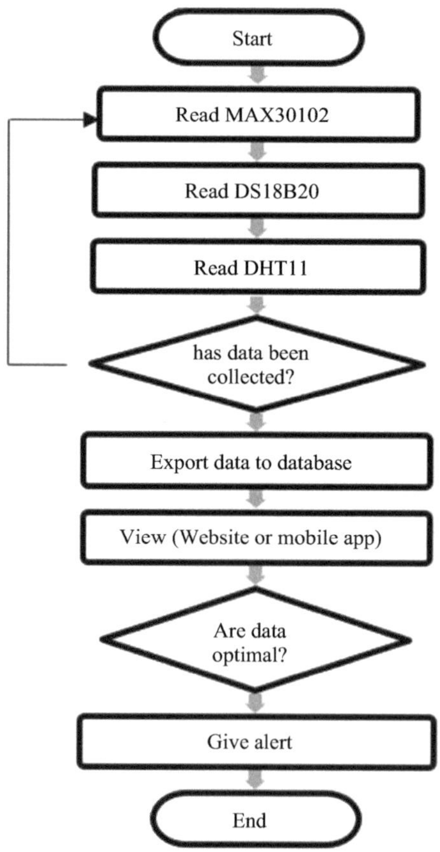

Figure 5.6 Flowchart of the system

visual interface (website or mobile app). Figure 5.7 shows a block diagram of the system.

5.3.4.1 Web software interface (GUI)

In order to access the health data registered in the database, first of all, it is necessary to be authorized to access the designed site (Figure 5.8). After logging into the system with a user name and password, the vital data of the relevant patient can be observed instantly and historical records can be followed.

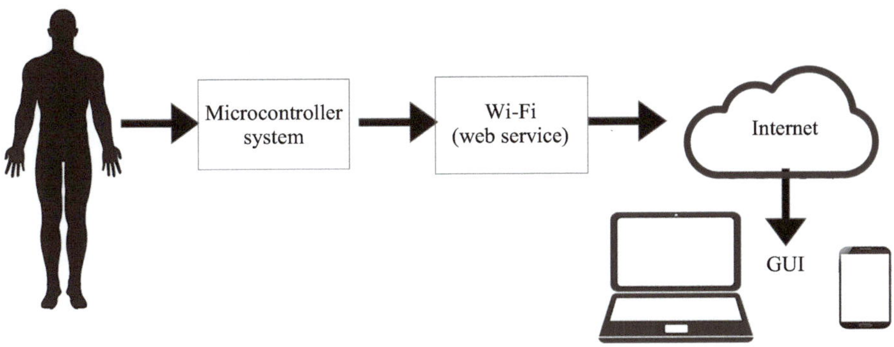

Figure 5.7 System block diagram

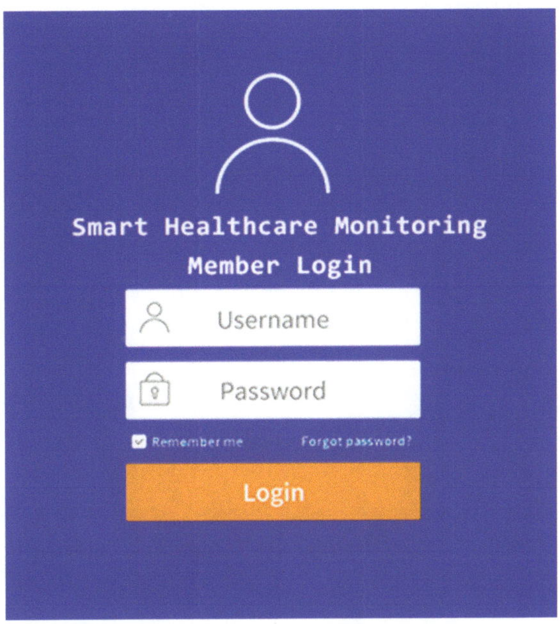

Figure 5.8 Website interface

5.3.4.2 Mobile software (GUI)

The mobile application, which is another interface of the system, provides the measurement data taken from the patient to be viewed by smart devices by querying the database. These data can be viewed by both the patient and healthcare professionals.

After installing the application, you must first register. During the registration process, the individual selects one of the "Doctor" or "Patient" profiles in the system and performs the registration from the screen in Figure 5.9(a).

After the registration screen, the login is made from the screen that appears for login. After specifying the doctor or patient status, the system can be entered in-line with the information in the system.

In logins made with the "Doctor" user type, a doctor can see the list of patients he has added himself. By selecting any of these patients, it can also check the historical measurement data of the patient. When the lower and upper limit values of the measured values are exceeded, a warning notification is sent to the doctor by the platform.

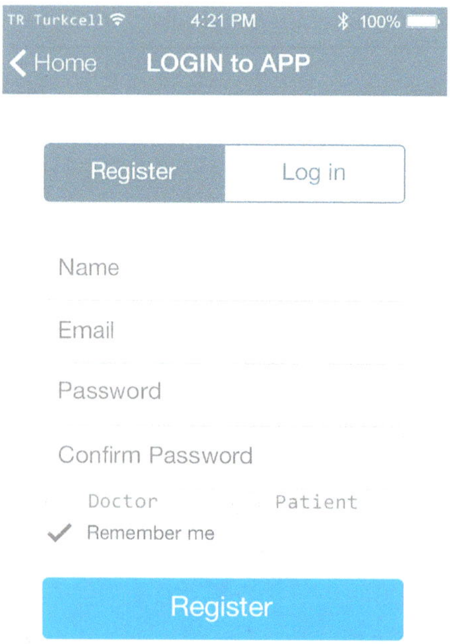

(a)

HR	SpO_2	Body Temperature
72	95	36.5
75	92	37
71	92	36.5
73	95	37
68	94	36.5
74	96	36.5
75	95	36.5
68	93	37
72	92	37
70	91	37
72	92	36.5
72	95	37
71	92	36.5
70	94	37
67	95	37

(b)

Figure 5.9 (a) Mobile application registration screen, (b) patient screen

When logging in with the "Patient" user type, he or she can see the values of past health measurements from the device, which are regularly made, as well as his personal information (Figure 5.9(b)). In addition, the patient can view the doctor who added himself, and a warning notification is sent to the patient by the platform when the lower and upper limit values of the measured values are exceeded, just as in the doctor's entrance. In this way, conditions that may continue and pose a risk in the patient will be controlled remotely, and this will create a facilitating factor for early action.

5.3.4.3 Implementation of the system

The integrated system hardware with microcontroller created within the scope of this study processes the data obtained from the sensors in the patient's body and sends it to a server system in the Internet environment. The patient who will use the system should place the sensors in the system in the correct parts of his body. After the sensors are placed properly, the patient can continue with his daily life activities. After the system starts to work, the data read from the sensors are transferred to the database via the ESP-8266 and through the developed web services. Both web-based and mobile-based application software can be used to view the records on the database server.

5.4 Result and discussion

In the designed system, three vital patient data such as body temperature, oxygen saturation and heart rate and simultaneous data of two ambient information such as ambient humidity as well as ambient temperature are presented in graphical interfaces. Vital values taken from the person's body have been tried to be measured with full and precise accuracy. If a problem occurred with any of the parameters, the values were tried to be obtained again quickly. Because these measured values are fully converted into data packets suitable for transfer, incomplete data loss for system continuity is prevented. In order not to cause any complexity in data packets, data are sent to the network device at certain time intervals (four data packets per minute). It has been observed that the information obtained from the sensors during the test stages can transmit more than four times per minute. However, it has been determined that four data packets per minute are more suitable for the system to read the relevant values and transfer data to the Arduino Uno microcontroller and from there to the Arduino Wi-Fi network.

5.4.1 Room temperature

The ambient temperature of the patient is important for human health. It is especially important to monitor the ambient temperature of people in sensitive periods such as the elderly, infants and children.

There are three pins on the DHT11 sensor, which can operate with 5-V supply, as positive (+) terminal, negative (−) terminal and data pin. The measured data are

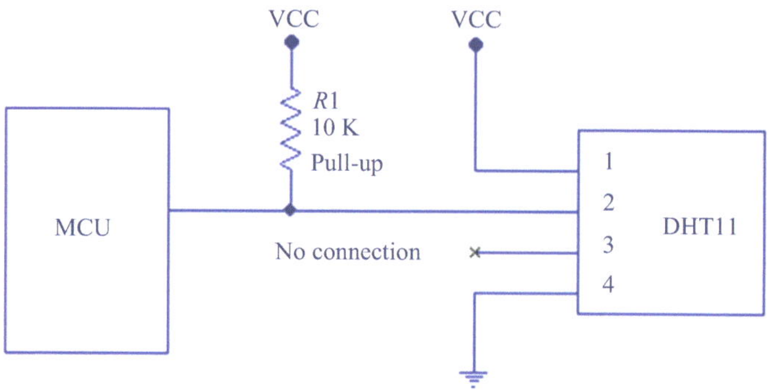

Figure 5.10 Microcontroller connection of a DHT11 sensor

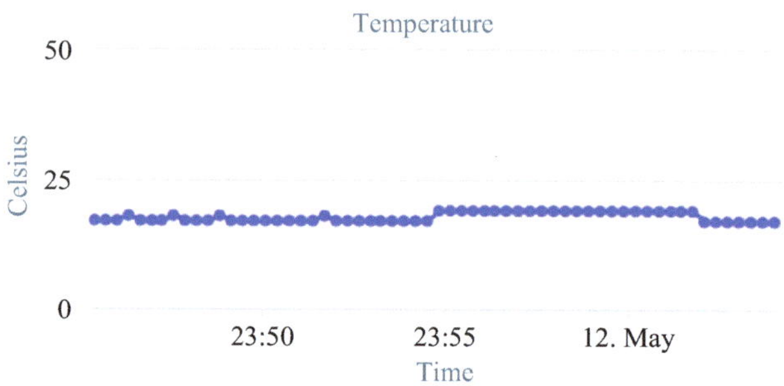

Figure 5.11 Temperature values received from the DHT11 sensor by the ThingSpeak platform

transferred by connecting the sensor's data pin to the digital pin number 3 on the Arduino Uno microcontroller. These pin connections are shown in Figure 5.10.

The data read from the DHT11 sensor were transferred to the microcontroller unit via digital pin number 3 and sent to the Arduino Wi-Fi wireless transmission unit. It was transferred to the Internet environment after the wireless transmission unit and presented in a graphical display in Celsius as in Figure 5.11.

5.4.2 Humidity

For people with certain diseases, the humidity of the environment is as important as the temperature. Ambient humidity is especially important for asthma patients. The DHT11 sensor placed on the patient's body transmits the humidity information of the patient's environment to the microcontroller system via digital pin number 3. It was transferred to the Internet environment after the wireless transmission unit and presented in a graphical representation in % as in Figure 5.12.

5.4.3 Body temperature

Body temperature gives important clues in the diagnosis of some diseases and in determining the general condition of the patient. In the designed microcontroller

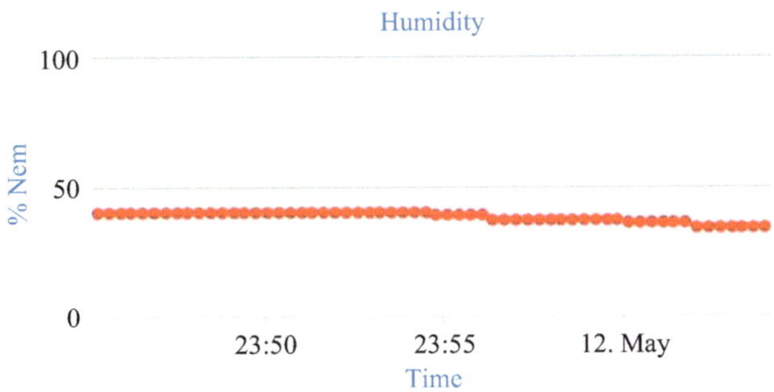

Figure 5.12 *Humidity values received from the DHT11 sensor by the ThingSpeak platform*

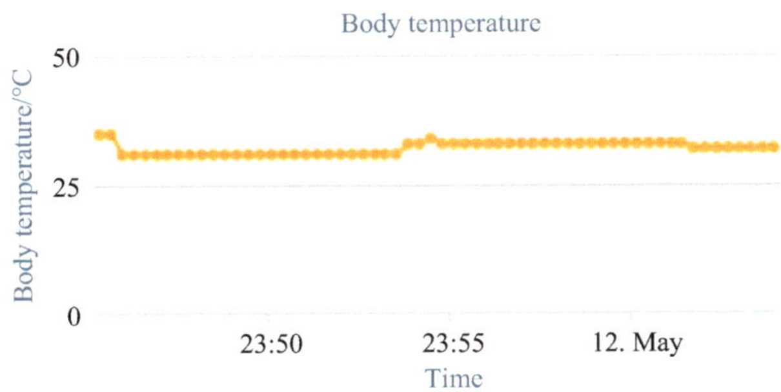

Figure 5.13 *Body temperature values taken from DS18B20 sensor by ThingSpeak platform*

system, DS18B20 digital temperature sensor was used to measure the patient's body temperature. This value was measured in Celsius temperature units. The designed body temperature-time graph is shown in Figure 5.13.

5.4.4 Heart rate

Heart rate is also often referred to as pulse rate. It can give important clues in determining the degree of some disorders. In the designed microcontroller system, the patient's average heart rate per minute was calculated and made suitable for graphical display. The MAX30102 heart rate sensor is used to detect heartbeats in the system. This sensor can detect the heartbeat from areas such as fingertips or earlobes. In the application system, the person was asked to make fingertip measurements.

There is an LED on the heartbeat sensors that emits infrared light waves. The infrared rays emitted by this LED reflect back in direct proportion to the rate of blood passing through the vein and fall on the infrared light sensor. In this way, the heart rate is monitored by calculating the back reflection rate. The designed heart rate–time graph is shown in Figure 5.14.

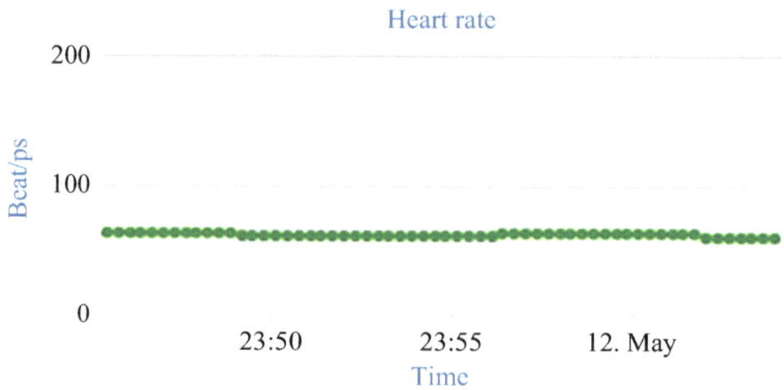

Figure 5.14 Heart rate values received from the MAX30102 sensor by the ThingSpeak platform

5.4.5 Oxygen saturation

Today, oxygen saturation in the blood (pulse oximetry) is a noninvasive method that is frequently used as an important tool for monitoring vital parameters. Pulse oximetry devices enable the diagnosis of asthma, pneumonia, sleep apnea, chronic obstructive pulmonary disease and bronchitis, pulmonary edema and congestive heart failure.

Oxygen is carried to all living tissues of the body by the hemoglobin protein in red blood cells and oxygenated hemoglobin (HbO_2) absorbs infrared light more, while red light is absorbed by deoxygenated hemoglobin (Hb). This basic principle allows the indirect determination of blood oxygen saturation level (SpO_2) by optical techniques [52]. An optically based SpO_2 sensor assembly consists of infrared and red diodes (usually at wavelengths of 650 and 950 nm, respectively), an optical receiver and complementary electronic circuits. The working principle of the transducer is based on two different methods: transmission or reflection [53]. In the transmission-based method, the targeted body area is placed between the red and infrared light sources and the optical receiver, and SpO_2 measurements are performed depending on the transmitted light intensity. The measurement areas where sensors based on this method can be placed are very limited: fingertip, earlobe or toe, etc. From the reflection method, the light sources and the optical receiver are placed side by side and SpO_2 measurements are calculated from the reflected light intensity. Sensors using the transmission method allow measurement from areas such as fingertips, earlobes, toes, as well as flat surfaces such as forehead, wrist or chest area.

Reflective-type optical SpO_2 sensors are very popular today because they can be used in many different body parts and this feature allows for many different innovative designs. In the designed microcontroller system, the oxygen saturation value in the patient's blood per minute was calculated and made suitable for graphical display. The MAX30102 sensor was used to measure the oxygen saturation in the system. In the application system, the person was asked to make fingertip measurements. The designed oxygen saturation–time graph is shown in Figure 5.15.

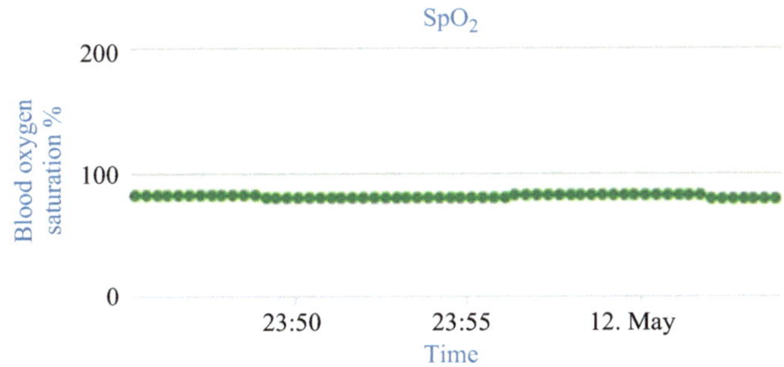

Figure 5.15 Oxygen saturation values from the MAX30102 sensor by the ThingSpeak platform

Table 5.3 Devices used in the system and measured values

No	Sensor	Measured data
1	MAX30102	Heart rate (pulse rate)
2	MAX30102	Oxygen saturation in the blood
3	DS18B20	Body temperature
4	DHT11	Ambient temperature
5	DHT11	Ambient humidity

In the designed patient monitoring system, a total of five data, three patient vital data and two environmental information were received over a single microcontroller circuit and transferred to the Wi-Fi module over the network. The devices used in the system and the measured values are given in Table 5.3.

When the studies in the literature were examined, it was seen that various vital data such as body temperature, blood pressure, heart rate, oxygen ratio in the blood, respiratory rate and ECG were measured. A holistic smart patient monitoring system using all of these data has not been found. It has been observed that different sensors are used according to the disease state (emotion perception, stress perception, diabetes, Parkinson's, etc.) [54,55]. However, one of the generally neglected cases is that the ambient values from which these measurements are obtained are also important. According to the environment in which people are located, body temperature, pulse, oxygen saturation, etc. values may differ. In the developed system, a holistic smart patient monitoring system was developed by taking at least three vital data as well as data from two different environments where the user is located.

Another feature of the system is the transfer of vital data to the Internet environment via the Wi-Fi module by utilizing the IoT technology. Regardless of the environment in which the patient is located, a wide range of motion is provided according to the coverage areas of wireless technologies, the Arduino Wi-Fi network unit. Another advantage of the system is that it has dimensions and lightness that can be carried on the patient. In this respect, it is thought that ease of use is provided.

5.5 Conclusion and future scope

Today, which we describe as the age of information communication and change, there are rapid developments in science and technology. Accordingly, a continuous improvement is observed in the field of health. The aim in health services is to provide benefits by combining rapidly advancing communication technologies, information technologies, web technologies and all other technologies that can contribute so that they can be received quickly and in a quality way when necessary. With the IoT and wearable technological devices that have just started to enter our lives, better health services can be provided to patients. It is aimed to increase the quality and effectiveness of health services with these technologies used. With wearable technologies that continue to develop today, the quality of health services will increase in the future and access to health services will no longer be a problem.

The scope of work: First of all, a model, including health data to be monitored by the system and sensors to provide these data, is designed for recording and monitoring patient health data on the IoT platform. In this model, the collected health data were re-examined by health professionals at the desired time and place, thanks to the data recorded anywhere, not only in the hospital environment.

This system, which was developed in the field of health and includes the IoT, ensures the reusability of the data regarding the measurements performed by the patients in different environments and also supports interoperability. With the developed system, an approach has been followed that will facilitate the daily life processes of both healthcare professionals and patients and strengthen the relationship between them. The notification feature in the case of exceeding the upper and lower values offered by the system facilitates immediate intervention, and it is thought that vital situations can be prevented, even if a little.

Today, there are many studies on recording and examining some physiological data. One of the common goals of these studies is to save time. In addition, these portable devices provide convenience to both the patient and the doctor. In this study, real-time ECG, EMG, SpO_2 and heart rate data obtained from the person with the e-Health sensor platform, which is a completely portable system, are displayed, recorded, graphed and displayed when requested. In addition, the patient's data are sent to the relevant physician, and a feedback is given about the physiological values measured in the light of purely medical data.

References

[1] Lee I. and Lee K., 'The Internet of Things (IoT): Applications, Investments, and Challenges for Enterprises'. *Business Horizons*, 2015; 58(4): 431–440.

[2] Qi J., Yang P., Amft O., Dong F., and Xu L., 'Advanced Internet of Things for Personalized Healthcare Systems: A Survey'. *Pervasive and Mobile Computing*, 2017; 41: 132–149.

[3] Başçiftçi F. and Gündüz K. A., 'Nesnelerin İnterneti Uyumlu Mikrodenetleyiciler Üzerine Bir Araştırma'. *Selçuk Üniversitesi Sosyal ve Teknik Araştırmalar Dergisi*, 2019; 18: 62–71.

[4] Laplante P. A. and Laplante N., 'The Internet of Things in Healthcare Potential Applications and Challenges'. *IT Professional*, 2016; 18(3): 2–4.

[5] Islam S. M. R., Kwak D., Kabir M. D. H., Hossain M., and Kwak K. S., 'The Internet of Things for Health Care: A Comprehensive Survey'. *IEEE Access*, 2015; 3: 678–704.

[6] Raj P., Chatterjee J. M., Kumar A., and Balamurugan B. (Eds.), *Internet of Things Use Cases for the Healthcare Industry*, Springer Nature, Berlin, 2020.

[7] Sujatha R., Nathiya S., and Chatterjee J. M., 'Clinical Data Analysis Using IoT Data Analytics Platforms'. *Internet of Things Use Cases for the Healthcare Industry*, Springer, Berlin, 2020. pp. 271–293.

[8] Choudhuri A., Chatterjee J. M., and Garg S., 'Internet of Things in Healthcare: A Brief Overview'. *Internet of Things in Biomedical Engineering*, Elsevier, Amsterdam, 2019. pp. 131–160.

[9] Chien C. N., Hsu H. W., Jang J. K., Rau C. L., and Jaw F. S., 'Microcontroller-Based Wireless Recorder for Biomedical Signals', *Engineering in Medicine and Biology 27th Annual Conference*; Shanghai, China, 2005.

[10] Baş Ş., *Kişisel Alan Ağları Ve Giyilebilir Bilgisayarların Kullanımıyla Gerçekleştirilecek Bir Hasta Izleme Sistemi Önerisi*, Ege University FBE Computer Engineering Department Master Thesis; 2011.

[11] Catarinucci L., Donno D., Mainetti L., *et al.*, 'An IoT-Aware Architecture for Smart Healthcare Systems'. *IEEE Internet of Things Journal*, 2015; 2(6): 515–526.

[12] Saha J., Saha A. K., Chatterjee A., *et al.*, 'Advanced IoT Based Combined Remote Health Monitoring, Home Automation and Alarm System', *8th Annual Computing and Communication Workshop and Conference*; Las Vegas, NV, USA, 2018.

[13] Köksal G. M., Dikmen Y., Utku T., *et al.*, 'Perioperatif Hasta Sıcaklık Takibi Ve Isıtılması: Anket Çalışması'. *Turkish Journal of Anaesthesiology & Reanimation*, 2013; 41: 49–155.

[14] Jubran A., 'Pulse Oximetry'. *Critical Care*, 1999; 3: 11–17.

[15] Ward M. and Langton J. A., 'Blood Pressure Measurement'. *Continuing Education in Anaesthesia, Critical Care & Pain*, 2007; 7(4): 122–126.

[16] Steven J. B., '11 – Pulse Oximetry' in Ehrenwerth J., Eisenkraft J. B., and Berry J. M. (Eds.). *Anesthesia Equipment*, W.B. Saunders, Philadelphia, PA, 2021. pp. 253–270.

[17] Takano H. and Ohta Y., 'Heart Rate Measurement Based on a Time-Lapse Image'. *Medical Engineering & Physics*, 2007; 29(8): 853–857.

[18] Akbulut P. F. and Akan A., 'Akıllı Giyilebilir Hasta Takip Sistemleri', *2015 Medical Technologies National Conference (TIPTEKNO)*; Bodrum, Turkey, 2015.

[19] Barnes K., *Health Wearables: Early Days*. PwC Health Standards, PwC Health Research Institute Report, 2014.
[20] Khan S. F., 'Health Care Monitoring System in Internet of Things (IoT) by Using RFID', *The 6th International Conference on Industrial Technology and Management*; Cambridge, UK, 2017.
[21] Lebepe F., Niezen G., Hancke G. P., and Ramotsoela T. D., 'Wearable Stress Monitoring System Using Multiple Sensors', *IEEE 14th International Conference on Industrial Informatics*; Poitiers, France, 2016.
[22] Alexander A. and Arun C. S., 'Mobile ECG Monitoring Device Using Wearable Non-Contact Armband', *International Conference on circuits Power and Computing Technologies*; Kollam, India, 2017.
[23] Puente S. T., Úbeda A., and Torres F., 'e-Health: Biomedical Instrumentation With Arduino'. *IFAC-PapersOnLine*, 2017; 50(1): 9156–9161.
[24] Kaplan M., Berk T. N., Çemrek B., Şahin S., and Fidan U., 'Mobile Physiological Signal Monitoring System for Family Medicine', *Medical Technologies National Congress*; Trabzon, Turkey, 2017.
[25] Delrobaei M., Memar S., Pieterman M., Stratton T. W., McIsaac K., and Jog M., 'Towards Remote Monitoring of Parkinson's Disease Tremor Using Wearable Motion Capture Systems'. *Journal of the Neurological Sciences*, 2018; 384: 38–45.
[26] Chen B.-R., Shyamal P., Buckley T., *et al.*, 'A Web-Based System for Home Monitoring of Patients with Parkinson's Disease Using Wearable Sensors'. *IEEE Transactions on Biomedical Engineering*, 2011; 58(3): 831–836.
[27] Otto C., Milenkovic A., Sanders C., and Jovanov E., 'System Architecture of A Wireless Body Area Sensor Network For Ubiquitous Health Monitoring'. *Journal of Mobile Multimedia*, 2006; 1(4): 307–326.
[28] Almotiri S. H., Khan M. A., and Alghamdi M. A., 'Mobile Health (M-Health) System in The Context of IoT', *4th International Conference on Future Internet of Things and Cloud Workshops*; Vienna, Austria, 2016.
[29] Sung M., Marci C., and Pentland A., 'Wearable Feedback Systems for Rehabilitation'. *Journal of Neuroengineering and Rehabilitation 2.1*, 2005; 17: 2–17.
[30] Lukowicz P., Anliker U., Ward J., Troster G., Hirt E., and Neufelt C., 'AMON: A Wearable Medical Computer for High Risk Patients', *6th International Symposium on Wearable Computers*; Seattle, USA, 2002.
[31] Fua Y. and Liub J., 'System Design for Wearable Blood Oxygen Saturation and Pulse Measurement Device'. *Procedia Manufacturing*, 2015; 3: 1187–1194.
[32] Ahn B. G., Noh Y. H., and Jeong D. U., *Smart Chair Based On Multi Heart Rate Detection System*, IEEE Sensors; Busan, Korea (South), 2015.
[33] Gupta P., Agrawal D., Chhabra J., and Dhir P. K., 'IoT Based Smart Healthcare Kit', *International Conference on Computational Techniques in Information and Communication Technologies (ICCTICT)*; New Delhi, India, 2016.

[34] Sahoo P. K., Mohapatra S. K., and Wu S. L. 'Analyzing Healthcare Big Data With Prediction for Future Health Condition'. *IEEE Access*, 2016; 4: 9786–9799.

[35] Nagavelli R. and Guru Rao C. V., 'Degree of Disease Possibility (DDP): A Mining Based Statistical Measuring Approach for Disease Prediction in Health Care Data Mining', *International Conference on Recent Advances and Innovations in Engineering (ICRAIE-2014)*; Jaipur, India, 2014.

[36] Xu B., Xu L. D., Cai H., Xie C., and Hu J., 'Ubiquitous Data Accessing Method in IoT-Based Information System for Emergency Medical Services'. *IEEE Transactions on Industrial Informatics*, 2014; 10(2): 1578–1586.

[37] Arduino, *Arduino Platform*, [online]. 2021. Available from https://www.arduino.cc/en/guide/introduction [Accessed 25 Apr 2021].

[38] Louis L., 'Working Principle of Arduino and U Sing It'. *International Journal of Control, Automation, Communication and Systems*, 2016; 1(2): 21–29.

[39] Banzi M. and Shiloh M., *Make: Getting Started With Arduino the Open Source Electronics Prototyping Platform*, 3rd ed., Maker Media, Inc., Sebastopol, CA, 2014. p. 262.

[40] Wardana H., Indahwati E., and Fitriyah L., 'Measurement of Non-Invasive Blood Glucose Level Based Sensor Color TCS3200 and Arduino'. *IOP Conference Series: Materials Science and Engineering*, 2019; 336(1): 12–19.

[41] Galadima A. A., 'Arduino as A Learning Tool', *11th International Conference on Electronics, Computer and Computation*; Abuja, Nigeria, 2014.

[42] Ya'acob N., Adnan S. F. S., Yusof A. L., *et al.*, 'RFID Lab Management System Using Arduino Microcontroller Approach Associate with Webpage'. *Journal of Scientific Research and Development*, 2016; 3(2): 92–97.

[43] Nayyar A. and Puri A., 'A Review of Arduino Boards, Lilypad's & Arduino Shields', *3rd International Conference on Computing for Sustainable Global Development*; New Delhi, India, 2016.

[44] Djajadi A. and Wijanarko M., 'Ambient Environmental Quality Monitoring Using IoT Sensor Network'. *Internetworking Indonesia Journal*, 2016; 8(1).

[45] Kodali R. K. and Soratkal S., 'MQTT Based Home Automation System Using ESP8266', *2016 IEEE Region 10 Humanitarian Technology Conference*; Agra, India, 2016.

[46] Thaker T., 'ESP8266 Based Implementation of Wireless Sensor Network with Linux Based Web-Server', *2016 Symposium on Colossal Data Analysis and Networking*; Indore, India, 2016.

[47] Wibowo S. F. and Pribadi A. B., 'Internet of Things Experiment Using Esp8266 Wi-Fi Module, ThingSpeak Channel and Delphi Interface', *International Symposium for Modern School Development, Social Science and Applied Technologies*; Yogyakarta: Samudra Biru, 2016.

[48] Samsugi S., Ardiamsyah A., and Kastura D., 'Arduino Dan Modul Wi-Fi Esp8266 Sebagai Media Kendali Jarak Jauh Dengan Antarmuka Berbasis Android'. *Jurnal Teknoinfo*, 2018; 12(1): 23–27.

[49] Puput Dani P. A. and Kitagawa A., 'A Study of LoRa Performance in Monitoring of Patient's SpO_2 and Heart Rate based IoT'. *International*

Journal of Advanced Computer Science and Applications, 2020; 11(2): 238–251.

[50] Prahl S., *Tabulated Molar Extinction Coefficient for Hemoglobin in Water*, [online]. 1998. Available from http://omlc.org/spectra/hemoglobin/summary.html [Accessed 28 Feb 2021].

[51] Divya M., Subhash N., Vishnu P., and Tejesh P., 'Smart Health Care Monitoring Based on Internet of Things (IoT)'. *International Journal of Scientific Research and Engineering Development*, 2020; 3(1): 409–414.

[52] Cohen A. and Wadsworth N., 'A Light Emitting Diode Skin Reflectance Oximeter'. *Medical and Biological Engineering*, 1972; 10: 385–391.

[53] Jawahar Y., *Design of an Infrared Based Blood Oxygen Saturation and Heart Rate Monitoring Device*. Electrical and Biomedical Engineering Project Report, 2009.

[54] Yang G., Xie L., Mantysalo M., *et al.* 'Zheng Industrial Informatics'. *IEEE Transactions on Industrial Informatics*, 2014; 10(4): 2180–2191.

[55] Babu M., Raju R., Sylvester S., Mathew T. M., and Abubeker K. M., 'Real Time Patient Monitoring System Using LabVIEW Parameters'. *International Journal of Advanced Research in Computer and Communication Engineering*, 2016; 5: 505–507.

Chapter 6

Development of a secured IoMT device with prioritized medical information for tracking and monitoring COVID patients in rural areas

P.K. Jawahar[1], K. Indragandhi[1], G. Kannan[1] and Yiu-Wing Leung[2]

Abstract

Quality medical care and remote monitoring will significantly mitigate the mortality rate of rural people during the COVID outbreak. Individual care and diagnosing are challenging in a short period during the pandemic situation in the hospital. An exhaustive survey on the technologies and wearable devices used on the Internet of Medical Things (IoMT) to combat COVID-19 is done in this chapter. The security threats at different levels of IoMT are also discussed. This chapter also proposes a low-cost secured IoMT device to monitor the quarantined COVID patients in rural areas. The essential medical parameters like body temperature, oxygen level, heart rate, and glucose level have been measured and securely transmitted to the cloud. Any abnormal condition will be identified and informed to the medical data center with high priority using a priority-based preemptive real-time operating system scheduling algorithm. The medical information collected from the IoMT device is securely transmitted and stored in a cloud using Advanced Encryption Standard. Further, the device will also track an unauthorized movement of the quarantined patient and intimate the local administrative officer to prevent the COVID-19 spread.

Keywords: Internet of Medical Things; Security; LoRaWAN; Real-time operating system (RTOS); Sensors; COVID; Contact tracing

6.1 Introduction

The world is moving toward automation of all systems. Internet of Things (IoT) has become an inevitable technology in the field of automation. From M2M (machine

[1]Department of Electronics and Communication Engineering, B.S. Abdur Rahman Crescent Institute of Science and Technology, Chennai, India
[2]Department of Computer Science, Hong Kong Baptist University, Kowloon Tong, Hong Kong

to machine) concept, the cyber-physical systems take IoT to all domains across the world. By 2025, several IoT devices across all fields in the world will reach 3 trillion, as per Gartner's report [1]. All the gadgets at home started communicating with each other with the support of IoT. Hence, automation of medical devices is not an exception. In the healthcare sector, IoT has played a prominent role as the Internet of Medical Things (IoMT). The advantages of IoMT are remote monitoring, mitigation of diseases, cost reduction, medical data accessibility, improved healthcare, and treatment management [2].

IoMT is an integration of medical devices with sensors through the Internet allowing the local/remote healthcare center to diagnose, track, and monitor physiological parameters.

If the regional center cannot process the cloud data, it can be processed at a distant center through a gateway [3]. Figure 6.1 defines the IoMT. Telemedicine systems have already been prevailing in many multispecialty hospitals, interconnecting patients from one part of the world and specialized physicians and surgeons on the other side [4]. As is suited for a specific diagnosis, a unique infrastructure is required. Hence, telemedicine systems are heterogeneous, addressing a particular diagnosis. It is not suitable for multiple therapies as it requires expensive infrastructure. IoMT is more scalable and reliable, dynamic, and generic. Devices in IoMT are heterogeneous, but the system is homogenous and supports interoperability [5,6].

The growth of IoMT is drastic and may reach US$72 billion. By the end of 2021, IoMT will interconnect healthcare centers with 32 billion medical devices. About 64% of IBM, Cisco, and Apple technologies are used for telemonitoring [7]. Table 6.1 shows the comparison of telemedicine and IoMT. One of the restrictions in IoMT is dynamic bandwidth delaying the diagnosis as the data are transmitted from an edge device (sensors with devices connected to the patient) to a head device (remote hospital) through a cloud. The gateway may be used between these

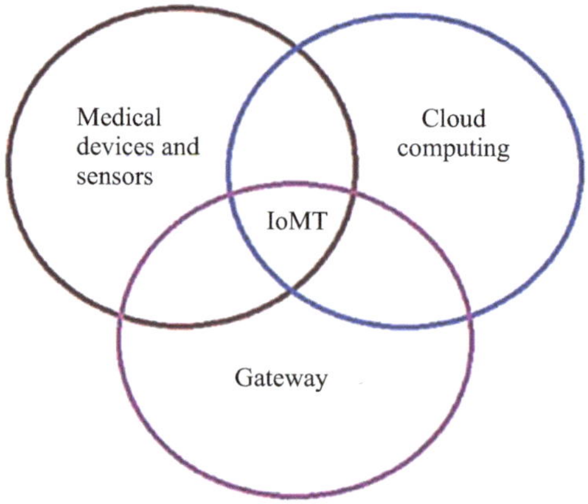

Figure 6.1 IoMT representation

Table 6.1 Comparison of telemedicine and IoMT

Telemedicine	IoMT
Uses dedicated network and centralized control	Uses open network and control is decentralized
Expensive infrastructure	Cost-effective infrastructure
Wide bandwidth	Dynamic bandwidth
Data size is huge	Small data size
Critical data are shared	Hospitals can share any physiological data
Uses developed technology	Technology is evolving
More secured and private	Security and privacy are the challenges
Rarely uses cloud services	Often uses cloud services
Edge computing is not preferred	Edge computing is application based
Delay in communication and processing is significantly less	Prominent delay due to Internet services

devices, and edge devices must be capable of computing to act. But for critical care, edge computing is a bottleneck.

Edge computing enables all data processing and computation at the edge (end) of the network, on behalf of cloud services at the sender end, and receiver data on IoT services. End devices (EDs) can use computation-intensive processors to reduce the overhead. In the latter part of this chapter, we will discuss edge computing in detail.

The chapter is organized as follows. Section 6.1 will deal with the different versions of IoT, the architecture of IoMT, technology, and sensors used in IoMT. Section 6.2 deals with security threats involved in IoMT. Existing solutions are also discussed. Section 6.3 deals with the introduction to COVID, and Section 6.4 covers the implementation of IoMT for tracking and monitoring of COVID-19 patients [8–10] in rural areas. Section 6.5 concludes the chapter. While the mitigation of COVID in urban areas is complex, tracking and monitoring COVID-19 patients in rural areas is a big challenge for healthcare workers and the government. We discuss contact tracing and monitoring a patient using preemptive scheduling in this section with results.

6.1.1 Different versions of IoT

IoT has taken different dimensions within two decades from its inception by Kevin Ashton based on the application and implementation [11]. Interconnection of multiple media devices with the Internet has become the Internet of Multimedia Things. It will be helpful for media channels to share emergency information instantaneously over high-speed Internet. IoMT is another version of IoT, which is the core discussion of this chapter. Internet of Robotic Things is another area used for confidential, remote, defense applications using robots. Even beyond earth, IoRT can be extended. Artificial Intelligent Internet of Things is booming in recent years as artificial intelligence and machine learning have found an essential requirement to predict the future. In industries, IoT, with the help of digital twins, has emerged as the Industrial

Internet of Things. With application-specific integrated circuit (ASICs), other parameters can be customized, including latency, power, security, etc., in addition to physiological parameters. Interconnecting underground, underwater things with the Internet of Under Ground Things, Internet of Under Water Things, Internet of Aviation, Internet of Nano Things, etc. [12] are about to come soon.

6.1.2 IoMT architecture and framework

As mentioned earlier, IoMT interconnects medical devices and sensors from a patient's place to a hospital located at a remote place. Gateways are used to connect the EDs at the patient's location. Cloud may be used to collect, store, and process patients' data if the ED is not capable. Else, EDs with the help of a local server can process the data collected and transmitted to the physician's location. Figure 6.2 shows the traditional architecture of IoMT. Depending upon the application, the nature of connectivity between gateway and Internet may vary. Figure 6.3 shows the layered approach of IoMT.

The TCP/IP suite can be related to the layers of IoMT. TCP/IP or Internet Suite has five layers against OSI/ISO reference model having seven layers. In IoMT, the physical layer is known as the perception layer [12]. The physical layer is hardware-based, and it provides all the physical connectivity with the gateway/edge server. The healthcare devices with sensors (Table 6.2) to measure the physiological parameters are responsible for communicating with the gateway/edge server [13]. Five factors are considered to develop an IoMT device. They are (1) connectivity which is reliable, (2) privacy and secrecy of personal medical data, (3) optimal performance of the device, (4) user-friendly front-end application, and (5) competent analysis of patient's data [14]. The

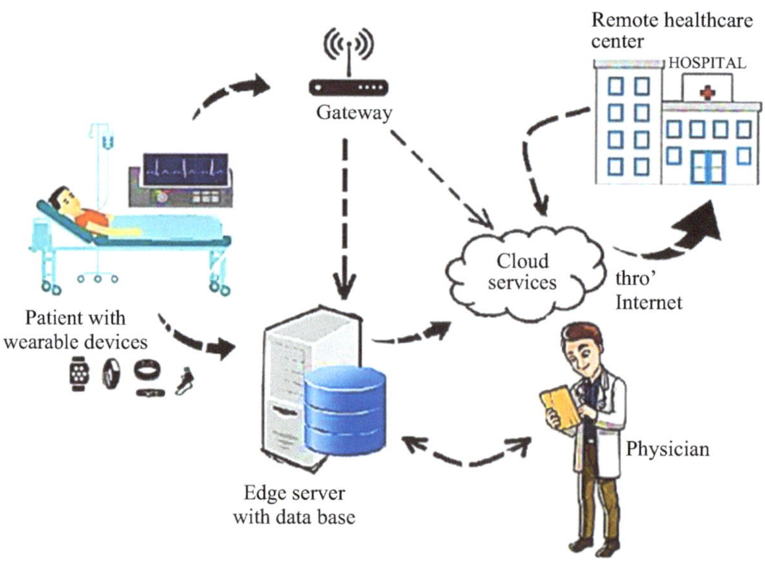

Figure 6.2 Architecture of IoMT

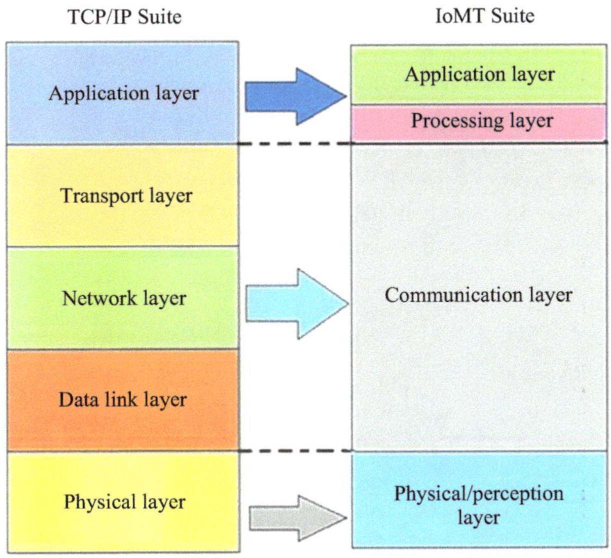

Figure 6.3 Layered approach of IoMT

Table 6.2 Devices used in physical/perception layer

Name of the IoMT device	Purpose
Temperature sensor	Measure the body temperature
Blood pressure sensor	Monitor the blood pressure (BP) of a person
GPS sensor	Locate the place of a patient
Pulse oximeter	Measure oxygen saturation level (SpO_2) and BP
Heartbeat sensor	Monitor heartbeats
ECG sensor	Monitor electrocardiogram of a patient
Accelerometer and gyroscope	Monitor the movements of a patient and his activities and postures (sitting, lying, standing, walking, or running)
Biometric sensor	Identify patient's identity using unique features like thumb impression, Iris

devices used in the physical layer are listed in Table 6.2. Figure 6.4 shows the classification of IoMT devices. Medical devices are classified as implantable, stationary, and ambient devices. Implantable devices are placed inside the body of the patient for diagnosis.

One implantable device called "swallowable camera capsule" is shown in Figure 6.4. It consists of LEDs, a CMOS imager, an ASIC transmitter, and an antenna. The dimension of the capsule is 11 mm $\times$ 26 mm and weighs approximately 3 g.

Stationary devices are imaging equipment like MRI, CT scanner, and X-ray scanner available at the hospital. Both doctors and patients can carry wearable devices. Figure 6.5 shows the classification of IoMT devices.

For instant diagnosis, tracking, monitoring, and treatment, these wearable devices help healthcare workers. Ambient devices are used at the hospital, including pressure, temperature, door status, motion, daylight, and vibration sensors. These sensors highly help the healthcare workers to monitor patients' activities.

The communication layer of IoMT performs the functions of datalink, network, and transport layers of the TCP/IP suite. Communication protocols like BLE, Zigbee, Wi-Fi, etc. (discussed in detail in the later section) are responsible for error-free communication, security, authentication, and patient data privacy. The

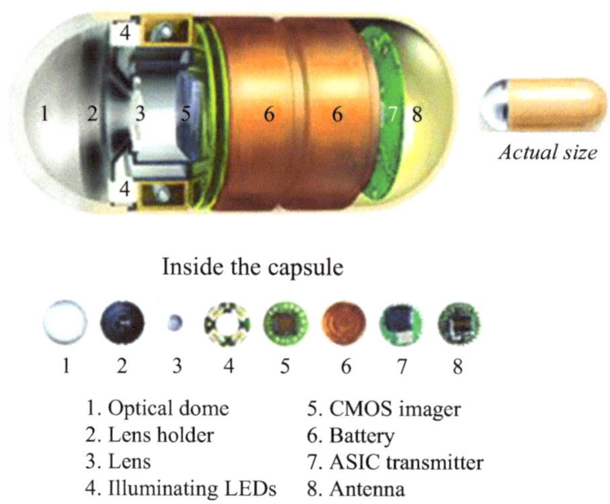

Figure 6.4 Swallowable camera capsule

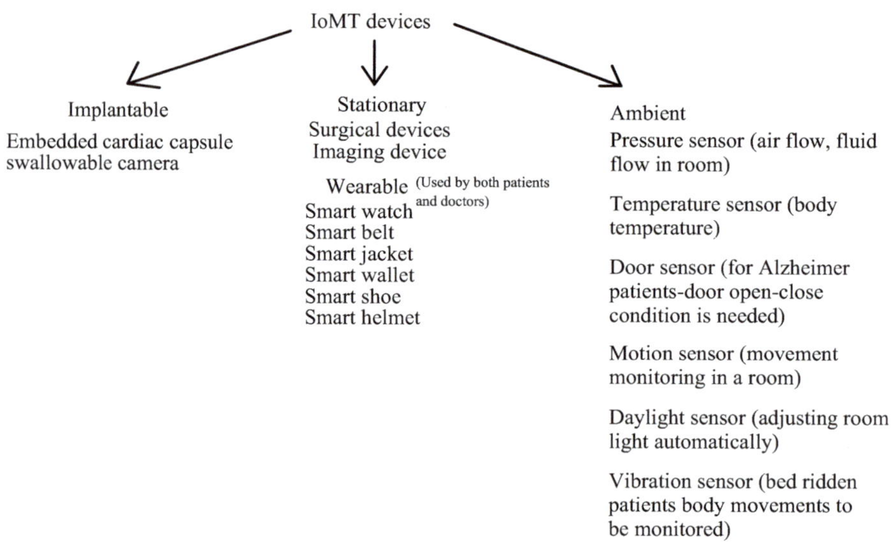

Figure 6.5 Classification of IoMT devices

processing layer is concerned with data aggregation and data processing for further analysis to be done by physicians. The processing layer is divided into three sublayers: medical service sublayer, service management sublayer, and user sublayer.

User sublayer deals with data collection from the patient, data cleaning, conversion, aggregation, and service management sublayer responsible for efficiently managing data [11]. The electronic health record (EHR) of a patient is created by a medical service sublayer based on the data collected from the user sublayer.

The application layer acts as an interface with the application programs and end-users. End-users include both patients and doctors. Mobile apps and apps running on computers are available to view and study physiological parameters like BP, heart rate, body temperature, oxygen saturation level, ECG, and the patient's location.

6.1.3 Technologies

All the medical devices with sensors communicate gateway/local server through any one or multiple technologies depending upon the nature of sensors used for a patient. IoMT can use radio frequency (RF) technology, sensor positioning technology using GPS in addition to 3G/4G/5G mobile network technology to contact patients, healthcare workers, clinics, intensive care units, and operation theaters. Widely used communication technologies are RFID, Bluetooth (now comes with low energy–BLE), Zigbee, Wi-Fi, 3G/4G GSM (5G is yet to come), LoRaWAN (long-range wide area network), SigFox, 6LoWPAN, and LTE. Narrow-band IoT (NB-IoT) is also competing with these technologies [15].

The edge devices connected with the patient may collect the data, process it, and communicate to the gateway/local server [16]. In such a case, edge computing will be more beneficial for the physician to diagnose the disease quickly. But in reality, many of the EDs have low-power and low-speed controllers and sensors that cannot react rapidly in processing the collected data to diagnose a disease. In such a case, cloud computing is preferred, where the EDs can collect the data and forward it to the cloud. The servers at the cloud will process and communicate with the doctors for further analysis and diagnosis. Cloud services are offered to many organizations like Google, Amazon, and Apple. Table 6.3 shows the differences between edge computing and cloud computing [17].

Table 6.3 Edge computing vs. cloud computing

Edge computing	Cloud computing
Decentralized processing	Centralized processing
Low bandwidth is required	Wide bandwidth is required
Delay is low	Delay is more
Offers real-time services	All the services are non–real time
Highly secured	Security is the threat
The cost of computation is less	The cost of computation is high
Fast data processing	Slow data processing
Power consumption is less	Power consumption is more
Reliability is less	Reliability is high

Cloud servers have highly computation-intensive processors with colossal memory, which can analyze the data and prepare the patient's EHR with statistics of all parameters collected; the doctors can use that for treatment. The cloud servers offer services to different healthcare centers simultaneously, which is not possible with edge computing [18].

Table 6.4 lists the specifications and their features of the various technologies used in IoMT. Many devices use Bluetooth technology as a well-established and proven technology for short-distance communication [15]. For edge computing, Bluetooth, Zigbee will be helpful for the transmission of data. RFID can be a non-contact automatic identification device. RFID has three parts: RF tag, reader, and data management system. RFID tag; the core of RFID is used to store the data like BP, SpO_2, ECG, breath rate, and contact with the transceiver [17]. A low-cost RFID tag antenna can monitor medication doses [19]. But the limitation is the coverage range.

Wi-Fi, LoRaWAN, GSM, SigFox, 3G/4G/5G, LTE, NB-IoT use for cloud computing. These technologies support long-distance communication of patient's data. As the patient's data size is small (BP, SpO_2, heart rate), they can be transmitted to the cloud servers, whereas ECG, EEG, EMG, MRI, CT scan image, X-ray image require more packets with wide packet size. They need high-speed devices for processing at the cloud for immediate and live diagnosis.

6.1.3.1 Long-range wide area network

In recent days, the spread of COVID-19 resulted in a pandemic globally, which results in low-cost technology in the healthcare sector. LoRa has a high communication range with a low data rate, suitable for healthcare as it ensures interoperability between IoT devices [11]. The architecture of LoRaWAN is shown in Figure 6.6. All the medical devices with sensors are called EDs. EDs are connected to the Internet through the LoRa gateway. Healthcare workers can access the data through apps running on mobile phones, laptops, and cloud servers at the remote healthcare center. Table 6.4 shows that it consumes less power and inexpensive with a large coverage area. LoRa device is classified as class A, B, and C. The lowest power LoRa EDs are class A LoRa devices. They are battery-operated.

Class B devices have low latency and communicate bidirectionally. Class C devices have the lowest latency among all the LoRa class EDs for data communication between server and ED and consume more power. It can communicate bidirectionally [20].

6.1.4 Sensors used in IoMT

The core element of any Internet of Things is a sensor. Many transducers are available to sense the variations of physical/physiological parameters. In IoMT systems, wearable sensors are prevalent [21] and play a significant role in acquiring, measure patient data for decision-making [22].

Table 6.5 shows few popular wearable sensors used in IoMT. Wearable low-cost pulse oximeters are available in the market, using which a patient can read his/her heart rate, SpO_2. Maxim-Integrated IC MAX30102 (Figure 6.7) is used in this.

Table 6.4 Communication technologies used in IoMT

	Distance	Application	Power	Security	Challenges	Frequency
Bluetooth	20 m	Heart rate monitor, speedometer	3 mW	Less secured, not preferred for critical data	Speed, range, compatibility, and security	ISM band
Zigbee	10–100 m	Home automation, industrial automation, smart meters, smart grid monitoring	10–100 mW	Less secured	Security, power consumption and data rate	ISM band
Wi-Fi	50 m	Wireless Internet access, remote CCTV access	100 mW	More vulnerable to attackers	Coverage, security, usage, and cost	ISM band
GSM	25 km	Tracking and monitoring	2 W	More secured	Intruders	850/900/1 800/1 900 MHz
LoRaWAN	5–10 km	IIoT, smart city, smart home, smart farming, building automation, smart grid, smart hospitals	25 mW	More secured	Scalability, interference, capacity, and coverage	ISM band
SigFox	25 km	Low power smart metering, healthcare, smart watch	25 mW	Secured	Noise interference, not yet implemented in many countries	ISM band
LTE	2 km	Wireless broadband communication	200 mW	More secured	Interoperability, sniffing, eavesdropping, traffic management	600 MHz to 2.5 GHz
5G	2 km	High-speed wireless broadband communication	250 mW to 120 W (based on cell size)	More secured	Deployment, coverage, cost, and maintenance	28 and 39 GHz
NB-IoT	10–15 km	Smart metering, healthcare monitoring, alarms	200 mW	Vulnerable to DoS attacks	Battery life, coverage, lack of security standards	815–1 980 MHz (up) 860–2 170 MHz (down)

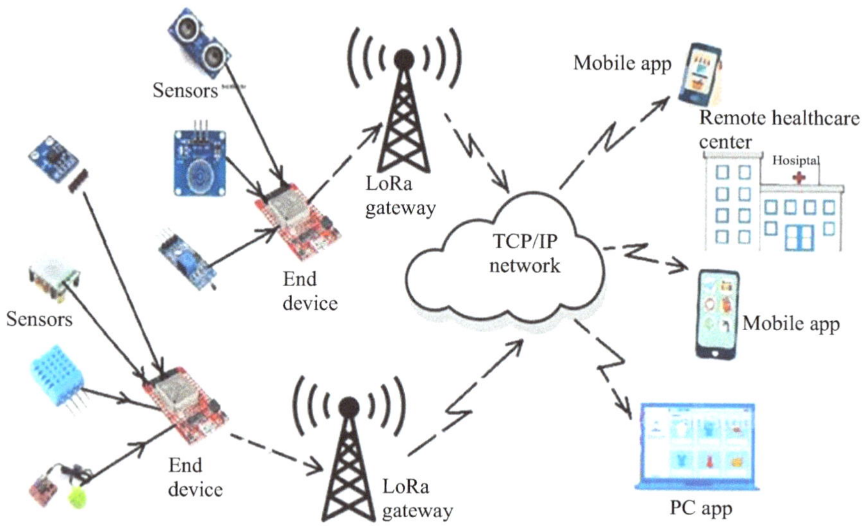

Figure 6.6 LoRaWAN architecture

It has red LED operating at a wavelength of 660 nm, an infrared LED operating at 880 nm, and a photodetector to approximate blood oxygen content and heart rate pulses. The sensor can be placed on the wrist/finger or another area with a significant blood flow. It operates at 3.3–5 V, consuming 6-mA current.

In a wristwatch, belt, jacket, helmet, wristband, and shoes, sensors can be fitted to sense physiological data [21]. They can be communicated to a server/gateway using one or multiple technologies discussed earlier through the controllers. Figure 6.8 shows an OLED-based ECG monitor with its electrodes. With this, we can also measure the heart rate of a person.

6.1.4.1 Limitations in wearable sensors

Wearable medical sensors have low computational capability and operate with meager power supply because of security vulnerability [23]. They are small devices. Many sensors are mobile and dynamic. Patients have to go to a restricted healthcare center for diagnosis, during which they have to leave the allotted place from where they are monitored. They need to remove the sensors as the area is restricted and secured. Continuous monitoring is not possible in such a situation that creates vulnerable points in the system for the intruders to attack the device and manipulate the critical data. The accuracy of the data collected from the wearable sensors is also a concern.

6.2 Security threats in IoMT

As medical devices access and process critical information of a person, they have to be secured for confidentiality. Security is mandatory for two reasons: (1) the data

Table 6.5 Wearable sensors

Device	Figure	Application
Pulse oximeter—MAX30102	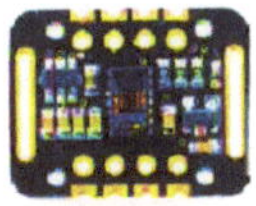	Measure oxygen saturation level (SpO_2), heart rate
Skin patch	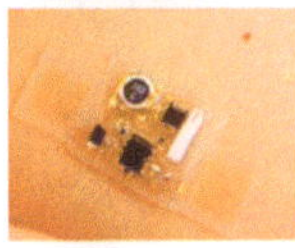	Measure ECG
Wrist band	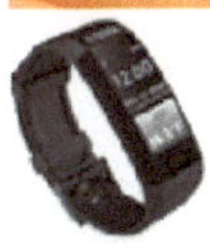	Measure body temperature, location tracker, and heart rate
Smart helmet	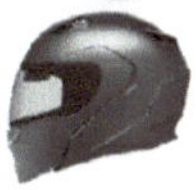	Tracking and monitoring, Bluetooth communication
Wearable skin sensor	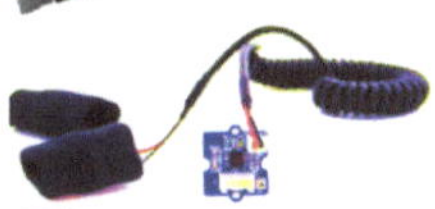	To study emotional changes
Headband	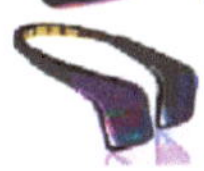	To measure brain activities using EEG
Smart shoe	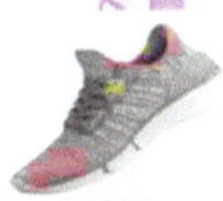	Measure the calorie burnt, distance walked, track location
Smart jacket	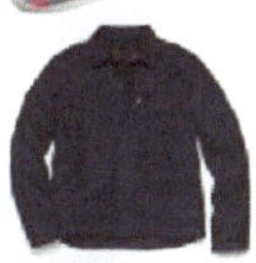	Body temperature, BP, muscle activity, pulse rate
Smart belt	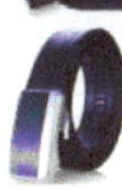	Fitness tracker

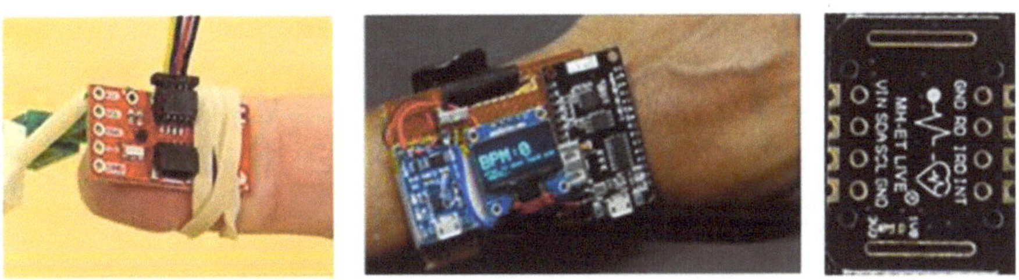

Figure 6.7 MAX30102 pulse oximeter

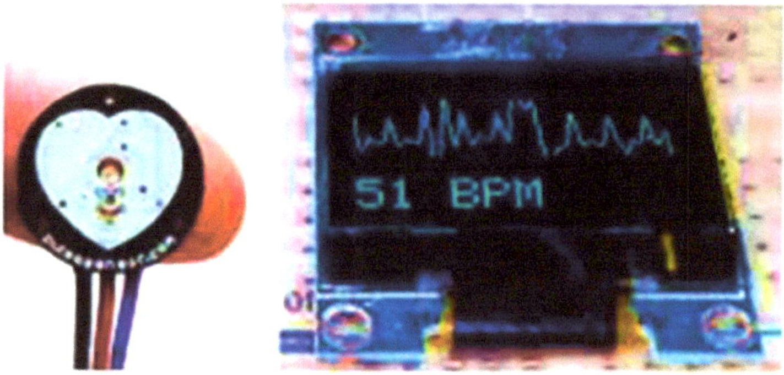

Figure 6.8 OLED-based ECG display

Table 6.6 Security levels

Level	Nature of security
Data	Confidentiality, integrity, availability, authentication, nonrepudiation, and authorization
Sensor	One time programmable (OTP) hardware, over the air programmable (OTAP) hardware, self-recovery, upward and downward compatibility
Local server (Edge)	Device authentication, user authentication, patient anonymity
The remote server (head level, i.e., healthcare center)	Access control, key management, trust management, and DoS resistance

can be easily leaked and misused during the life cycle of medical data and (2) exposing personal data may lead to abuse and even social discrimination against patients [24]. As the devices are tiny, computation power and security features will also be less. Secure communication in such a scenario is a very challenging task. The impact will result in eavesdropping, delayed detection of critical parameters due to denial-of-service attacks. To ensure the integrity of the data, user and device authentication are essential [25]. As wearable and implantable devices consume low power and less computation-intensive, many IoMT systems allow cloud computing than edge computing. Privacy of individual's data at cloud servers requires more security as they face more threats by malicious attackers [26].

Security can be provided in IoMT systems at three different levels: (1) data level, (2) sensor level, and (3) server level (Table 6.6). At the data level, authentication, confidentiality, integrity, nonrepudiation (authenticated user responsible for their action and any communication cannot be denied), authorization, and data availability need to be maintained [1,19]. At the sensor level, tamperproof hardware, localization of sensors, self-recovery of the system, over the air programming of the hardware are required.

At the server level, applications' upward and downward compatibility is expected [26,27]. If the firmware is updated, the hardware should work with the existing interfaces at the local server and the server present in the medical center [22].

Hackers can attack medical things like the way they attack desktop computers, servers in computer networks. Manufacturers of intelligent medical devices should ensure minimum security standards to overcome attacks. Different types of malware affect medical things like spyware, keylogger, Trojan horse, virus adware, ransomware, and rootkit [1]. "Wannacry" was a famous ransomware attack demanding lump sum money by the attacker in 2017. For IoMT, such an attack will affect a patient who cannot afford massive money during a critical condition, and the hospital also cannot bear the amount [7].

The expectations in IoMT security are (1) frequency of security patches and updates by the manufacturer; (2) detection strategy of the security threats; (3) security with interoperable, scalable devices; and (4) service destruction like denial of service (DoS) [7]. Table 6.7 shows various threats and attacks happening in IoMT protocols [26]. The security risks occur due to the exchange of sensitive data of a person, incompatibility between devices, and many smart devices used in an IoMT system [28]. Privacy and secrecy are also not maintained. Many Bluetooth-based

Table 6.7 Security threats in IoMT protocols

Protocol	Threat	Possible attacks
RFID	Active and passive systems suffer from weak signals	Side-channel attack
Bluetooth	Partial encryption of the payload, capturing frequency hops, and data address validation	DDoS, sniffing, Brute-force, and device replication
Wi-Fi	Device authentication, denial of service, and service integrity	DoS, replay, channel collision, and spoofing
Zigbee	Insecure key transportation for pre-shared keys, no integrity checks, insufficient registration of network keys, the lack of authentication of IDs	Fitting default link keys, sending security information in auxiliary frames, flooding leading to DoS, key negotiation, energy-consuming attacks
LoRaWAN	Resetting frame counters without rekeying, caching, and replay of ACKs, forged gateway beacons to sensors	Replay attacks, hacking of passwords, malicious message alteration, battery exhaustion, and DDoS
HL7	Message sources, HL7 messages not validated	Spoofing and flooding attacks
HTTP	Message communication without encryption	Eavesdropping, theft breach, and flooding attacks
CoAP	Proxies decide if DTLS implementation is unicast or multicast, or unicast	Parsing, cache, spoofing. cross-layer attacks
MQTT	No data encryption mechanism and insecure IP broker	Port obscurity, Botnet

devices are used in IoMT. They are quickly attacked by sniffers so that device duplication is possible. DoS and spoofing attacks happen in any system that uses Wi-Fi whether it is an IoMT system or a simple computer network [29].

Constrained application protocol (CoAP) is a unique protocol used for constrained devices in IoT. MQTT (Message Queuing Telemetry Transport) is a lightweight IoT protocol running over Internet protocol. HL7 is Health Level 7, an ANSI standard that provides solutions for health data interoperability globally. At every layer also, security threats are present.

Table 6.8 shows the threats at various layers of IoMT and their risk level [30]. Though attacks occur in the physical layer with a high-risk group, they can be controlled by the users at the physical layer. In contrast, communication layer attacks cannot be prevented, and the user must implement a specific algorithm to foil these attacks.

Table 6.9 shows how the security threats can be overcome at each layer [31].

In wired IoMT systems, wired equivalent privacy encryption standards can be implemented to ensure security. In wireless systems, Wireless Protected Access and

Table 6.8 Security threats at various layers

Layer	Nature of attack	Risk level
Physical/perception layer	Side-channel attack: attacker exploits collected data and applies reverse engineering to encrypt secured data	High
	Sensor attack: attacker tracks a sensor when a user accesses a webpage, sending queries to sensors	High
	Tag cloning: attacker creates a new reprogrammed clone by capturing data from a node in a network	Low
Communication layer	Sinkhole: attacker enters a network by collecting routing table through a fake node	High
	DoS (denial of service): attacker denies all the services or resource access to the original node temporarily or permanently	High
	Man in the middle: attacker changes the connection between two nodes that are involved in communication	High
	Session hijacking: attacker hides as a regular user in a network by sending commands through an active connection based on source initiated routing packets	High
	Cross-site scripting: attacker injects malicious scripts into a reliable website	Medium
	Cross-site request forgery: attacker makes an authenticated software to execute automatically	High
Application layer	Ransomware: malware penetrates a PC as a Trojan using vulnerable points in that machine and detains the PC until the PC owner pays ransom money	High
	Brute-Force: attacker accesses the node using password by guessing using key extraction software	High
	Account hijacking: gain control over a banking/financial account—one of identity thefts	High

Table 6.9 Protection techniques at various layers

Implementation layer	Security approach	Outcome
Physical layer	Data collection and access control	Prevent data leakage and attack on IoMT
Communication layer	Access control	Use lightweight IoMT, data storage in IoMT with adaptive access control
	Identification authentication	Ensure patient identification and integrity of data, prevent authenticated patients from accessing the unauthenticated insecure server
Processing layer	Data encryption	Guarantee data security of data communication, lightweight IoMT device communication
	ID authentication and data encryption	Secured cryptosystem with mutual authentication in IoMT

Wireless Protected Access II encryption standards are used nowadays. Extensible Authentication Protocol (EAP) provides standard functions and negotiation of authentication methods. EAP proposes 40 different ways of authentication [32].

6.3 Introduction to COVID-19

COVID-19 is a respiratory illness caused by severe acute respiratory syndrome corona virus (SARS-CoV2) that belongs to single-stranded positive-sense RNA virus. In December 2019, the virus was first reported in Wuhan City, China. About 213 countries are affected by COVID-19. In 2021, the second wave of COVID-19 caused a significant pandemic, with massive deaths within few days of infection. It could not be prevented amidst the introduction of vaccines in different countries.

Symptoms of COVID-19 are illustrated in Table 6.10. If COVID-19 is diagnosed at an earlier stage, quick recovery is possible [33]. But diagnosis at an earlier stage is a challenge. Figure 6.9 shows the precautionary steps to avoid COVID-19. Three steps need to be followed: (1) wear a mask, (2) maintain social distancing of about 6 ft, (3) wash your hands with soap or sanitizer frequently, and (4) without washing, do not touch nose, eyes, and mouth [34].

Once a patient is diagnosed with COVID-19, he must be isolated so that his family and neighbors are not infected. If an external person infects the patient, contact tracing is essential, and identifying those who are all in contact with the infected person must be tested, isolated, and treated. One of the ways to track the patient is using the Markov model [35]. The patient may be at different postures inside as well as outside his home. Based on the poses of the patient, he can be tracked, and contact tracing can also be done,

The five-stage transition diagram is shown in Figure 6.10 to implement the Markov model. The numbers indicate the probability of moving from one posture to another.

Table 6.10 COVID-19 symptoms

Most common	Fever, fatigue, dry cough, continuous sputum discharge
Least common	Discomfort in breathing, headache, sore throat, chills, arthralgia
Rare	Diarrhea, nausea, nasal congestion, hemoptysis, conjunctival congestion

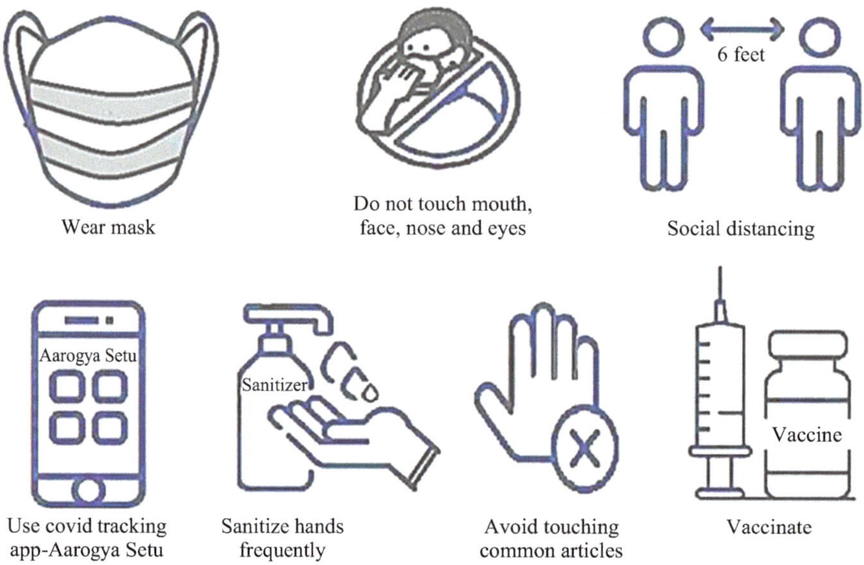

Figure 6.9 Precautionary steps to prevent COVID-19

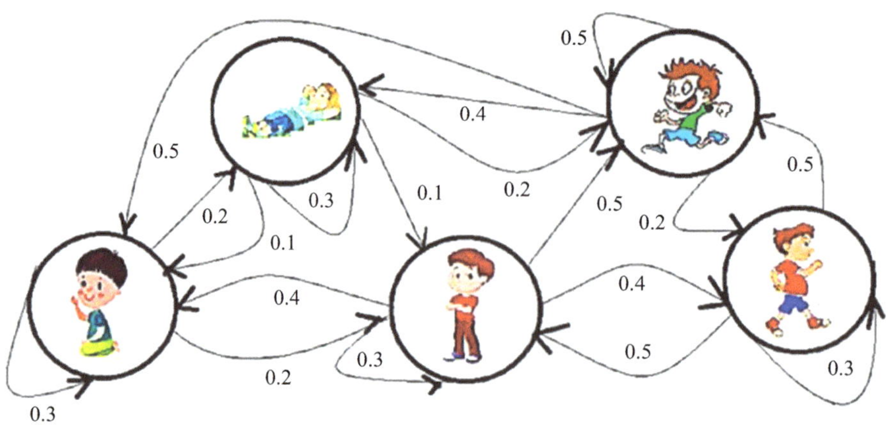

Figure 6.10 Markov model to track a COVID patient

Table 6.11 Different technologies evolved till COVID-19

Technology	Application	Disease and year
Internet of Things	Early symptoms diagnosis by measuring blood pressure, body temperature, heart rate, SpO_2, proximity detection, location detection, contact tracing, social distancing	SARS (2002)
AI-based IoT	Infection evaluation, prediction, treatment monitoring, disease outbreak	SARS (2002), MERS (2012) COVID (2019)
Big Data–based IoT	Health analysis, diagnosis, outbreak tracking, CT imaging manifestation, and pathogen detection	Ebola (2014), COVID (2019)
Cloud-based IoT and blockchain–based IoT	Infection administration, disease prevention, outbreak detection, and application-based management like Amazon AWS, Azure	COVID (2019)

To mitigate COVID-19, different technologies are used in IoMT. Table 6.11 shows the evolution of various technologies used till COVID-19 spread across other countries [36–38].

Social media can create awareness about the importance of social distancing. Smartphone apps can be used to monitor the social distancing and contact tracing of patients. In different countries, various smartphone application programs are used. In Singapore, a BLE-enabled mobile app called "Trace together" is used [37]. In European countries like German, France, and Italy, BLED-enabled smartphone app called "Pan-European Privacy-Preserving Proximity Tracing" (PEPP-PT) is used. In India, "Aarogya Setu" is used [39]. In BLE-based apps, both centralized and decentralized approaches create a problem [40]. If a patient has no smartphone or no Bluetooth, tracing is difficult. Two types of data are collected using these apps: location and proximity. Both may cause false alarm, false-negative alarm, and false-positive alarm if a person comes in contact by location information or contact information when the infected person left the place [36].

In addition to a mobile app, drones, Big Data, artificial intelligence, virtual meetings, and wearable smart devices can help to improve social distancing. For data extraction, Twitter, Facebook types of social media are used. To measure temperature, a smart helmet, thermal imager, noncontact thermopile sensors can also be used [33]. GPS mobile and wearable trackers can be used to locate a patient. Table 6.12 shows the contact tracing technologies used for COVID-19 [41].

6.3.1 Implementation of blockchain in IoMT systems

Blockchain technology has the features like (1) immutability—falsification of data is difficult, (2) nonrepudiation is ensured, (3) traceability, (4) decentralization

Table 6.12 Technologies used for COVID-19 contact tracing

Technology	Application
GIS	Corona watch, SMC COVID-19 tracker
Bluetooth	Trace together, Stanford's COVID watch, MIT's Pact
GPS	India's Aarogya Setu, HaMagen, MIT's private kit, Europe's PEPP-PT, Tabaud
Blockchain	CIVITAS, TRACY

Table 6.13 Blockchain-based IoMT

Blockchain-based IoMT implementation	Uses
Noncontact thermopile sensors, thermal cameras, RNA test	Pandemic regions can be traced quickly, and origin can also be identified
Wristband sensors	Quarantine and social distancing monitoring
RFID, NFC tags for asset management	Smart hospital
Wearable sensors	Telehealth and remote healthcare

reduces the cost of blocks. One of the applications of blockchain technology is COVID prevention. A blockchain technology can be implemented to limit the pandemic by integrating different data sources, which can be analyzed to extract features for the healthcare team and government [42].

Core applications and technologies of blockchain help (1) early disease detection and diagnosis, (2) observation and management, (3) contact tracing, (4) projection of infected person and mortality prediction, (5) medication and vaccine development, and (6) disease prevention. Table 6.13 shows how blockchain can be implemented with various sensors to build an IoMT application.

The strategy is to strengthen and reorganize healthcare, tracking, screening, and prioritize the patient's need and treatment based on severity [43]. Deployment of wearable and noninvasive technology with mobile health technology is a promising solution to combat this pandemic. BP, SpO_2, heart rate, and body temperature using wearable sensors provide a prompt alert to abnormal changes in these parameters. Asymptotic carriers of COVID are highly prevalent during an explosive stage [44–46].

6.4 Proposed system architecture

Figure 6.11 represents the framework of secured IoMT system architecture and integrates embedded systems, IoT technology, and cloud computing for healthcare applications. This system is dedicatedly developed for home quarantined COVID patients living in rural areas [47]. During the global pandemic, a massive number of

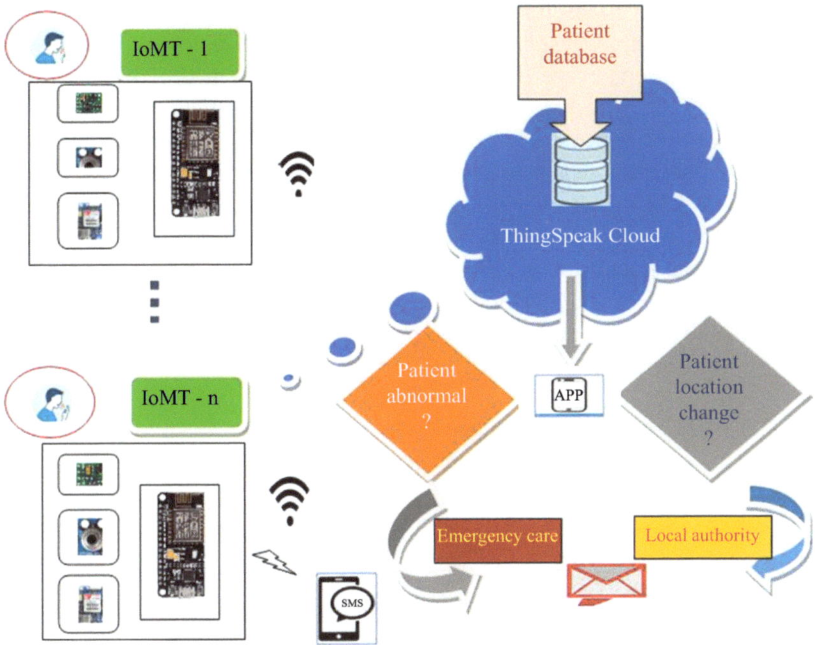

Figure 6.11 Secured IoMT system architecture

people may be affected by the virus spreading. So it is impossible to provide treatment for all the people in the rural area hospitals.

This work suggests that most infected patients can be admitted to the hospital, and with mild symptoms, patients can be remotely monitored with the help of the proposed IoMT device. An IoMT device has a feature to monitor the location of the home quarantined patient to avoid the virus spreading among the innocent public. The patient clinical data measured from the IoMT device are transferred to the ThingSpeak cloud lively. The local authority can visualize the home quarantined patient location remotely from the cloud, and it also sends an alert mail in the case of unauthorized movement. The healthcare experts remotely monitor the patient's vitals through a cloud and mobile app to assist them constantly. In the case of any abnormality, an alert mail is sent to the medical emergency center. Short message service (SMS) is also provided for easy access to the authorities.

6.4.1 IoMT device

Figure 6.12 represents significant components used in the IoMT device. The NodeMCU ESP8266 development board with a Wi-Fi network facility is the heart of the IoMT device. It has a Tensilica Xtensa 32-bit RISC processor with adjustable operating frequency ranging from 80 to 160 MHz [48]. It also supports real-time operating system (RTOS) features and various low power operating modes, making this board more suitable for prototyping the IoMT device. MAX30102 pulse oximeter sensor, MLX90614 temperature sensor, and SIM808 GPS/GPRS/GSM module are interfaced with NodeMCU ESP8266 [48]. Blood oxygen level and heart rate are measured using a MAX30102 pulse oximeter sensor. This sensor operates at 1.8 V and has an ADC with an 18-bit resolution. The MLX90614 temperature sensor is used to measure the object temperature ranging from −70°C to +380°C. It provides high accuracy with 16-bit ADC. The unique feature of this sensor is to measure the temperature without physical contact as it operates based on infrared waves. Both the sensors are communicating with ESP8266 through the I2C protocol [49]. Table 6.14 represents the clinical parameters and their range. An SIM808 module is a combination of GPS and GSM/GPRS technology. It

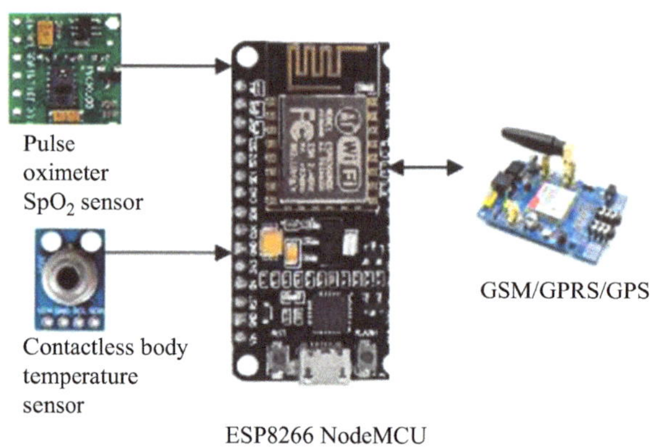

Figure 6.12 IoMT device components

Table 6.14 Clinical parameters and its state

Blood oxygen level (SpO_2)	
Range (%)	State
95–100	Good
94	Normal
90–94	Low
Below 90	Very low
Heart rate	
Range (BPM)	State
60–100	Normal
>100	High
<60	Low
Body temperature	
Range (°C)	State
36–37.5	Normal
>37.5	High
<36	Low

supports a quad-band frequency of 850/900/1 800/1 900 MHz. The tracking sensitivity of GPS is −165 dBm. GPS coordinates, latitude, and longitudes are obtained using an SIM 808 module. An SMS service is provided in the IoMT device using an SIM 808 module.

The pseudocode of the scheduling algorithm for the proposed IoMT device is shown in Figure 6.13. RTOS helps to build a deterministic system that is very much essential for remote healthcare monitoring systems [50]. RTOS is used in a multitasking environment, where all the tasks are executed based on priority. The proposed method used open-source RTOS, namely, FreeRTOS. In IoMT, the

```
Pseudo code : IoMT
Input:
Heart rate-H,Blood oxygen-BO,Body temperature-BT,Threshold-T,GPS latitude-
LT,GPS longitude-LG, Medical Emergency Care-MEC, Local authority-LA,Priority-
P-Highest number yield highest priority
Include FreeRTOS libraries
Task_Scheduler() //Preemptive priority scheduling
Task1_cloud( ); //Task decleration
Task2_SMS( );
 Task3_AES( );
Task creation
Task_Create(Task1_cloud, P=2)
Task_Create(Task2_SMS,P=5)  //highest priority
Task_Create(Task3_AES P=1)

init_Task()  //startup task
{Read →H,BO,BT
Read →GPS coordinates-LT,LG}

Task1()
{
ThingSpeak Channel ←unique write API key
 H,BO,BT,LT,LG  →channel}

Task2 ()
{
10 samples →H,BO,BT→mean
If(H,BO,BT)<T
 SMS →MEC
If(LT & LG=out of range)
SMS →LA}

Task3 ()
{
Secrect Key
AES →Encrypt→H,BO,BT,LT,LG +Secret Key
Mail →Medical data base }
```

Figure 6.13 Pseudocode—IoMT device scheduling algorithm

software module is programmed with multiple tasks having different priority levels. A *preemptive priority scheduling algorithm* is implemented using FreeRTOS [51]. In the IoMT system, three tasks are created. Kernel's initial task is reading the sensor and GPS coordinates data and configuring the cloud with a unique channel using the write API key. Task1 function is to send data from the IoMT node to the ThingSpeak cloud. Task2 is assigned the highest priority among other tasks. Its role is to send the SMS whenever abnormal in medical parameters and the unauthorized movement of the patient to the concerned authorities. Task3 function is to encrypt the data using Advanced Encryption Standard (AES) with a 128-bit secret key. AES employs symmetric key encryption and uses a single pass with different lengths like 128, 192, and 256 bits for encryption and decryption. This work uses AES with a 128-bit secret key, as shown in Figure 6.14 with sample data.

Each patient IoMT device sends the medical data and GPS latitude and longitude data to the ThingSpeak cloud platform. ThingSpeak is cloud-based data aggregation, visualization, and analytics IoT platform. It supports many embedded devices. A ThingSpeak platform provides a list of channels with a unique ID. The channel is accessed using read and write API keys. Each channel supports up to eight fields, so eight different parameters are visualized in the cloud from an embedded device. Each embedded device is programmed with a unique channel using the API key. It allows us to visualize the data from the embedded device lively in the cloud and act on the specific value of data. Figure 6.15 shows the pseudocode of the proposed system on the cloud. An authenticated person only able to access the ThingSpeak cloud. Data are streamed live to the cloud from the different IoMT devices. GPS coordinates, latitude, and longitude are received from the edge device and programmed to visualize a patients' exact location using the Google Maps. In the cloud, data are analyzed, and an alert mail is sent to the authorized person. Device failure is also indicated through the alert mail.

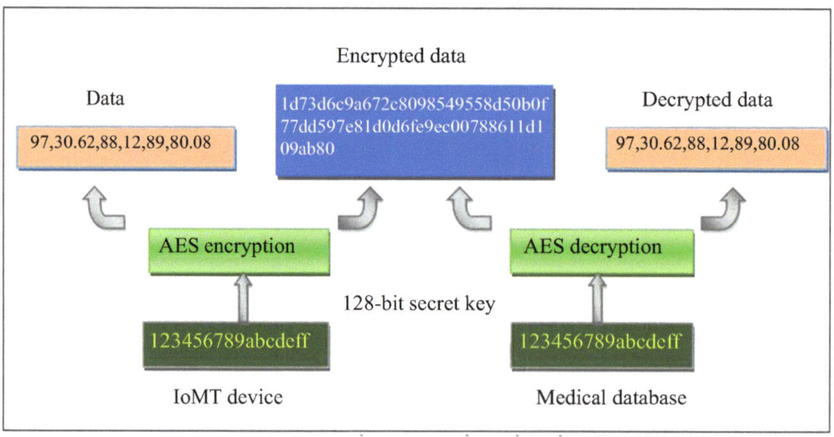

Figure 6.14 Implementation of AES algorithm

```
Pseudo code: Cloud
Create a unique channel for each IoMT
Set the field in the channel
IoMT→Visualize H, BO, BT, LT, LG data
Cloud→Mobile app
 Map the LT and LG in Google map
If (LT & LG not in range)
Alert mail →LA
If (H, BO, BT< T)
Alert mail →MEC
If (no data ←IoMT)
Alert mail →LA
```

Figure 6.15 ThingSpeak cloud programming

6.4.2 Results and discussion

The IoMT device is periodically sending clinical data and GPS coordinates to the ThingSpeak cloud platform. The medical parameters, namely, blood oxygen level, heart rate, and body temperature, are measured through MAX30102 pulse oximeter and MLX90614 contactless IR temperature sensors [52]. The sensors' values are transmitted to the cloud through a live data stream and visualized as shown in Figure 6.16.

Figure 6.16(a)–(c) represents blood oxygen level (SpO_2), body temperature (°C), and heart rate (BPM) of the patient, respectively. From the IoMT device, GPS coordinates of the patient location are also transferred to the cloud lively. With the help of the MATLAB® visualization app in the ThingSpeak cloud platform, GPS latitude and longitude values are processed and visualized as a Google Map, as shown in Figure 6.17. Figure 6.17(a) and (b) represents the GPS latitude and longitude received from the IoMT device. Figure 6.17(c) represents Google Map visualization of a patient's location. This patient tracking system will be helpful for

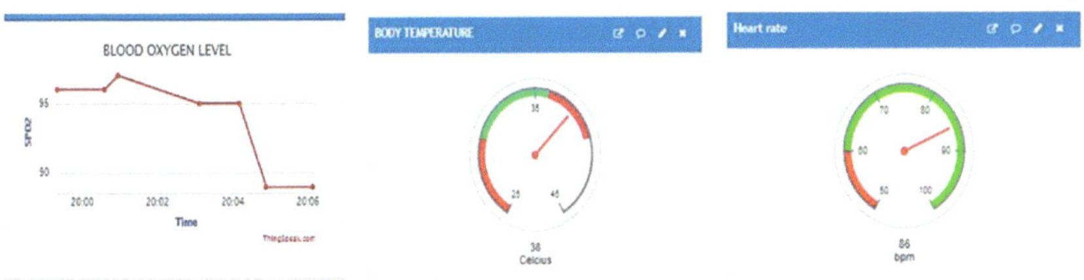

(a) (b) (c)

Figure 6.16 Live visualization of patient's medical data on a ThingSpeak cloud platform: (a) blood oxygen level, (b) body temperature, (c) heart rate

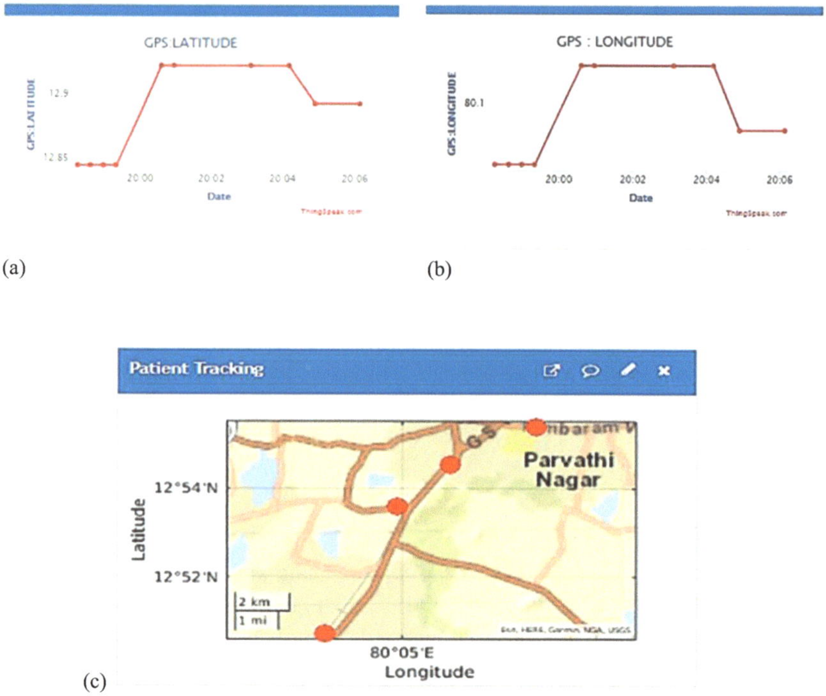

Figure 6.17 Patient tracking through GPS coordinates on cloud platform: (a) GPS latitude, (b) GPS longitude, (c) Google Map

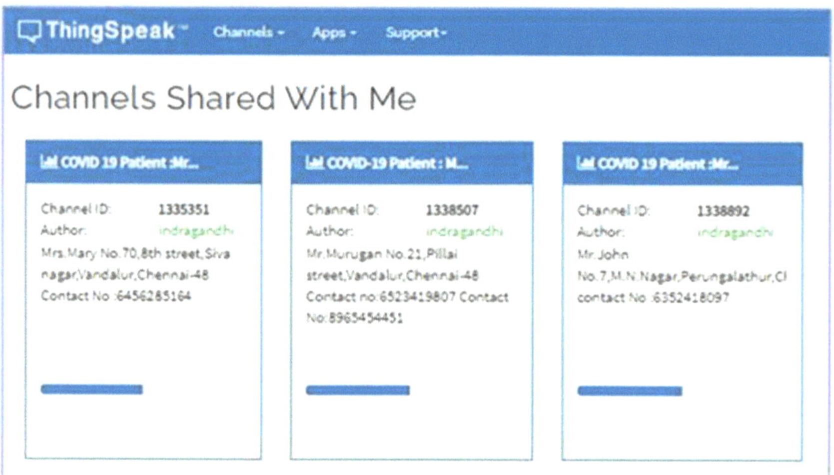

Figure 6.18 Channels shared with the authorized person

the local authority to monitor the unauthorized movement of the home quarantined patient [51]. This mechanism will significantly reduce the chance of spreading the COVID-19 virus among the public.

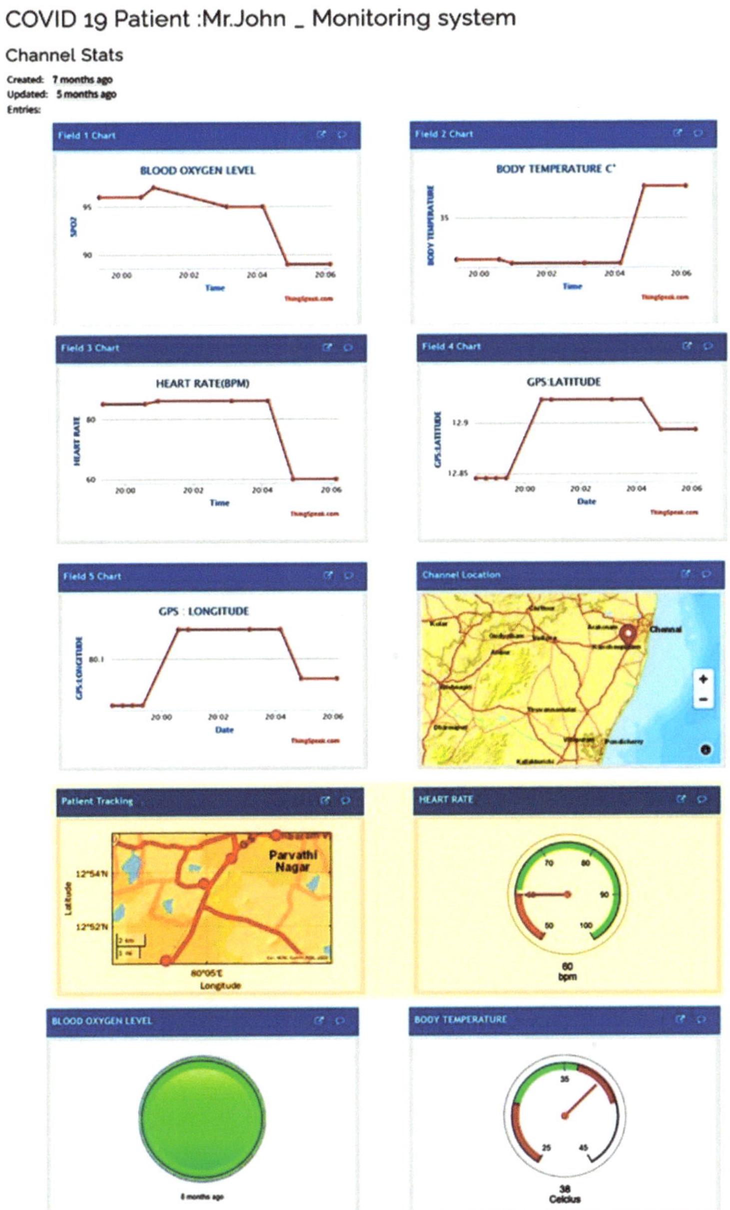

Figure 6.19 Patient information from a single channel

Each IoMT device is linked with a unique channel in the ThingSpeak platform using the API keys. Only the authorized person would be able to access the different patient data. For analysis, three patient details are shared with the qualified person, as shown in Figure 6.18.

The authorized person can monitor each patient's live status from the unique channel as shown in Figure 6.19.

Each person's location is configured in the channel. If the patient location is out of range, an alert mail is sent to the local authority to take necessary action. Figure 6.20 represents Mr. John out of range indication along date and time.

Figure 6.21 represents alert mails sent to the medical emergency center whenever the patient's medical parameters become abnormal as programmed in the ThingSpeak cloud platform.

Suppose the data have not arrived continuously from any IoMT devices due to malfunction or power failure. In that case, the ThingSpeak cloud will send an alert mail to the concerned authority, as shown in Figure 6.22.

As an alternate method, the SMS service facility is also supported in the IoMT device to communicate with the local authority and medical emergency center, as shown in Figure 6.23(a) and (b). This feature is provided to mitigate the issues in Internet connection failure.

Figure 6.24 represents the mobile app view of different patients. Figure 6.24(a) represents the patient's details, and (b) shows individual patient's clinical data. This mobile app helps the authorities to access the patient data at any time remotely.

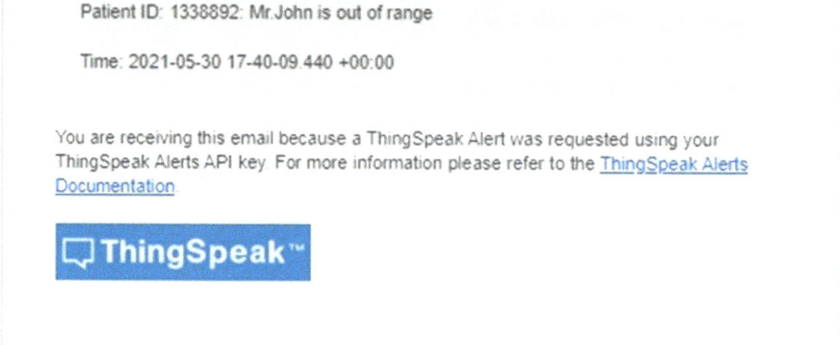

Figure 6.20 Alert mail for unauthorized movement of a patient

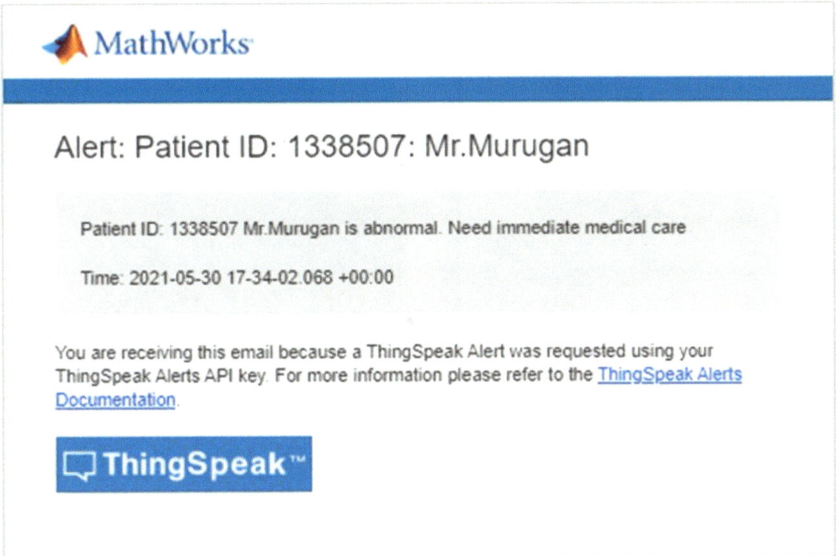

Figure 6.21 Medical emergency indication of patient

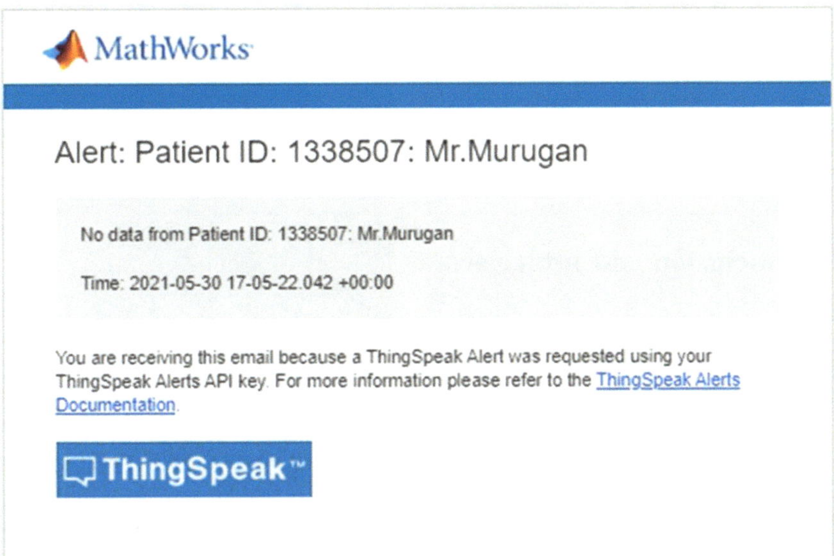

Figure 6.22 Indication of inactive IoMT device

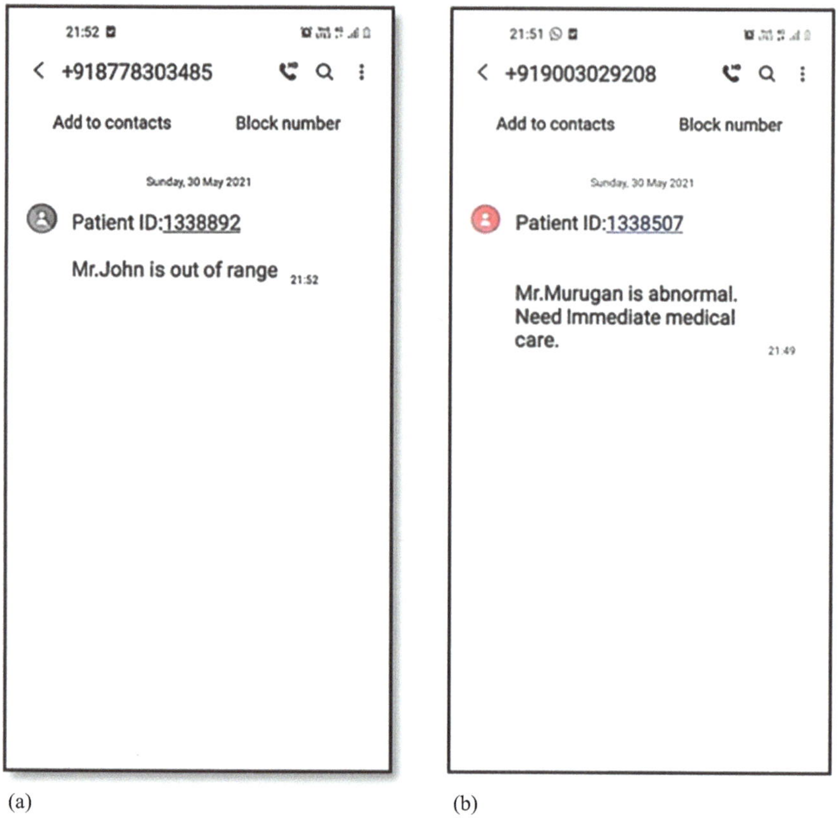

Figure 6.23 SMS from IoMT device: (a) alert SMS to local authority and (b) alert SMS to medical emergency center

6.5 Conclusion and future scope

The emerging IoT technology facilitates healthcare providers to extend their service to hospitals in rural areas. The proposed IoMT device plays a prominent role in the medical system by observing COVID patients who stay in the home quarantine. The device senses, measures, and processes real-time clinical data such as heart rate, blood pressure, body temperature, and patient location, which would be forwarded as a continuous stream of data to the medical center and local authorities through a cloud platform. Based on the sensor values, the patient abnormality could be diagnosed, and the treatment could be suggested accurately by the physicians through a remote device. High priority is assigned for critical and abnormal information using the preemptive algorithm, and the patient-sensitive information

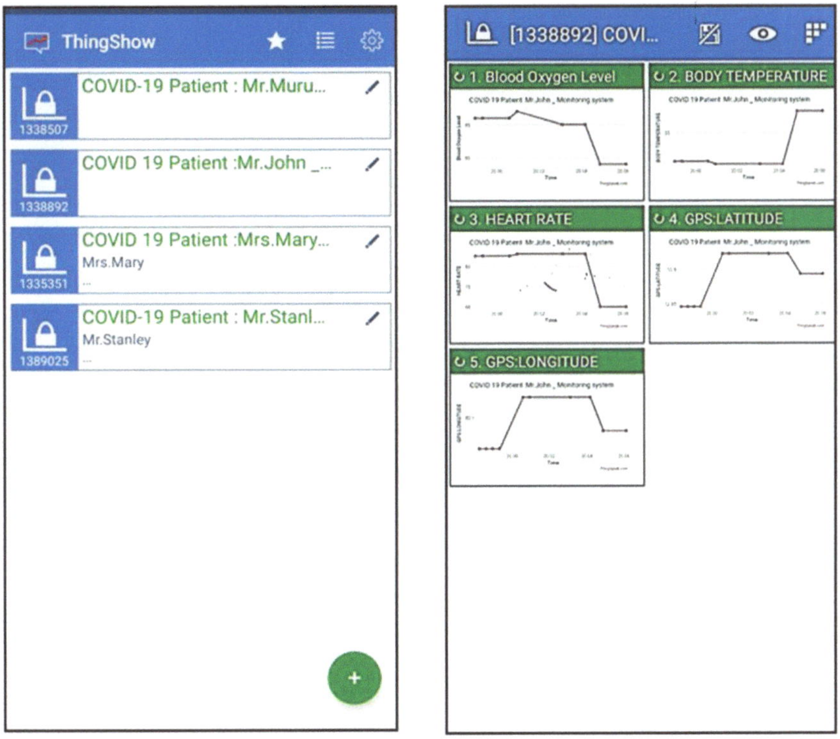

(a) (b)

Figure 6.24 ThingSpeak mobile app view: (a) list of patients and (b) details of individual patient

is securely transferred using the AES algorithm. The experimental results demonstrated the observations made in various stages of this proposed system. Consequently, the proposed framework will play a vital role in preventing and combating the COVID-19 spread. In the future, more clinical data can be sent over 5G integrated IoMT devices to enable high-speed data transfer.

References

[1] M. Wazid, A.K. Das, J.J.P.C. Rodrigues, S. Shetty and Y. Park, "IoMT Malware Detection Approaches: Analysis and Research Challenges," *IEEE Access*, Vol. 7, 2019, pp. 182459–182476.

[2] Y. Myrka, "Advantages and Disadvantages of Implementing IoT in Healthcare", Available at https://iotforall.com/iot-healthcare-advantages-disadvantages, 2020, Accessed on June 6, 2021.

[3] A. Limaye and T. Adegbija, "HERMIT: A Benchmark Suite for the Internet of Medical Things," *IEEE Internet of Things Journal*, Vol. 5, No. 5, 2020, pp. 4212–4222.
[4] A. Gatouillat, Y. Badr, Bertrand M., *et al.*, "Internet of Medical Things: A review of Recent Contributions Dealing With Cyber-Physical Systems in Medicine," *IEEE Internet of Things Manual*, Vol. 5, No. 5, 2018, pp. 3810–3822.
[5] D. YokeshShelke and A. Sharma, "Internet of Medical Things," Thematic report, Technology Intelligence and IP Research, Aranca, 2016.
[6] J.N.S. Rubi and P.R.I. Gondim, "IoMT Platform for Pervasive Healthcare Data Aggregation, Processing, and Sharing Based on One M2M and Open HER," *Sensors Journal*, 2019, p. 4283.
[7] J. Fiaidhi and S. Mohammed, "Security and Vulnerability of Extreme Automation Systems: The IoMT and IoA Case Studies," *IT Professional*, Vol. 21, 2019, pp. 48–55.
[8] R. Sujath, J.M. Chatterjee and A.E. Hassanien, "A Machine Learning Forecasting Model for COVID-19 Pandemic in India," *Stochastic Environmental Research and Risk Assessment*, Vol. 34, 2020, pp. 959–972.
[9] C. Iwendi, A.K. Bashir, A. Peshkar, *et al.*, "COVID-19 Patient Health Prediction Using Boosted Random Forest Algorithm," *Frontiers in Public Health*, Vol. 8, 2020, p. 357.
[10] S. Dhamodharavadhani, R. Rathipriya and J.M. Chatterjee, "COVID-19 Mortality Rate Prediction for India Using Statistical Neural Network Models," *Frontiers in Public Health*, Vol. 8, 2020.
[11] N. Misran, K. Beng Gan, M. Shahidul Islam and N. Amin, "IoT Based Health Monitoring with LoRa Communication Technology", *International Conference on Electrical Engineering and Informatics (ICEEI)*, July 2019, Bandung, Indonesia.
[12] K. Li-Minn Ang and J. KahPhooi Seng, "Application Specific Internet of Things (ASIoTs): Taxonomy, Applications, Use Cases and Future Directions," *IEEE Access*, Vol. 7, 2019, pp. 56577–56590.
[13] R. Barry, "5 Key factors to consider when developing a medical (IoMT) device", Available at https://polymorph.co.za/5-key-factors-to-consider-when-developing-a-medical-(IoMT)-device/, Accessed on June 6, 2021.
[14] F. Alshehri and G. Muhammed, "A Comprehensive Survey of the Internet of Things (IoT) and AI-Based Smart healthcare," *IEEE Access*, Vol. 9, 2021, pp. 3660–3678.
[15] R. Barry, "IoT connectivity comparison", Available at https://polymorph.co.za/iot-comparison-table, Accessed on June 6, 2021.
[16] W. Yu, F. Liang, X. He, *et al.*, "A Survey on the Edge Computing for the Internet of Things," *IEEE Access*, Vol. 6, 2017, pp. 6900–6919.
[17] W. Shi, J. Cao, Q. Zhang, Y. Li and L. Xu, "Edge Computing: Vision and Challenges," *IEEE Internet of Things Journal*, 2016, DOI:10.1109/JIOT.2016.2579198.

[18] L. Sun, X. Jiang, H. Ren and Y. Guo, "Edge-cloud computing and Artificial Intelligence on Internet of Medical Things: Architecture, Technology, and Application," *IEEE Access*, Vol. 8, 2020, pp. 101079–101092.

[19] P. Dang, Z. Ning, M.S. Obaidat, X. Jiang, *et al.*, "Edge Computing-Based Health Care Systems: Enabling Decentralized Health Monitoring on Internet of Medical Things," *IEEE Network*, 2020, pp. 254–261.

[20] I.U. Din, A. Almogren, M. Guizani and M. Zuhair, "A Decade of Internet of Things: Analysis in the Light of Healthcare Applications," *IEEE Access*, Vol. 7, 2019, pp. 89967–89979.

[21] W. Ayoub, A.E. Sambat, F. Nouvel, M. Mroue and J.C. Prevotet, "Internet of Mobile Things: Overview of LoRaWAN, DASH7, and NB-IoT in LPWANs standards and Supported Mobility," *Communication Surveys and Tutorials*, Vol. 21, No. 2, 2019, pp. 1561–1581.

[22] S. Seneviratne, Y. Hu, T. Nguyen, *et al.*, "A Survey of Wearable Devices and Challenges," *IEEE Communications Surveys & Tutorials*, Vol. 19, No. 4, 2017, pp. 2573–2620.

[23] Y. Sun, F.P.W. Lo and B. Lo, "Security and Privacy for the Internet of Medical Things enables healthcare Systems: A Survey," *IEEE Access*, Vol. 7, 2019, pp. 183339–183355.

[24] X. Li, H. Dai, Q. Wang, M. Imran, *et al.*, "Securing the Internet of Medical Things With Friendly-Jamming Schemes," *Computer Communications*, Vol. 160, 2020, pp. 431–442.

[25] A. Ghubaish, T. Salman, M. Zolanvari, *et al.*, "Recent Advances in the Internet of Medical Things (IoMT) Systems Security," *IEEE Internet of Things Journal*, 2020, DOI:10.1109/JIOT.2020.3045653.

[26] R. Pratap Singh, M. Javid, A. Haleem, R. Vaishya and S. Ali, "Internet of Medical Things (IoMT) for Orthopedic in COVID-19 Pandemic: Roles, Challenges, and Applications," *Journal of Clinical Orthopedics and Trauma*, Vol. 11, 2020, pp. 713–717.

[27] M. Alex, "Threat Intelligence and Internet of Medical Things (IoMT)," *International Journal of Engineering Trends and Application*, Vol. 7, No. 3, 2020.

[28] A.A. Mawgoud, A.I. Karadawy and B.S. Tawfik, "A Secure Authentication Technique on Internet of Medical Things Through Machine Learning," *Cryptography and Security*, 2019, DOI:10.6084/m9.figshare.13311479.v2.

[29] D. Koutras, G. Stergiopoulos, T. Dasaklis, *et al.*, "Security in IoMT Communications: A Survey," *Sensors Journal*, 2020, p. 4828.

[30] A. Hafizah Mohd Aman, W. Haslina Hassan, S. Sameen, *et al.*, "IoMT Amid COVID-19 Pandemic: Application, Architecture, Technology and Security," *Journal of Network and Computer Applications*, Vol. 174, No. 102886, 2021, pp. 1–19.

[31] I.D. Morais Barraoca Filho, G. Aquino, R. Malaquias, G. Girao and S.R. Menezes Melo, "An IoT-Based Healthcare Platform for Patients in ICU Beds During the COVID-19 Outbreak," *IEEE Access*, Vol. 9, 2021, pp. 27262–27277.

[32] R. A/L Jegatheswaran, I. J. Sakira, and N. A. Abd Rahman, "A Review on IoMT Device Vulnerabilities and Countermeasures," *Journal of Physics Conference Series*, Vol. 1712, 2020, 012020.

[33] Laird Connectivity, "Connectivity choices for your Medical Device and IoMT application", white paper, Laird Connectivity, Available at https://lairdconnect.com/resources/white-papers/connectivity-choices-your-medical-device-and-iomt-application, 2019, Accessed on June 6, 2021.

[34] V. Chamola, V. Hassija, V. Gupta and M. Guizani, "A Comprehensive Review of the COVID-19 Pandemic and the Role of IoT, Drones, AI, Blockchain, and 5G in Managing Its Impact," *IEEE Access*, Vol. 8, 2020, pp. 90225–90265.

[35] F. Aydemir, "Can IoMT Help to Prevent the Spreading of New Coronavirus?," *IEEE Consumer Electronics Magazine*, 2021, pp. 66–71.

[36] K. Wei, L. Zhang, Y. Guo and X.I. Jiang, "Health monitoring on Internet of Medical Things: Architecture, Enabling Technologies, and Applications," *IEEE Access*, Vol. 8, 2020, pp. 27468–27478.

[37] B. Benreguia, H. Moumen and M. Amine Merzoug, "Tracking COVID-19 by Tracking Infectious Trajectories," *IEEE Access*, Vol. 8, 2020, pp. 145242–145255.

[38] N. Ndiaye, S. Syewobi, A.M. Abu-Mahfouz, *et al.*, "IoT in the Wake of COVID-19: A Survey on Contributions, Challenges, and Evolution," *IEEE Access*, Vol. 8, 2020, pp. 186821–186839.

[39] M. Abdel Basset, V. Chang and N.A. Nabeeh, "An Intelligent Framework Using Disruptive Technologies for COVID-19 Analysis," *Technological Forecasting and Social Change*, Vol. 163, 2021, 120431, pp. 1–14.

[40] M.T. Rahman, R.T. Khan, M.R.A. Khandaker, M. Sellathirai and M.S.A. Salan, "An Automated Contact tracing Approach for Controlling Covid-19 Spread Based on Geolocation Data From Mobile Cellular Networks," *IEEE Access*, Vol. 8, 2020, pp. 213554–213565.

[41] L. Garg, E. Chukwu, N. Nasser, C. Chakraborty and G. Garg, "Anonymity Preserving IoT based COVID-19 and Other Infectious Disease Contact Tracing Model," *IEEE Access*, Vol. 8, 2020, pp. 159402–159414.

[42] A.A.R. Alsaeedy and E.K.P. Chong, "Detecting Regions at Risk for Spreading COVID-19 Using Existing Cellular Wireless Network Functionalities," *IEEE Open Journal of Engineering in Medicine and Technology*, Vol. 1, 2020, pp. 187–189.

[43] A. Roy, F.H. Kumbhar, H.S. Dhillon, *et al.*, "Efficient Monitoring and Contact Tracing for COVID-19: A Smart IoT Based Framework," *IEEE Internet of Things Magazine*, 2020, pp. 17–23.

[44] H.-N. Dai, M. Imran and N. Haider, "Blockchain-Enabled Internet of Medical Things to Combat COVID-19," *IEEE Internet of Things Magazine*, 2020, pp. 52–57.

[45] S.S. Vedaei, A. Fotovvat, M.R. Mohebbiah, *et al.*, "COVID-Safe: An IoT-Based System for Automated Health Monitoring and Surveillance in Post-Pandemic Life," *IEEE Access*, Vol. 8, 2020, pp. 188538–188551.

[46] X. Ding, D. Clifton, N. Ji, *et al.*, "Wearable Sensing and Telehealth Technology With Potential Applications in the Coronavirus Pandemic," *IEEE Reviews in Biomedical Engineering*, Vol. 14, 2021, pp. 48–70.

[47] M. Talal, A.A. Zaidan, B.B. Zaidan, *et al.*, "Smart Home-based IoT for Real-Time and Secure Remote Health Monitoring of Triage and Priority System Using Body Sensors: Multi-Driven Systematic Review," *Journal of Medical Systems*, Vol. 43, No. 42, 2019.

[48] R. Basatneh, B. Najafi and D.G. Armstrong, "Health Sensors, Smart Home Devices, and the Internet of Medical Things: An Opportunity for Dramatic Improvement in Care for the Lower Extremity Complications of Diabetes," *Journal of Diabetes Science and Technology*, Vol. 12, No. 3, 2018, pp. 577–586.

[49] J. Shilpa V and P.K. Jawahar, "Efficient Algorithm Design on Hybrid CPU-FPGA Architecture for High-Performance Computing," *International Journal on Systems, Control, and Communications*, Vol. 12, No. 1, 2021, pp. 28–45.

[50] K. Indragandhi and P.K. Jawahar, "An Application-based "Efficient Thread Level Parallelism" (ETLP) Scheme on Heterogeneous Multicore Embedded System for Real-Time Image Processing," *Scalable Computing Practice and Experience*, Vol. 21, No. 1, 2020, pp. 47–56.

[51] S. Abhishek, "IoT Enabled Smart Hospital Management System for Covid-19 Patients," *Turkish Journal of Computer and Mathematics Education (TURCOMAT)*, Vol. 12, No. 10, 2021, pp. 4500–4506.

[52] J. Gang, X. Zhang, W. Fan, Y. Liu and P. He, "Design of Non-Contact Infra-Red Thermometer Based on the Sensor of MLX90614," *The Open Automation and Control Systems Journal*, Vol. 7, No. 1, 2015, pp. 6–18.

Chapter 7

An IoT-based system for a volumetric estimation of human brain morphological features from magnetic resonance images

S.N. Kumar[1], A. Lenin Fred[2], L.R. Jonisha Miriam[2], H. Ajay Kumar[2], I. Christina Jane[2], Parasuraman Padmanabhan[3] and Balázs Gulyás[3]

Abstract

Medical imaging is the noninvasive technique employed for disease diagnosis and therapeutic planning. Computer-aided algorithms play a pivotal role in the medical field for automatic processing of data, and the IoT role is inevitable in telemedicine. This chapter proposes an IoT-based system for a volumetric estimation of human brain morphological features from magnetic resonance images (MRIs). Brain age prediction paves the way toward the diagnosis of neurological disorders. The input T1-weighted MRIs are subjected to improved fuzzy *C*-means clustering for the extraction of white matter (WM), gray matter (GM), and cerebral spinal fluid (CSF). The volumetric estimation of morphological features helps one to distinguish the normal and abnormal brain images. The T1-weighted MRIs are used in this work, and for volumetric estimation of morphological features, the pixel counting technique is employed to estimate the WM, GM and CSF values. The Raspberry Pi processor was used for the IoT-based system design and the programs were developed in Python.

Keywords: Automatic processing; Brain age prediction; Brain image; Cerebral spinal fluid; Clustering; Fuzzy *C*-means clustering; Gray matter; IoT; Intensity inhomogeneity; Medical imaging; Morphological features; MR image; Neurological disorders, Pixel counting technique; Python; Raspberry Pi; Telemedicine; Volumetric estimation; White matter

[1]Department of Electrical and Electronics Engineering, Amal Jyothi College of Engineering, Kottayam, India
[2]Department of Electronics and Communication Engineering, Mar Ephraem College of Engineering and Technology, Elavuvilai, India
[3]Cognitive Neuroimaging Centre (CONIC), Lee Kong Chian School of Medicine, Nanyang Technological University, Singapore, Singapore

7.1 Introduction

Medical imaging in three-dimensional (3D) format gains importance in accurate disease diagnosis and treatment planning like chemotherapy. The accurate region of interest (ROI) extraction and tumor stage classification is a challenging task owing to the complex neuron structures [1]. The advancement in imaging technology enables the automatic quantitative measurements of 3D and volume measurement of brain regions, especially when the morphological changes in the brain tissues remain constant, same and difficult to be predicted by clinical examination [2,3].

The morphological features of gray matter (GM) and white matter (WM) are unique for each person and play a significant role in brain age prediction [4]. The purpose of volumetric imaging is to facilitate 3D analysis of brain structures and cell populations in the intact brain [5]. The clinical whole-brain 3D imaging provides valuable insights in early detection, diagnosis and interpretation of neurodegenerative diseases in humans [6,7].

A new volumetric feature extraction technique using seed point selection to make smooth boundaries with a decrease in the overall energy was proposed in [8], which is applied in the extraction of hippocampi from magnetic resonance (MR) brain images with good accuracy. A normative volumetric brain MR database created using 194 T2-weighted MR images (MRIs) was proposed in [9] based on multispectral segmentation by ANALYZE. The database comprises the cerebral spinal fluid (CSF), subarachnoid CSF, total brain volume (TBV), total ventricular volume, and white and gray matter volume as a reference for future studies. Initially segmented GM, WM and CSF using 3DVIEWNIX software system from MR data sets were reviewed by a neuroradiologist. The brain tissues are then subjected to the fuzzy domain to create the brain volume [10,11]. Several brain volume estimation tools are put forward in [12] for analyzing the brain tissues that rely on anatomical atlas. The BAMM software is used in the mapping of GM and WM volume in MRI brain, and variance is analyzed using a multiple analysis of covariance (MANCOVA) to study the volumetric differences and is utilized for the diagnosis of autism [13]. A convolution of 3D Gaussian surfaces (Co3DGS) technique for the volumetric intensity inhomogeneity estimation and correction in 3D MR T1 and T2 images was proposed in [14]. The changes in the brain volume of the HIV-infected patients are accessed using deformation-based morphometry, voxel-based morphometry and cortical modeling and statically by voxel-wise general linear models and compared with the neuropsychological performance between HIV-infected and HIV-uninfected subjects [15]. In [16], an algorithm was developed from enhanced 3D multichannel, FLAIR, T2 and T1C MRIs to generate the 3D model, which unambiguously highlights the glioblastoma multiforme tumor region. FreeSurfer software suite v.5.1.0 was used for the volumetric segmentation of an MR brain image for analyzing the volumetric changes in MRI, predicted with machine learning analysis. The functioning of the brain was analyzed with SVM in bipolar disorder [17].

The brain volume changes due to multiple sclerosis in 3D T1w images are calculated by segmentation-based techniques like SIENAx, FreeSurfer, Statistical Parametric Mapping (SPM), MINC and registration-based techniques like SIENA, and longitudinal FreeSurfer pipeline [18]. A hybrid segmentation algorithm comprising chicken swarm optimization for selecting threshold values in the Otsu algorithm for calculating the cerebral hemorrhage volume in the MRI brain images was proposed in [19]. The brain and CSF volume was estimated from the transaxial magnetic resonance images using a semi-automatic algorithm, subtraction of proton-weighted from T2-weighted images were used to highlight CSF [20]. The MRI studio was used for the brain volume assessment based on the duration of illness and frequency of attacks in migraine patients and healthy subjects. The changes in volume structures in the brain frontal, parietal, occipital and temporal lobes were assessed and statically analyzed using SPSS 15.0 (Statistical Product and Service Solutions) [21]. A web-based brain volume calculation tool that classifies and calculates TBV and intracranial volume was discussed in [22]. A detailed review of the different types of segmentation algorithms used for the brain volume measurement by the computer-aided design system for the better understanding and diagnosis of abnormalities in MR brain images was carried out in [23,24]. Section 7.2 highlights the improved fuzzy *C*-means (FCM) algorithm for the ROI extraction in MRIs, Section 7.3 portrays the results and discussion, and finally conclusion is drawn in Section 7.4.

7.2 Materials and methods

The apparent signal in brain MR imaging is represented as a product of the original signal plus a spatially changing component known as the bias field. If the *c*th pixel intensities of A_c and B_c are true and recorded, the bias field is H_c, and the total number of pixels in the MR brain image is M.

$$A_c = B_c H_c, \quad 1 \le c \le M \tag{7.1}$$

The gradual and steady fluctuation in signal intensity is called intensity inhomogeneity or bias [25]. If the magnitude is 40 percent in bias field, the values ranging from 0.8 to 1.2 is multiplied with the field signal. The artifact may be represented as an additive bias field by adding a logarithmic modification to the intensities [26], as shown in the following:

$$a_c = b_c + \beta_c, \quad 1 \le c \le M \tag{7.2}$$

The bias field is calculated using a linear combination of a series of foundation functions as follows:

$$x_c = \sum_{1}^{N} \overline{u}_c h_c(c) = \overline{u}^S H(c) \tag{7.3}$$

where $\overline{u}^S = (\overline{u}_1, \overline{u}_2, \ldots, \overline{u}_N)S$ is the coefficients of the combination. The basic function used is $H(c) = (h_1(c), h_2(c), \ldots, h_N(c))S$.

Noise generates unwanted visual quality and reduces the appearance of small contrasting items. Hence image denoising is one of the major processes in numerous applications. Its goal is to estimate the original image as accurate as possible from its noisy version. Image filtering can increase the performance of segmentation algorithms [27]. By averaging the pixel values of their adjacent pixels, linear low-pass filters modify the pixel value. These filters minimize noise but generate fuzzy pictures, and in the case of great noise, they do not maintain the edges. Nonlinear filters perform better in terms of edge preservation, but they impair fine structure, lowering picture resolution [28,29]. This issue can be solved using wavelet filtering. At high frequencies, wavelet processing generates strong spatial resolution whereas, at low frequencies, it produces average resolution. Different techniques of picture denotation have advantages and disadvantages concerning calculation costs, denoising quality and border conservation. Thus denoising remains an open question and needs to be improved.

7.2.1 Improved fuzzy C-means (FCM) clustering algorithm for the extraction of ROI

Images used are weighted sequences and they are segmented with FCM clustering algorithms to identify areas of WM, GM and CSF [30]. The cerebral volume is then calculated by the pixel-counting method. The clustering of fuzzy data depends on whether the pattern data only belong to one cluster or numerous clusters with various relationship degrees. By some defined criteria, FCM tries to split a whole collection of picture components into a collection of floating clusters. Each data point related to each cluster center is assigned a membership function based on the distance between the data point and the cluster center [31,32]. The cluster center is more closely connected with the data, the closer it is to the cluster core.

The following steps are used to describe the FCM clustering algorithm:

Step 1: Set cluster number and random points from the data set to establish the centers.

Step 2: Update membership grades using Step 1, if v_{nm} is the membership of nth and mth clusters, d_{nm} is the Euclidean distance of the nth and mth clusters:

$$v_{nm} = \frac{1}{\sum_{i=1}^{a} \left[\frac{d_{nm}}{d_{mi}}\right]^{(2/b-1)}} \tag{7.4}$$

Step 3: Use Step 2 to update the centers:

$$a_m = \frac{\sum_{n=1}^{N} \left(v_{nm}^b\right) \times x_n}{\sum_{n=1}^{N} v_{nm}^b} \tag{7.5}$$

Step 4: Steps 2 and 3 should be repeated, until convergence is achieved. When changing membership values are smaller than the center value, the convergence of this algorithm will be achieved.

A modified fast FCM (MFCM) algorithm is an automated way of determining initial central value and an adaptive way of integrating local spatial continuity into the MR brain image segmentation [33]. The desired feature of the updated FCM algorithm is

$$B = \sum_{a=1}^{d} \sum_{c=1}^{N} \left[(1-\alpha)\mu_{ac}^{e}(v_c - k_c - u_a)^2 + \alpha \sum_{g \epsilon N_c} \mu_{ac}^{e} \omega_{cg} \left(v_g - k_g - u_a\right)^2 \right]$$
$$+ \sum\nolimits_{c=1}^{N} \alpha_c \sum\nolimits_{a=1}^{d} \mu_{ac}\left(1 - \mu_{ac}^{e-1}\right) \tag{7.6}$$

where ω_{cg} denotes the weight of pixels in the cth pixel's neighborhood and α_c is the term's control parameter that promotes crispness membership degrees. This method uses histogram to automatically initialize the centroid and offers an adaptive strategy to add local spatial continuity to efficiently reduce noise and eliminate edge distortion. A linear combination of the fundamental function is used to determine intensity inhomogeneity, and an objective function is added to decrease the number of iterations. The partition matrix and cluster's center and bias fields are calculated as follows:

$$\mu_{ac} = \left(\sum_{b=1}^{d} \left(\frac{(1-\alpha)h_{ca} + \alpha \sum_{g \epsilon N_c} \omega_{cg} h_{ga} - \alpha_c}{(1-\alpha)h_{ca} + \alpha \sum_{g \epsilon N_c} \omega_{cg} h_{ga} - \alpha_c} \right) \right)^{-1} \tag{7.7}$$

$$u_a = \frac{\sum_{c=1}^{M} \mu_{ac}^{e}(1-\alpha)(v_c - k_c) + \alpha \sum_{g \epsilon N_c} \omega_{cg}\left(v_g - k_g\right)}{\sum_{c=1}^{N} \mu_{ac}^{e}} \tag{7.8}$$

$$k_c = \sum_{c=1}^{M} \overline{\omega}_c f_c(c) = \overline{\omega}^T F(c) \tag{7.9}$$

where $h_{ca} = \left(v_g - k_g - u_a\right)^2$, $\overline{\omega} = (\overline{\omega}_1, \overline{\omega}_2, \ldots, \overline{\omega}_M)^T$, and $F(C) = (f_1(c), f_2(c), \ldots, f_M(c))^T$, and $c = 1, 2, \ldots, M$ are the combination coefficients. The orthogonal polynomials are employed as the basis functions, and they must fulfill the following condition:

$$\int_{\Omega} f_a(y) f_b(y) = \delta_{ab} \tag{7.10}$$

where $\delta_{ab} = 0$, $a \neq b$, $\delta_{ab} = 1$, $a = b$. At the same time, the MFCM approach eliminates three significant artifacts in brain images. The centroids' starting values are computed automatically. Approaches based on FCM are updated by the inclusion of spatial limitation into the FCM objective function. These methods are used to adjust intensity inhomogeneity and segment partial volumes of brain MRIs.

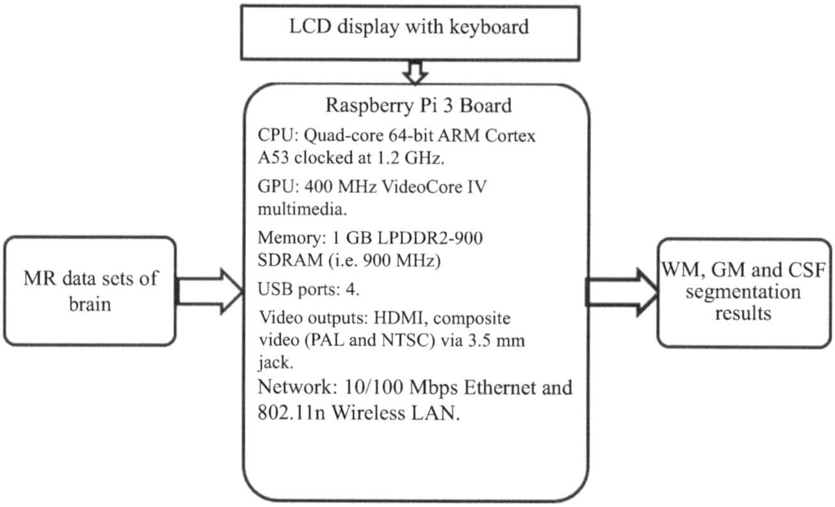

Figure 7.1 Flow diagram of a hardware implementation of IoT-based system for ROI extraction

Bias-corrected FCM (BCFCM) compensates for intensity inhomogeneity by altering the objective function of FCM. But it takes a lot of time since, at each iteration stage, BCFCM calculates the neighborhood term. It, therefore, substitutes kernel-induced distance for the similarity measurement in FCM. Improved and updated FCM clustering algorithms were used to speed up the segmentation process and precise intensity inhomogeneity during segmentation. Fuzzy spatial relation is integrated into deformable models for brain MRI [34] segmentation.

7.2.2 IoT-based system for the extraction of ROI

The hardware implementation of the ROI extraction using improved FCM was carried out on Raspberry Pi B+ embedded board. The flow diagram of the hardware implementation of IoT-based system for ROI extraction is depicted in Figure 7.1. The algorithm is developed in Python and MRIs in DICOM (digital imaging and communications in medicine is the standard for the communication and management) format are used as input. The characteristics of the Raspberry Pi board are also depicted in Figure 7.1, the system generates the WM, GM and CSF outputs. For hardware implementation, many embedded processors are there; however, in terms of cost and features, the Raspberry Pi B+ was proficient. The medical data are stored and analyzed for diagnosing health issues and play a vital role in today's scenario, thereby facilitating the telediagnosis [35,36].

7.3 Results and discussion

The segmentation algorithms are developed in Python 2.7 and implemented in the Raspberry Pi–embedded processor. The front and rear view of the portable

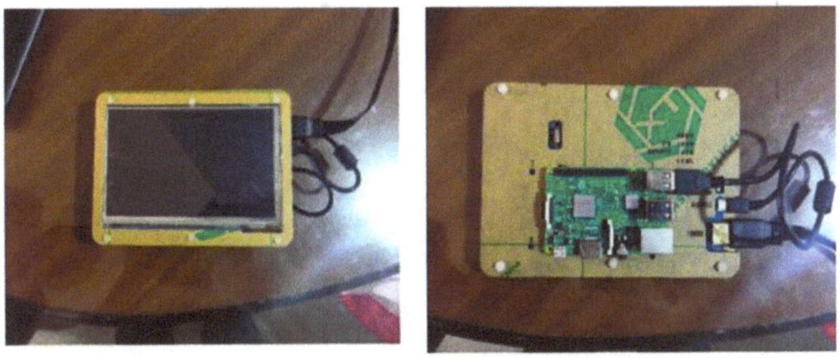

(a) (b)

Figure 7.2 (a) Front view of the portable IoT-based system and (b) back view of the proposed IoT-based system

IoT-based system is shown in Figure 7.2(a) and (b). The user interface is done with the help of a keyboard. The LCD touch screen is also there; however, the cost will be a little high. A standard LED computer monitor can also be interfaced through the HDMI port on the Raspberry Pi. The USB port facility helps us to load the images into the system.

The sample input images from 8-MR brain data sets are represented in Figure 7.3. The data sets are represented as D1–D8. The clustering algorithm parameters are as follows: the number of clusters-3, fuzzy membership value-3, number of iterations-20. The fuzzy membership value usually ranges from 2 to 3 and the number of iterations is a user-defined parameter. The number of clusters is also a user-defined parameter; however, in this research work, it is tuned to 3, since three regions WM, GM and CSF have to be extracted.

The ROI extraction results of the improved FCM algorithm are depicted in Figure 7.4. The WM extraction results are represented in Figure 7.5. The GM extraction results are represented in Figure 7.6 and CSF extraction results are represented in Figure 7.7.

The WM, GM and CSF voxel count values are represented in Table 7.1. The automated pixel counting procedure is employed in this work for the estimation of WM, GM and CSF count. A method of tessellation is used to estimate volume via the region of concern. Pixel counting is easier and more robust in the calculation of the volume of the human brain compared to the Tessellate approach.

The WM/CSF, GM/CSF and GM/WM values of the data sets are depicted in Table 7.2. In the case of an organ, multiple section images are taken from different viewpoints such as sagittal, coronal and axial. Each slice depicts the tissues in the cross section of the image. The slice thickness is a parameter that is set by the radiologist, and lower slice thickness gives the detailed anatomy of an organ.

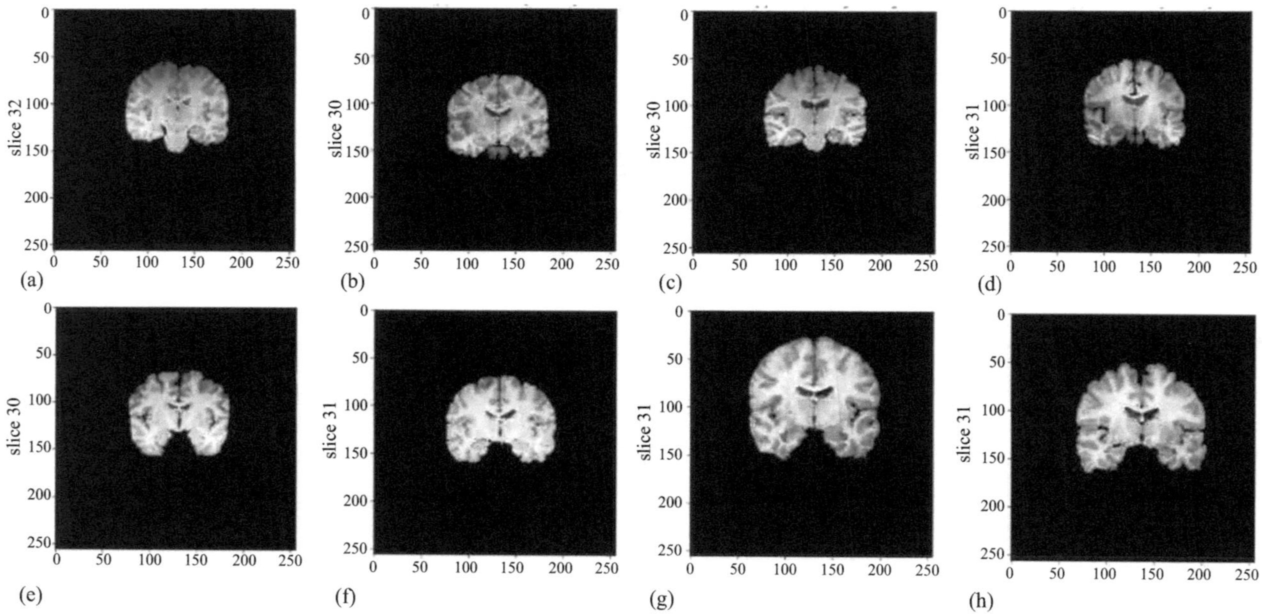

Figure 7.3 Input MR DICOM brain data sets (D1–D8)

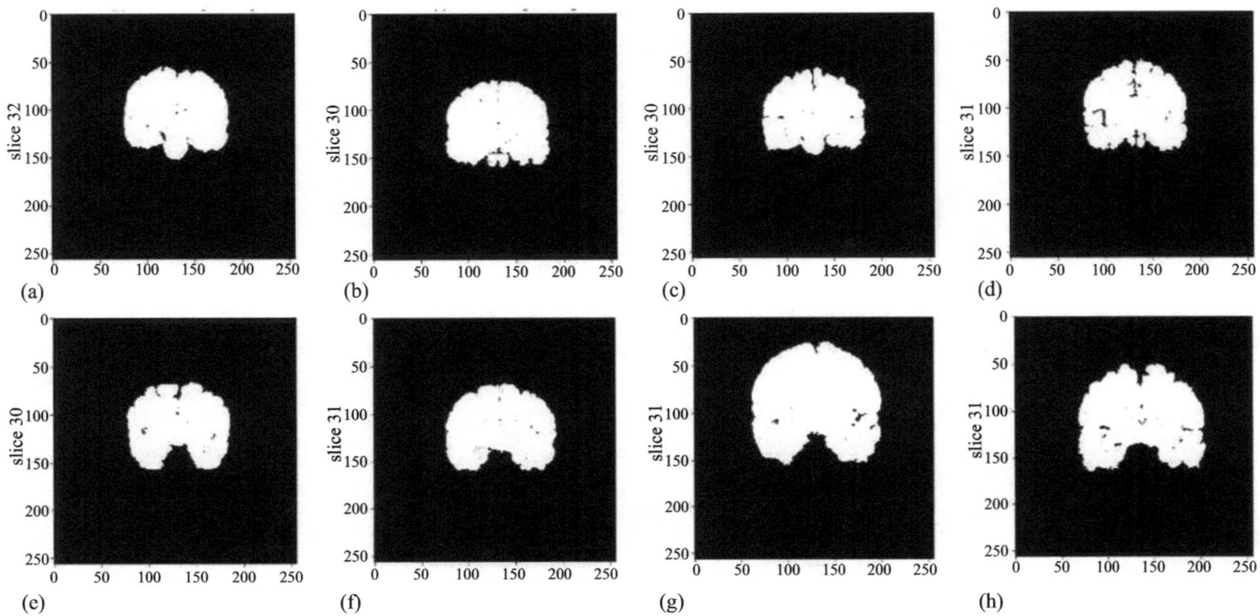

Figure 7.4 ROI extraction results of the improved FCM algorithm corresponding to MR brain data sets (D1–D8)

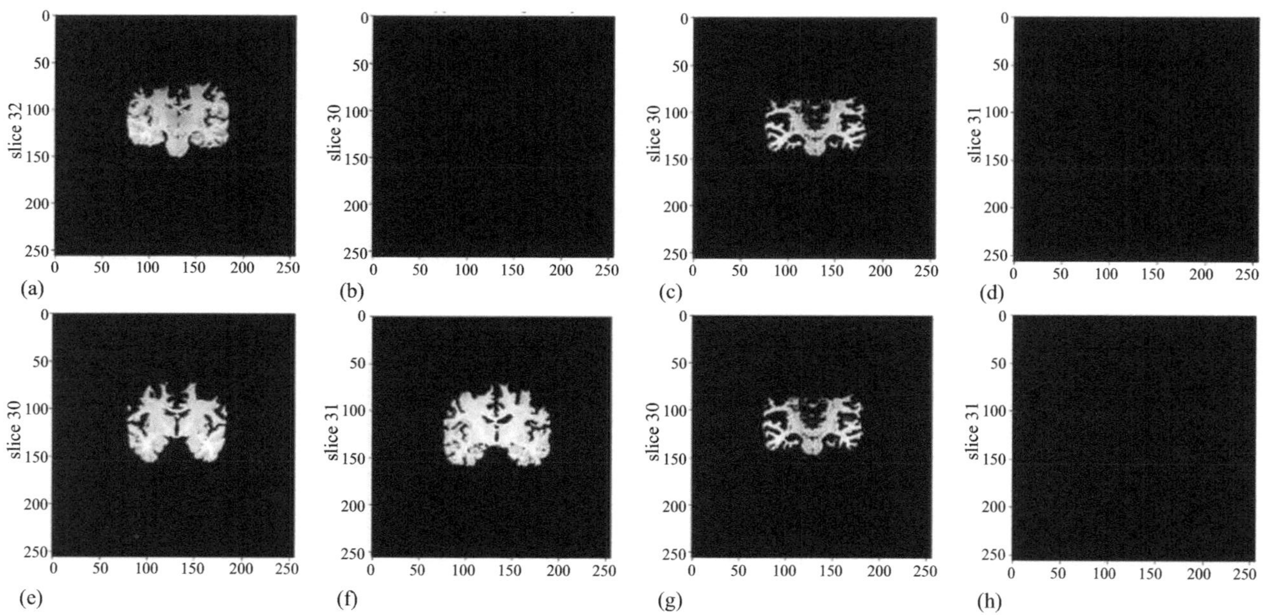

Figure 7.5 White matter extraction results of MR brain data sets (D1–D8)

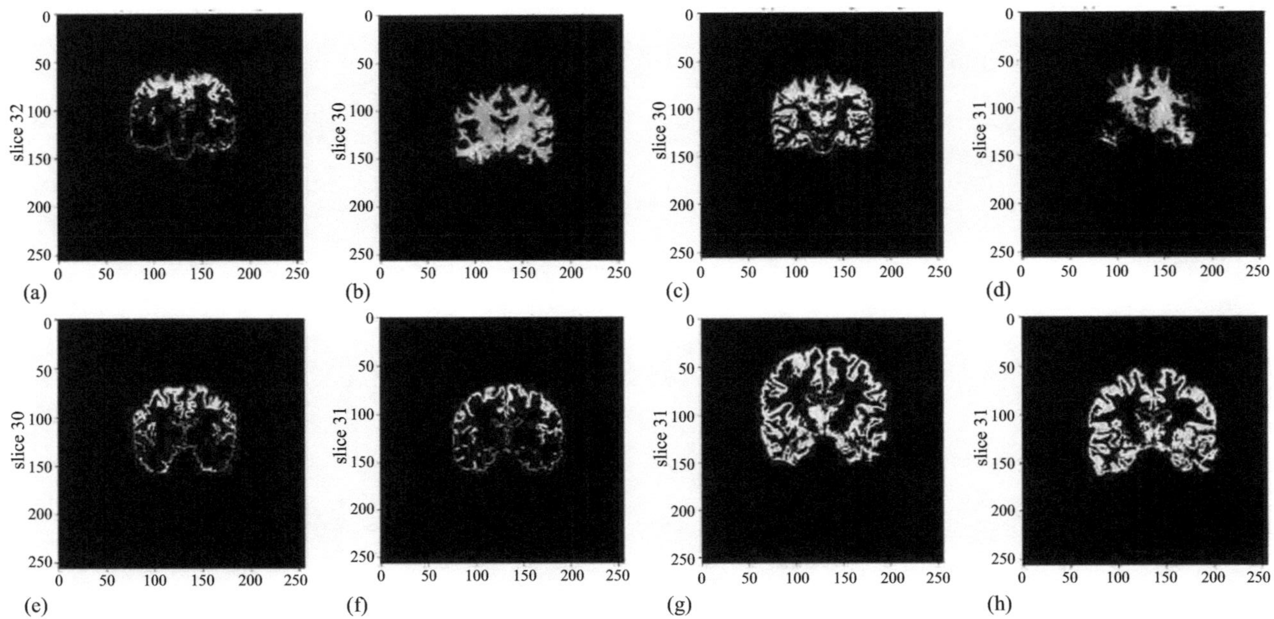

Figure 7.6 Gray matter extraction results of MR brain data sets (D1–D8)

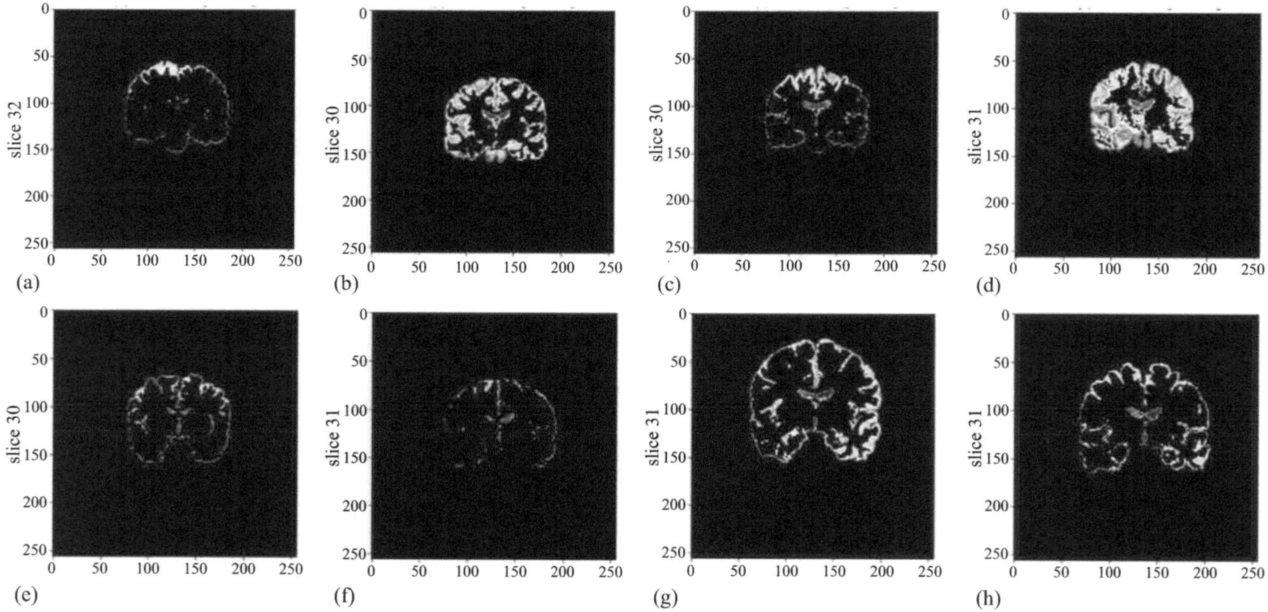

Figure 7.7 Cerebrospinal fluid extraction results of MR brain data sets (D1–D8)

Table 7.1 White matter, gray matter and CSF voxel count

Data set ID	Total voxels	White matter voxels	Gray matter voxels	CSF voxels
D1	310 908	85 644	134 633	90 631
D2	320 335	49 368	148 599	122 368
D3	291 695	78 882	129 460	83 353
D4	356 557	76 244	132 975	147 338
D5	323 103	116 604	142 552	63 947
D6	335 016	125 441	138 315	71 260
D7	550 042	191 761	234 306	123 975
D8	505 911	168 288	224 941	112 682

Table 7.2 WM/CSF, GM/CSF and GM/WM values of data sets

Data set ID	Vol. of WM/CSF	Vol. of GM/CSF	Vol. of GM/WM
D1	0.94	1.488	1.57
D2	0.40	1.21	3.01
D3	0.94	1.55	1.64
D4	0.51	0.90	1.74
D5	1.82	2.22	1.22
D6	1.76	1.94	1.10
D7	1.54	1.88	1.22
D8	1.49	1.99	1.33

7.4 Conclusion and future scope

This chapter proposes hardware implementation of IoT-based system for the extraction of morphological features from MR brain images. The WM, GM and CSF extraction was done by an improved FCM algorithm. The pixel counting technique was utilized for the volumetric estimation. The Raspberry Pi B+ processor implementation provides a cost-effective solution and the volumetric estimation of morphological features aids the detection of neurological disorders. The future work focuses on the hardware implementation for the analysis of neurological disorders based on morphological features.

Acknowledgments

The authors would like to acknowledge the support provided by DST under IDP scheme (no. IDP/MED/03/2015). Parasuraman Padmanabhan and Balazs Gulyas also acknowledge the support from Lee Kong Chian School of Medicine and Data Science and AI Research (DSAIR) center of NTU (Project Number ADH-11/2017-DSAIR) and the support from the Cognitive NeuroImaging Centre (CONIC) at NTU. The author S.N. Kumar would also like to acknowledge the support provided by Schmitt Centre for Biomedical Instrumentation (SCBMI) of Amal Jyothi College of Engineering.

References

[1] Weese J, Kaus M, Lorenz C, Lobregt S, Truyen R, and Pekar V. Shape constrained deformable models for 3D medical image segmentation. In *Biennial International Conference on Information Processing in Medical Imaging* 2001 Jun 18 (pp. 380–387). Springer, Berlin, Heidelberg.
[2] El-Dahshan ES, Mohsen HM, Revett K, and Salem AB. Computer-aided diagnosis of human brain tumor through MRI: a survey and a new algorithm. *Expert Systems with Applications*. 2014; 41(11): 5526–45.
[3] Chatterjee K, Carman-Esparza CM, and Munson JM. Methods to measure, model and manipulate fluid flow in brain. *Journal of Neuroscience Methods*. 2020; 333: 108541.
[4] Liu F, Guo W, Yu D, *et al.* Classification of different therapeutic responses of major depressive disorder with multivariate pattern analysis method based on structural MR scans. *PLoS One*. 2012; 7(7): e40968.
[5] Renier N, Adams EL, Kirst C, *et al.* Mapping of brain activity by automated volume analysis of immediate early genes. *Cell*. 2016; 165(7): 1789–802.
[6] Fischl B, Salat DH, Busa E, *et al.* Whole brain segmentation: automated labeling of neuroanatomical structures in the human brain. *Neuron*. 2002; 33(3): 341–55.
[7] Rajagopal S and Gopal B. "Effective and Accurate Diagnosis Using Brain Image Fusion. *Applications of Deep Learning and Big IoT on Personalized Healthcare Services*. IGI Global, Pennsylvania, USA, 2020. 197–217.
[8] Ashton EA, Parker KJ, Berg MJ, and Chen CW. A novel volumetric feature extraction technique with applications to MR images. *IEEE Transactions on Medical Imaging*. 1997; 16(4): 365–71.
[9] Blatter DD, Bigler ED, Gale SD, *et al.* Quantitative volumetric analysis of brain MR: normative database spanning 5 decades of life. *American Journal of Neuroradiology*. 1995; 16(2): 241–51.
[10] Ge Y, Grossman RI, Babb JS, Rabin ML, Mannon LJ, and Kolson DL. Age-related total gray matter and white matter changes in normal adult brain. Part I: volumetric MR imaging analysis. *American Journal of Neuroradiology*. 2002; 23(8): 1327–33.
[11] Khan H, Srivastav A, and Mishra AK. "Use of Classification Algorithms in Health Care." *Big Data Analytics and Intelligence: A Perspective for Health Care*. Emerald Publishing Limited, 2020. England.
[12] Shinohara RT, Oh J, Nair G, *et al.* Volumetric analysis from a harmonized multisite brain MRI study of a single subject with multiple sclerosis. *American Journal of Neuroradiology*. 2017; 38(8): 1501–9.
[13] McAlonan GM, Cheung V, Cheung C, *et al.* Mapping the brain in autism. A voxel-based MRI study of volumetric differences and intercorrelations in autism. *Brain*. 2005; 128(2): 268–76.

[14] Kahali S, Adhikari SK, and Sing JK. Convolution of 3D Gaussian surfaces for volumetric intensity inhomogeneity estimation and correction in 3D brain MR image data. *IET Computer Vision*. 2018; 12(3): 288–97.

[15] Sanford R, Cruz AL, Scott SC, *et al.* Regionally specific brain volumetric and cortical thickness changes in HIV-infected patients in the HAART era. *Journal of Acquired Immune Deficiency Syndromes*. 1999. 2017 Apr 15; 74(5): 563.

[16] Mitra S, Banerjee S, and Hayashi Y. Volumetric brain tumour detection from MRI using visual saliency. *PLoS One*. 2017; 12(11): e0187209.

[17] Sartori JM, Reckziegel R, Passos IC, *et al.* Volumetric brain magnetic resonance imaging predicts functioning in bipolar disorder: a machine learning approach. *Journal of Psychiatric Research*. 2018; 103: 237–43.

[18] Derakhshan M, Caramanos Z, Giacomini PS, *et al.* Evaluation of automated techniques for the quantification of grey matter atrophy in patients with multiple sclerosis. *NeuroImage*. 2010; 52(4): 1261–7.

[19] Wang N, Tong F, Tu Y, Chen H, Zhou Y, and Tang J. Extraction of cerebral hemorrhage and calculation of its volume on CT image using automatic segmentation algorithm. *Journal of Physics: Conference Series*. 2019; 1187 (4): 042088.

[20] Harris GJ, Rhew EH, Noga T, and Pearlson GD. User-friendly method for rapid brain and CSF volume calculation using transaxial MRI images. *Psychiatry Research: Neuroimaging*. 1991; 40(1): 61–8.

[21] Palanci Ö, Kalaycıoğlu A, Acer N, Eyüpoglu I, and Çakmak V. Volume calculation of brain structures in migraine disease by using MriStudio. *NeuroQuantology*. 2018; 16(10): 8–13.

[22] Karsch K, Grinstead B, He Q, and Duan Y. Web based brain volume calculation for magnetic resonance images. In *2008 30th Annual International Conference of the IEEE Engineering in Medicine and Biology Society* 2008 Aug 20 (pp. 1210–1213). IEEE.

[23] Roy S, and Bandyopadhyay SK. A review on volume calculation of brain abnormalities from MRI of brain using CAD system. *International Journal of Information and Communication Technology*. 2014; 4(4).

[24] Kamdar JH, Jeba Praba J, and George JJ. "Artificial Intelligence in Medical Diagnosis: Methods, Algorithms and Applications." *Machine Learning with Health Care Perspective*. Springer, Cham, 2020. 27–37.

[25] Guillemaud R, and Brady M. Estimating the bias field of MR images. *IEEE Transactions on Medical Imaging*. 1997; 16(3): 238–51.

[26] Gravel P, Beaudoin G, and De Guise JA. A method for modeling noise in medical images. *IEEE Transactions on Medical Imaging*. 2004; 23(10): 1221–32.

[27] Kang WX, Yang QQ, and Liang RP. The comparative research on image segmentation algorithms. In *2009 First International Workshop on Education Technology and Compute Science* 2009 Mar 7 (Vol. 2, pp. 703–707). IEEE.

[28] Pitas I, and Venetsanopoulos A. Nonlinear mean filters in image processing. *IEEE Transactions on Acoustics, Speech, and Signal Processing*. 1986; 34(3): 573–84.

[29] Andria G, Attivissimo F, Cavone G, Giaquinto N, and Lanzolla AM. Linear filtering of 2-D wavelet coefficients for denoising ultrasound medical images. *Measurement*. 2012; 45(7): 1792–800.

[30] Bezdek JC, Ehrlich R, and Full W. FCM: the fuzzy c-means clustering algorithm. *Computers & Geosciences*. 1984; 10(2–3): 191–203.

[31] Sikka K, Sinha N, Singh PK, and Mishra AK. A fully automated algorithm under modified FCM framework for improved brain MR image segmentation. *Magnetic Resonance Imaging*. 2009; 27(7): 994–1004.

[32] Dubey YK, and Mushrif MM. FCM clustering algorithms for segmentation of brain MR images. *Advances in Fuzzy Systems*. 2016; 2016.

[33] Yang MS, and Tsai HS. A Gaussian kernel-based fuzzy c-means algorithm with a spatial bias correction. *Pattern Recognition Letters*. 2008; 29(12): 1713–25.

[34] Khairandish MO, Sharma M, Jain V, Chatterjee JM, and Jhanjhi NZ. A hybrid CNN-SVM threshold segmentation approach for tumor detection and classification of MRI brain images. *IRBM*. 2021.

[35] Singla S. "Role of Ontology in Health Care." *Ontology-Based Information Retrieval for Healthcare Systems*. John Wiley & Sons, New York, 2020. 1–8.

[36] Trivedi SA, Patel M, and Patel S. Health care cube integrator for health care databases. In *Web Semantics* 2021 Jan 1 (pp. 129–151). Academic Press, New York.

Chapter 8

Healthcare monitoring through IoT: security challenges and privacy issues

S.O. Owoeye[1], A.S. Akinade[1], K.I. Adenuga[2] and F.O. Durodola[1]

Abstract

With a projected increase in world population to about 2.3 billion by the year 2050 and the corresponding challenges this increase would have on the provision of healthcare for the populace, there arises a need for a drastic improvement in the current state of the healthcare industry in order to overcome the challenges. A shift from the usual reactive approach to healthcare, in which health conditions would have deteriorated before treatment begins, to a more proactive methodology, which focuses on early diagnosis, identification and prevention of health conditions and wellness management is needed. This can be achieved by making health condition monitoring and well-being management a huge priority. Thus, considerations must be given to Internet of Things (IoT) technologies, as they can impact positively in designing, building and maintaining intelligent, interconnected and individually tailored healthcare services and products. With the aid of IoT technologies, individual physical conditions can be monitored continuously and remotely and actions are taken as necessary. Also, a proper record can be kept for individual health conditions and their progress levels monitored, thus, enabling healthcare providers to better evaluate and detect early symptoms of health problems. Although with the adoption of the IoT in healthcare, a lot of benefits are obtainable, there are still some concerns, including security, standards, scalability and privacy. These concerns seem to overwhelm the seemingly broad opportunities available in IoT and must be tackled to facilitate the application of IoT. This chapter aims to open up the techniques and advantages of IoT in personalized healthcare. It also opens up the challenges and possible solutions that can be adopted in tracking and monitoring health status.

Keywords: Diagnosis; Healthcare; Internet of Things; Security; Symptoms; Treatment; Privacy

[1]Department of Mechatronics Engineering, Federal University of Agriculture, Abeokuta, Nigeria
[2]Farnborough College of Technology, University Centre Farnborough, Farnborough, United Kingdom

8.1 Introduction

Over the past years, the usage of the Internet of Things (IoT) has continued to witness an exponentially increase in its application in the field of information and communication technology and is also tagged the future of the technical revolution. It is a popular belief that the total amount of devices currently connected over IoT (about 12 million devices) will witness an exponential increase in the nearest foreseeable future [1]. IoT is used to describe devices and equipment that are capable of communicating and interacting with the Internet through physical devices, sensors, microcontrollers and network connectivity to collect and exchange data. In a bid to ensure consistent real-time data collection, each device in the system is tagged with a unique identifier, which allows seamless communication between each machine, and the data collected from various devices in various locations around the globe are to be stored in cloud storage, thus making our systems more efficient and smarter. Smart objects, which are the fundamental foundation on which the process of refining the cyber-physical smart universal frameworks are implemented, were created by IoT. The IoT is targeted toward the interconnectivity of an unlimited amount of physical devices or equipment that would have various sensors and actuators embedded in them, being enabled by different access networks through the aid of technologies, including wireless sensor networks (WSN), radio-frequency identification (RFID), real-time and semantic web services [2]. It becomes obvious that the areas of application of IoT are limitless due to its ability to facilitate communication between different physical objects and allow an easy operation of devices over the Internet [3]. The role of sensors in detecting signals cannot be overlooked as their roles are found in numerous applications, including smart devices and systems, automotive systems, climate monitoring, industrial control, healthcare and so on.

The idea of the IoT took off recently and it is defined as the combination of devices that, by possessing network connectivity, can be monitored and controlled from a web platform and also provides real-time information for subsequent uses [4]. In another theory, the IoT is referred to as things, especially commonly used devices and equipment that are distinguishable, identifiable, addressable and controllable over the Internet by using either RFID, wireless LAN, wide area network or other methods [5]. Kevin Ashton first used the word IoT in the year 1998, when he observed that three models can be used to define the Internet, namely, the sensors-oriented semantics, Internet-oriented middleware and knowledge-oriented semantics. Although it is important to note that IoT is more versatile when working across these three models in its different application scenarios. The applications of IoT in the various facets of our lives include smart car parking systems, smart homes and cities, industrial automation, smart agriculture and healthcare processes. One major example of IoT application in healthcare is in real-time health status monitoring of patients [6]. In recent times, IoT has increased its usefulness in the health sector, through the use of sensors and microcontrollers in the collection and analysis of data and also transferring to the cloud for access by caregivers (doctors and nurses). When IoT features are integrated into equipment and devices used in the healthcare sector, the quality and value of care delivered to patients are greatly improved for different categories of patients with varying health conditions. Also, there is no restriction on the number of patients that can be monitored per time as patients' data are computerized, thus helping both patients and caregivers capture and monitor the data anytime from any location. These days, the majority of sensors used in the health sector are relatively small in size, making them wearable and closely connected to the patient for the doctor to monitor the patient's current condition irrespective of the time or location of the patient. This enables real-time diagnosis and prescriptions to be administered as and when necessary [1].

In many developing countries, their current infrastructure for supporting healthcare is not up to the minimum standard. To ensure that the general populace has unrestricted access to healthcare, the various wearable sensors can be equipped with communication capabilities with portable devices like smartphones and tablets, etc., which enables communication with the cloud and then the people can be provided with access to these devices to have access to real-time healthcare [7].

With the advent of IoT, medical records of patients are being transformed into data for smart healthcare delivery, thus making healthcare more technologically driven. IoT is capable of supporting applications that could potentially save lives in the healthcare sector by carrying out activities, including patient data and records collection from bedside and wearable devices, and real-time diagnosis of patients' conditions (see Figure 8.1).

Through the aid of IoT, caregivers or doctors do not need to pay a physical visit to the patient but can carry out monitoring, diagnosis and tracking of medical assets remotely. With the utilization of sensors and network connectivity, sensual

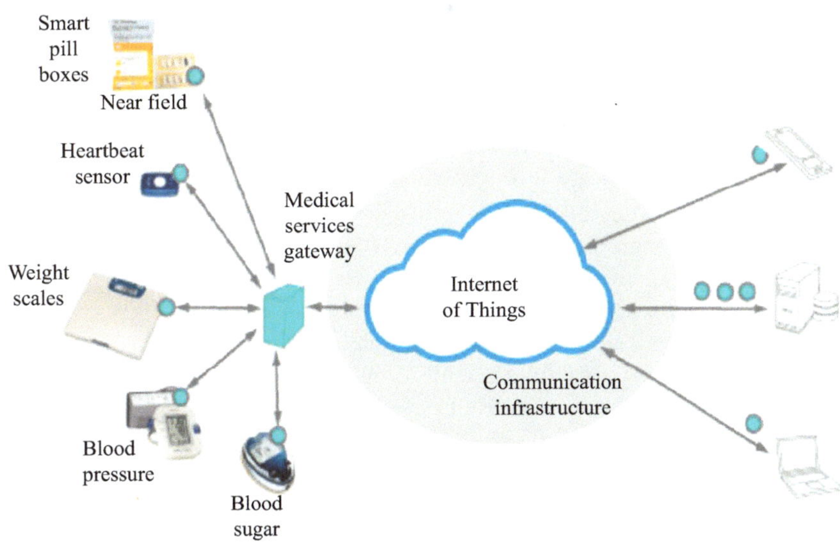

Figure 8.1 General IoT in healthcare [8]

information of patients can be retrieved from the necessary department, thus assisting the physician(s) to carry out more accurate diagnosis and treatment of patients, especially for those who are not physically available for on-the-spot operations.

In recent times, the number of people who are being diagnosed with chronic diseases is increasing daily, due to a lot of factors, including nutritional choices, physical inactivity, consumption of alcohol or toxic substances, environmental pollution, etc. According to the World Health Organization each year, an estimated 4.9 million people die as a result of the consumption of tobacco, 2.6 million deaths from overweight or obesity, 4.4 million from elevated cholesterol levels, 7.1 million deaths due to raised blood pressure (BP) and 1.9 million deaths due to lack of physical activity [9]. It is also forecasted that the number of deaths resulting from chronic diseases over the next 10 years will experience a drastic increase of 17%, resulting in about 64 million people deaths. Chronic diseases present a high level of variations in their symptoms as well as the way they evolve and techniques of treatment. Many of these diseases can lead to the death of the patient if not diagnosed and treated at their early stages. Some of the most chronic diseases that have possibilities of being treated include diabetes, BP and cardiac arrhythmia [9]. These chronic diseases often result in limitations to the physical mobility of patients that could also lead to socioeconomic and emotional related challenges [8]. In many cases, patients often find it hard to accept the reality of the long-term status of the disease, thus making adaptation difficult. This calls for constant monitoring by the doctor to constantly diagnose their health status and set treatment routines. In previous years, glucose and BP levels were measured by a physical examination in a specialized health facility, but with technological advancement, some sensors have been designed to do such measurements. Such sensors include a BP cuff, glucometer, heart rate monitor, etc.

One major concern in the evolution of humans is the health system with respect to technology development, the recent pandemic (COVID-19) shows a major example of how important standard healthcare is. In such situations, it is a better and safer approach to remotely monitor and diagnose patients, and healthcare systems equipped with the IoT could solve this challenge [10]. Remote patient monitoring enables the observational analysis of patients outside of the clinic environment and at their respective locations, thereby expanding access to healthcare services and reducing costs.

One common feature in the care delivered to critically ill patients is the repetitive measurement and diagnosis of patients body conditions, including heart rate and rhythm, respiratory rate, BP, blood oxygen saturation, blood sugar levels, etc. in instances where accurate and timely decision-making is required, electronic monitors play a crucial role in the collection and display of these data. Now, patients' data collection can be carried out using non-invasive sensors to record data that are routinely taken efficiently and detect conditions that could be life-threatening as quickly as possible [11].

The advent of IoT has allowed the number of people being cared for to increase and reduce overcrowding in healthcare facilities as the caregivers can attend to all patients placed under their care at any time and from any location without patients having to be physically present. For patients who require continuous monitoring, IoT would enable them only to visit the physician physically after the proactive intervention. Therefore, many of the challenges the healthcare system is currently facing will be addressed as a load of patients in the facilities would reduce, and also travel time of physicians will be reduced and also create more time to be devoted to the patients with critical needs.

It is important to also mention that current monitoring systems allow patients to be placed under continuous monitoring of vital signs, but this system allows sensors to be placed in such a way that restricts patients' mobility by being attached to bedside monitors. In this case, there might be a wireless connection between the sensors and the monitors [12], but it requires the patient to be within a specified distance from the monitor such that outside that range, data collection becomes impossible. Nowadays, an increase in the dominance of chronic diseases poses a major challenge on individuals and society at large. These diseases could require continuous and constant treatment in the hospital to keep important parameters under control. In a bid to improve the quality of life of such patients, employing automatic devices to monitor biological parameters in real-time takes it a step further. Thus, creating an integration of mobile communications into these wearable sensors has set the ball rolling for the migration of healthcare services from being clinic-centric to one that is more patient-centric [13].

During the recent decade, the demographic changes in developed countries resulting in a more elderly population and the increasing prevalence of chronic diseases have contributed to the need for constant monitoring of the state of patients' health. According to the World Health Organization [14], chronic diseases such as coronary heart disease, cancer, chronic obstructive pulmonary disease and diabetes mellitus type 2 constitute the leading cause of mortality in the world, representing about 60% of all deaths. Chronic diseases are primarily attributable to heart failure, currently the main cause of death in most Western countries. The 2016 report of the American Heart Association on the Heart Disease and Stroke Statistics showed that 15.5 million people in the USA suffer from cardiovascular disease, this prevalence increasing with age for both women and men [15]. Chronic diseases also have a negative impact on the quality of people's life. Patients suffering from these pathologies must, often, carry out a monitoring of physiological parameters such as heart rate and BP as well as take control of the main risk factors that can aggravate their state of health. In less dangerous cases, it is convenient to monitor patients outside the hospital. On the one hand, such patients can face their illness in a family context that helps to speed up their recovery time. On the other, this strategy implies a considerable saving of resources, allowing social health facilities and personnel to be assigned to patients with more severe diseases.

8.2 IoT applications in personalized healthcare

8.2.1 In-clinic care

This application involves utilizing an IoT-controlled sensor to continuously monitor the patient, for whom close attention is a necessity due to their physiological conditions. The condition of the patient is monitored with the aid of these sensors that use gateways to collect the needed physiological data and then stored in cloud storage for unrestricted access by caregivers and doctors who might require the data for further diagnosis as shown in Figure 8.2, thereby reducing the cost of healthcare for the patient and improving quality of care provided [16].

8.2.2 Remote monitoring

Generally, IoT applied to remote health monitoring systems operates by keeping a real-time track of crucial signs displayed by patients and providing a quick and proactive response in the advent of any problem with a patient's health. This device, when connected to the patient as shown in Figure 8.3, important information about patients' vital signs are transmitted from the patient's location to the hospital via a transmitter that establishes a connection over a telecom network [16].

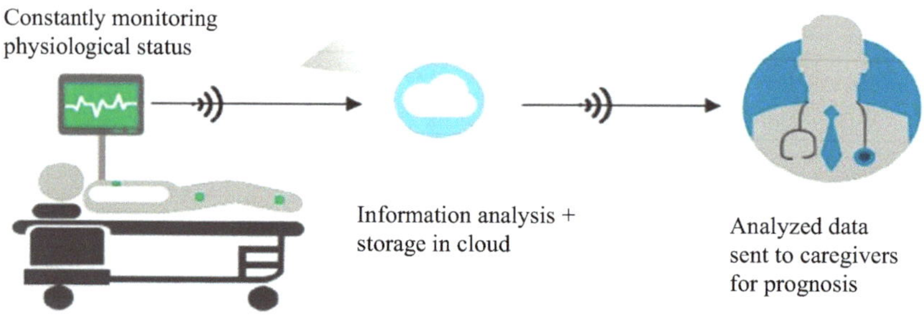

Figure 8.2 Clinical care system that constantly monitors the physiological status [17]

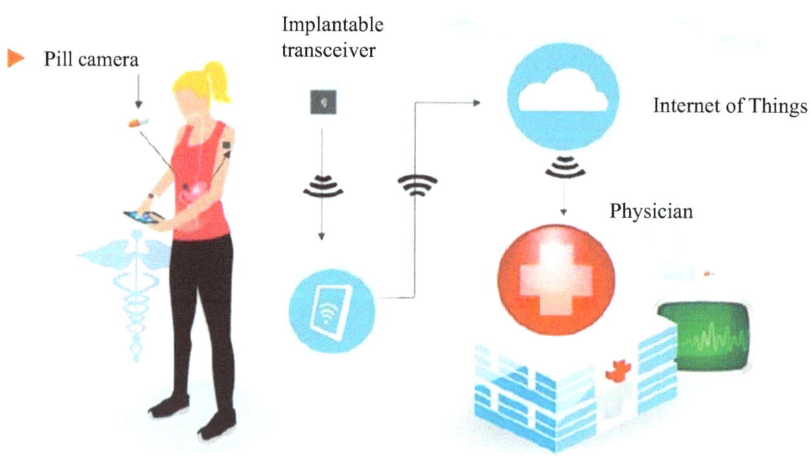

Figure 8.3 Remote health monitoring system [16]

In the hospital, there is a remote monitoring system that receives the data that has been transmitted and sends it securely to the caregivers.

8.2.3 Blood pressure monitoring

One important piece of physiological data that could be received from the human body is the BP and the most commonly used monitors are quite safe and easy to use [17]. With technological advancement in healthcare, the simple and electronic BP monitor is connected with an IoT sensor to enable real-time data collection and transmission of BP levels to the necessary quarters.

8.2.4 Rehabilitation system

A rehabilitation system is capable of restoring the lost functional abilities of people who are experiencing some form of disabilities, thereby improving the quality of their lives. It becomes very essential in mitigating challenges that are associated with the elderly ones, especially in cases of shortage of health personnel [10,17]. A convenient interaction and allocation of medical resources in respect to patient necessities can be done by an ontology-based automating designing method connected with an IoT-based smart rehabilitation system [18].

8.2.5 Oxygen saturation monitoring

To carry out continuous monitoring of a patient's blood oxygen saturation, in a non-invasive manner, a pulse-oximeter is used [17]. With the advancement in the field of communication technology, a lot of sensors used in the medical field are beginning to have low-power consumption and low-power loss, thereby making them very dominants. Pulse oximeters are employed for continuous monitoring in the medical field to keep track of the blood oxygen level and heart rate of patients. An IoT sensor, being attached to the body of the patient, will help to keep continuous track of these data in real-time [19].

8.2.6 Wheelchair management

When people suffer from a physical illness and find it difficult or unable to walk, the wheelchair becomes a saving grace. A sensor that senses humans could be connected over the Internet that detects when the human is falling off the wheelchair and can be monitored in real-time from the hospital. An acceleration sensor could be attached to the wheelchair to detect the falling of the wheelchair [20].

8.2.7 Healthcare solutions using smartphones

Healthcare professionals obtain numerous benefits from healthcare apps (Table 8.1) that provide on-the-go access to health records of patients, information about location and time of events or emergencies of patients, means of communication between doctors and patients and efficient and timely decision-making [21]. By using smartphone apps, in conjunction with sensors, the location and access to healthcare services have improved, thereby resulting in better results on patients' health conditions.

Table 8.1 General healthcare apps for smartphones [17]

Sl. No.	Healthcare app	Description
1	Calorie counter	Keeping track of the food that has been consumed and calculates the fat, weight as well as cholesterol present in the body
2	Heart rate monitor	It continuously monitors the heartbeat and collects relevant real-time information
3	Blood pressure monitor	It collects the blood pressure level of the patient, analyzes and records the data
4	Body temperature	Keeping track of the body temperature and alerting when the body temperature increased beyond set limits
5	Pedometer	It is used in recording the number of steps that have been walked and gives information about how many calories have been burned per unit of time
6	Water your body	The app is used to serve as a reminder to drink water every hour and also in tracking the human body water drinking habits
7	OnTrack Diabetes	It is used in the monitoring of the blood glucose level and administering proper medication in treating diabetes
8	Skin vision	It keeps on tracking the condition of the skin, thereby enabling us to identify early any skin disorder that occurs
9	Eye Care	It monitors the eyes vision and then is analyzed and tested
10	Asthma trackers and log	It monitors real-time information of the patients' asthma
11	CardioMobile	It monitors cardiac rehabilitation that is done remotely on a real-time basis and collects the data
12	Pill reminder	It serves as a reminder for the patient on the use of their medication at the appropriate time
13	Fall detector	This continuously monitors the rate of human activity and alerts in case there are issues

8.3 Challenges of IoT in personalized healthcare

The IoT exceeds a conventional computer-based model but is more of an interconnected model of distributed devices. Modern applications in IoT create an avenue for IoT services to integrate and use data from various devices. IoT builds a complex system with basic features for detecting the status of the environment, recording physiological data of humans, operational data of machines, detecting and differentiating between humans, animals, events and other nonliving objects in the environment, with additional capabilities of communicating with other devices [22]. In addition, the system can convert these data into instructions that drive automation and provide some form of feedback to the system via the specified communication networks to create actuation and control for other processes. Clearly, in this complex, interconnected and heterogeneous model, there is bound to be a lot of challenges associated with IoT. These challenges include, but are not limited to, the following:

1. Security and privacy: There could be a lot of situations that the devices connected in the IoT, such as smartphones, sensors, etc., could be exposed to risk

from hackers or hacking [1]. Thus, encryption must be carried out in instances when data are required to be exchanged between devices.

2. Integration: Another challenge faced by IoT in the healthcare sector is the integration of diverse protocols and different devices within the framework of the network. The numerous devices all collect data and transmit over different communication protocols in the same network, thereby making it complicated [23].
3. Technology adoption: In many cases, it is not enough to introduce a new technology that could help both patients and doctors, but more importantly its easy acceptance, adoption and usage are vital, which would help monetization easy in the healthcare system [24].

8.4 Security of IoT in personalized healthcare

With the increasing number of devices connected over communication networks in IoT, there is an increasing risk in their security as new challenges are posed. When a device is capable of Internet connection, there is a transfer of security risks faced by modern computing devices. Thus, there are basic security requirements that should be considered. These requirements include authorization, authentication, confidentiality, trust and data security. In other words, there should be a secure connection between devices over their dedicated networks, which has strict control and restricted access to only authorized users. The data that are of concern have to possess some level of security in collection, analysis, storage and transmission. Notwithstanding the risks associated with human–machine communications, there are also security risks in machine–machine communications. For instance, when there needs to be a form of access from human users to the devices, some security protocol has to be put in place. These protocols ensure that these devices are giving access to authorized personnel only and are not revealing private and confidential information to unauthorized users or for miscellaneous use.

8.4.1 The inherited security challenges in the IoT

In other terms, IoT can be referred to as Internet 2.0 or the future Internet. IoT is not a standalone form of communication or networks running differently or simultaneously with the Internet. Rather, it is an expansion of the Internet. This means that IoT inherits some of the security challenges of the Internet while also posing some new ones.

8.4.1.1 End-to-end security

As defined by Cisco, an end-to-end security system is a non-negotiable absolute prerequisite needed to achieve a secure communication process [25]. It entails keeping a layer of protection over the data transmitted from one end of the communication to the other without creating a chance of being read, eavesdropped on, tampered with or intercepted by unauthorized users. End-to-end security has been a major challenge for many devices in IoT and their applications. With the heterogeneous architecture and the number of devices that all are connected for information sharing and collaboration, there is a serious security challenge posed to end-to-end security. It becomes a lot more difficult to create secure communication when the devices possess varying attributes and employ different communication protocols (e.g., 802.11 vs. 802.15.4).

Again, most of the devices in the IoT have unequal capabilities. The majority of computers, smartphones and various types of computerized devices establish a connection with the Internet via HTTP, SMTP to carry out a lot of their actions, thereby using TLS and IPsec protocols for dynamic negotiation of session keys, and creating a level of security. But many other devices in the IoT cannot support these protocols as a result of their limitations in computing and power capacity. Also, embedded devices in the IoT may not have to use HTTP or IP for communicating, thus having limited connectivity.

8.4.1.2 Data security

Data security covers the protocols in place for protecting data during storage and communication. As defined by [26], data security involves putting measures in place to prevent unauthorized access to data by destructive bodies. In other terms, is referred to as information security, data security is very essential to the security of IoT and closely linked to its safety. Conventionally, the effect of breaches in the security of data has been confined within the scope of hacks of user personal information or uncensored access to critical information, e.g., financial information. But in recent times, these breaches could threaten the safety of humans. A major example is when unauthorized access to information transmitted from and to a self-driving car or a heart pacemaker could lead to a critical threat to the life of the user. In another view, when a breach occurs in an IoT-enabled forest fire detection system, the resulting event would be catastrophic.

8.4.1.3 Identity and access management

Cases of identity theft, impersonation, access credentials forgery, masquerading are examples of types of security attacks that face identity protection in IoT. The mechanism by which identification, representation, searching and accessing of things in IoT remain a mystery, thus, leaves devices vulnerable to attacks on their identity. There have been instances where a device in the IoT utilizes fake identities to gain access to services and information provided by another IoT device, a process referred to as a masquerade attack. In many cases, devices have to employ mechanisms with stricter and secure algorithms to be able to detect unauthorized access being sought by devices, thereby detecting imposters on short notice. Attacks that are targeted toward IoT include Spoofing, Masquerade, MiM and Smurf attacks.

8.4.1.4 Compliance

When preserving security in IoT systems, ensuring strict compliance with laid down government laws and regulations guiding the industry is an important factor to note. Devices that are interconnected in the IoT must ensure that they adhere to the necessary privacy policies and protection laws since IoT revolves around communication done autonomously by devices. This emphasizes the need to ensure adequate privacy and security.

8.4.1.5 Physical and DoS security risks

In conventional network devices, there are certain protection measures put in place to combat physical attacks or malicious access, for instance, securely storing routers in cabinets. Also, in IoT, the interconnected devices would need to have some form of protection mechanisms against attacks. Thus, implementing the physical security of devices is a vital consideration in IoT. In addition, denial of service (DoS) attacks are common in IoT. In its full activity, a typical DoS attack prevents the authorized users from getting access to the services of a server by bombarding the server with illegitimate service requests in a bid to fully exhaust the computational power of such server [27]. This possibility of experiencing DoS attacks also extends to WSNs.

Furthermore, the IoT, being heterogeneous in model and employing complex communications protocols, has an increased vulnerability to a distributed denial of service (DDoS) attack. The DDoS is a form of attack formulated by several agents in the network and initiated from different locations [28]. This makes such disruptive attacks, DoS and DDoS attacks a very great risk to the IoT as a lot of the devices have limited power, memory and processing abilities and can easily get all their available resources exhausted by a well-targeted attack [29].

In an attempt to counter DoS attacks, some protocols required the address of an initiating host to be verified before requests are responded to. Such protocols include DTLS, IKEv2, HIP and Diet HIP [29]. Other methods for creating resistance to DoS attacks include employing clustering techniques to detect DoS attacks in WSNs [30]. Other solutions revolved around designing intrusion detection systems, which could work specifically for WSNs [31].

8.4.2 IoT new security challenges

In IoT, fundamental issues of security, including authorization, authentication, integrity, trust and confidentiality are necessary to be tackled. But this security is often a challenge due to the unavailability of security protocols and infrastructure. This creates a lot of new security issues that are often more severe than the existing security challenges in the system.

The new security issues stem from the structure of IoT that is dynamic, the multiple forms of communication that are embedded and the properties of the devices that tend to make them low-cost. This reveals that these security challenges cannot be tackled using the existing security solutions since the architecture of modern IoT varies from that of the conventional Internet. With the continuous evolution of IoT and its ever-increasing complexity, there is also an increase in the complexity of these security challenges which is linked to two basic factors: low cost and heterogeneity.

With low cost, there is an increasing trend for large-scale deployment of IoT devices that have several constraints in their resources with devices having low-power capabilities, limited memory resources and inadequate computational abilities [32]. For instance, in a bid to implement some of the conventional Internet security techniques, such as public key infrastructure (PKI) and certificate authority (CA), the cost of IoT devices increases. When considering heterogeneity, diverse devices and communication protocols in IoT raise the amount and degree of complexity of security challenges. For instance, when WSNs are integrated into the Internet, newer security issues are created from the connection of the sensor node to the Internet device. In a more practical implementation of using communication devices having low power, such as ZigBee or IEEE 802.11ah, there is a need to create a link for secured communication with a high-power device like a smartphone and this requires employing necessary cryptographic techniques without utilizing a lot of energy and bandwidth. This becomes an additional feature to the basic security protocols already employed in establishing a secured connection to the Internet.

8.4.3 IoT security requirements

Authorization: In many smart IoT devices, conventional authorization techniques are used to satisfy this requirement. An administrator could be assigned to block unauthorized access in low-power devices such as ZigBee IP. This prevents these unauthorized requests from being routed to IoT devices.

Authentication: Authentication is a process that involves the verification of the identity of someone requesting access. This is mostly done by employing a username and password-based authentication protocol. However, this system has been proven not to have enough security as passwords usually require them to be changed frequently and also they cannot be used without keeping close attention to the device on which they are being used. Now, the Secure Sockets Layer protocol is commonly being used for authentication by websites. The process of authentication also involves requesting both senders and receivers to verify the origin of the information they are exchanging. This requirement is quite complex to satisfy as the things in the IoT may not have a dedicated IP address.

Integrity and freshness: Message integrity tries to ensure that messages have not been altered in any way. This is a very important requirement because IoT is all about information being transmitted to perform a particular operation. Freshness helps to ensure that only fresh messages are transmitted and not older messages being replayed.

Confidentiality: IoT must ensure that the personal and sensitive information of users is protected from unauthorized access by malicious entities.

Resilience to attacks: An IoT system must have the self-recovery capability in the advent of a crash. For instance, a server that works in an environment with multiple users must have enough intelligence and strength to protect itself from entities who might try to intrude or eavesdrop. In such a scenario, when it goes down, it would perform a self-recovery without users being conscious of its downtime conditions.

8.5 Privacy

IoT devices create links with insignificant strength that could be exploited by malicious entities and lead to events of a high volume of surveillance, tracing, tracking and monitoring of the activities and movements of users. This is due to the nature of the devices being distributed in large volumes [33]. Nowadays, several privacy threats are being introduced as a result of the proliferation of mobile devices, GPS devices and other modern technologies in humans. For example, the study in [34] revealed that the home location of a driver could be deciphered from the GPS information retrieved from his vehicle. Further revelation explains that the outer of an individual could be reconstructed so as to cater for the provision of a detailed profile of his movement that could enable interference. Another example is the indication of illness by recurring visits to a medical clinic, and consistent visits to activist organizations could signal political ideas [35]. This marks an indication that privacy incidents could have reasons to be on the increase as IoT continually finds expression in our everyday lives. Thus, privacy is fast becoming one of the major concerns as IoT undergoes increasing development.

In IoT, privacy is no longer being defined by anonymity [28]. Cases of profiling and mining of data in an IoT situation could lead to danger to the users as a result of data being collected and stored automatically, and the easy means of sharing and analyzing personal data. One interesting potential carried by IoT is the capability for devices to autonomously communicate with their environments by sensing and observations. This causes attackers to configure devices with an ability to autonomously carry out information retrieval about the environment of the system or the user in view [36]. The most pressing concern with devices in IoT is their autonomous exchanging of information between themselves. Another source of risk and vulnerability to user privacy are devices that are capable of logging data about their environment. This risk becomes a reality, especially the leakage of information when the devices begin to share data logs amongst themselves [37].

The enormous volume of data, belonging to a wide range of owners, including users, organizations and the general public, has been made available by the IoT [38], which could be a pointer to particular interests, destinations and intentions [39]. Although the opportunities provided are great, in terms of improving the quality of services, this must be considered also but not to jettison privacy preference. Users must have a level of trust in the services they use when putting regards to their privacy. Trust becomes a fundamental factor for users to consider while adopting new technology [40]. This is reflected in the reluctance of users to employ new technologies if there is not enough trust developed as regards their privacy, security and safety, which is more pronounced in the IoT [41,42].

A varying collection of data about users is retrieved by sensors, which then undergoes aggregation, analysis, processing, fusing and mining to allow the extraction of vital information for assistance in intelligent operations [43]. In 2006, Barnes [44] proposed a privacy paradox in which it stated that "adults are more worried about their privacy intrusion, while on the other hand teens tend to release information freely." In the year 2010, Mark Zuckerberg, the Facebook founder, justified the change in the default privacy setting by saying that "privacy is no longer a social norm," though this has been subjected to lengthy debates by academics.

Recently, in the report released by the Oxford Internet Institute, a new privacy paradox was proposed by [45] in which it was argued that younger people have a higher tendency to take definite actions to protect their privacy than older people. A more recent study carried out by Pew Research Center [46] revealed that 86% of the users of Internet services would have at a point taken deliberate actions to remove or cover their online tracks. Some of the actions taken include cookies clearing, employing pseudo-names, encryption of emails and hiding their IP addresses using virtual networks.

In distributed systems, one way of ensuring that trust is developed is by allowing users have more control over how their personal information is collected [35]. In previous projects, like the Platform for Privacy Preferences Project (P3P), users were given controlling access when the web browsers are being used. The P3P protocol, which was initiated by the World Wide Web Consortium in 2002, ensures that websites openly state their intention in the usage of information that is collected via their web browsers [47]. This is as a result of trying to translate website privacy policies into some form of information that could be read by the machine to enhance transparency and give users the opportunity to choose [48]. Although the project had to end prematurely, it had experienced some level of implementation [35].

8.5.1 Consent

As mentioned in the previous section, it is vital to create a balance between service optimization and personalization with privacy preference. One technique that could be adopted to attain this balance is to create an environment where users give consent for the collection, storage and sharing of data. But this creates another set of challenges. Traditionally, consent has been based on a transparent system in which the service provider explicitly states the kind, amount and use of the data being collected. Although there have been a lot of deliberations on the concept of having to present a user with numerous pages of details, various challenges are associated with the non-provision of an adequate interface on web pages to either offer or retract consent. These challenges do not only come to play in public places but also occur at homes that have embedded systems running IoT. An example is sensitive data retrieved from the pressure sensors, IR sensors, and RFID systems form enough source of information for monitoring and understanding the activities of humans in a home. A practical example is personal data that are retrieved from an IoT-enabled fridge that could be employed to predict the eating habits and the health conditions of the user, which might have an effect on the insurance policy with an insurance firm.

Privacy concerns related to the IoT also have effects in the industrial setting. With the enormous complexity of the industrial IoT than traditional ICT systems, there exists the potential for large-scale attacks as a result of its large attack surface with numerous potential attackers [49]. Thus, there needs to be a formulation of privacy requirements to prevent danger [50]. Looking beyond the risk of sensitive information of employees or clients being violated, the tendency to lose intellectual properties creates an avenue for competitors to reproduce the knowledge and the products of such an organization, leading to a potential loss of competitive advantage [49]. Although cases of industrial espionage could lead to theft of intellectual properties, compromising privacy could result in this intellectual capital leakage. For instance, if an event of data involving industrial orders is compromised, it could help the competitor in predicting the current state of goods and materials, and the futuristic supplies and innovations that are being developed. In another vein, when data protection is compromised, the financial performance and strength, together with the intellectual capacity of the industry, could be revealed, which could lead to severe financial implications in the long run.

8.6 Conclusion and future scope

Despite the fact that security and privacy issues have become key issues in our present world, the importance of incorporating IoT into our healthcare system cannot be overemphasized, as this will make healthcare accessible to more citizens especially those residing in the rural areas of the developing countries. Though there is a need to always create layers of security whenever IoT is being incorporated into our healthcare system in order not to compromise the patient's records.

References

[1] K. R. Darshan and K. R. Anandakumar, "A Comprehensive Review on Usage of Internet of Things (IoT) in Healthcare System," in *International Conference on Emerging Research in Electronics, Computer Science and Technology (ICERECT)*, Mandya, India, 2015.

[2] P. Gope and T. Hwang, "BSN-Care: A Secure IoT-Based Modern Healthcare System Using Body Sensor Network," *IEEE Sensors Journal*, vol. 16, no. 5, pp. 1368–1376, 2016.

[3] R. K. Kodali, G. Swamy and B. Lakshmi, "An Implementation of IoT for Healthcare," in *IEEE Recent Advances in Intelligent Computational Systems (RAICS)*, Trivandrum, India, 2015.

[4] J. Gómez, J. F. Huete, O. Hoyos, L. Perez and D. Grigori, "Interaction System Based on Internet of Things as Support for Education," *Procedia Computer Science*, vol. 21, pp. 132–139, 2013.

[5] N. I. Council, "Disruptive Technologies Global Trends 2025. Six Technologies With Potential Impacts on the US Interests Out to 2025," 2008.

[6] K. K. Raghavendra, P. S. Sharanya and P. Shaila, "An IoT Based Smart Healthcare System Using Raspberry Pi," *International Journal of Research and Scientific Innovation (IJRSI)*, vol. 5, no. 6, 2018.

[7] S. K. Dhar, S. S. Bhunia and N. Mukherjee, "Interference Aware Scheduling of Sensors in IoT Enabled Health-Care Monitoring System," in *4th International Conference of Emerging Applications of Information Technology*, Kolkata, India, 2014.

[8] J. Gomez, B. Oviedo and E. Zhumab, "Patient Monitoring System Based on Internet of Things," *Procedia Computer Science*, vol. 83, pp. 90–97, 2016.

[9] M. Swan, "Sensor Mania! The Internet of Things, Wearable Computing, Objective Metrics, and the Quantified Self," *Journal of Sensor and Actuator Networks*, vol. 1, no. 3, pp. 217–253, 2012.

[10] V. Prajoona, A. Tariq and H. Ali, "IoT Based Health Monitoring System," *Journal of Critical Reviews*, vol. 7, no. 4, pp. 739–743, 2020.

[11] R. M. Gardner and M. Shabot, "Patient-Monitoring Systems," in *Decision Support Systems in Critical Care*, Boston, Springer-Verlag, 1994.

[12] V. Shnayder, B. Chen, K. Lorincz, T. R. F. Fulford-Jones and M. Welsh, "Sensor Networks for Medical Care," in *3rd International Conference on Embedded Networked Sensor Systems*, New York, USA, 2005.

[13] S. Naddeo, L. Verde, M. Forastiere, G. De Pietro and G. Sannino, "A Real-Time m-Health Monitoring System: An Integrated Solution Combining the Use of Several Wearable Sensors and Mobile Devices," 2017.

[14] World Health Organization, "Chronic Diseases and Health Promotion," 2016.

[15] N. Townsend, L. Wilson, P. Bhatnagar, K. Wickramasinghe, M. Rayner and M. Nichols, "Cardiovascular Disease in Europe: Epidemiological Update 2016," *European Heart Journal*, p. 334, 2016.

[16] D. Niewolny, "How the Internet of Things Is Revolutionizing Healthcare, Freescale Semiconductors," 2013.

[17] S. M. R. Islam, D. Kwak, M. H. Kabir, M. Hossain and K. S. Kwak, "The Internet of Things for Health Care: A Comprehensive Survey," *IEEE Access*, vol. 3, pp. 678–708, 2015.

[18] Y. J. Fan, Y. H. Yin, L. Da Xu, Y. Zeng and F. Wu, "IoT-Based Smart Rehabilitation System," *IEEE Transactions on Industrial Informatics*, vol. 10, no. 2, pp. 1568–1577, 2014.

[19] C. Rotariu and V. Manta, "Wireless System for Remote Monitoring of Oxygen Saturation and Heart Rate," in *Federated Conference on Computer Science and Information Systems (FedCSIS)*, Wroclaw, Poland, 2012.

[20] L. Yang, Y. Ge, W. Li, W. Rao and W. Shen, "A Home Mobile Healthcare System for Wheelchair Users," in *IEEE International Conference on Computer Supported Cooperative Work in Design (CSCWD)*, Hsinchu, China, 2014.

[21] C. Lee, "MS Mobile Devices and Apps for Health Care Professionals: Uses and Benefits," 2014.

[22] M. Elkhodr, S. Shahrestani and H. Cheung, "A Semantic Obfuscation Technique for the Internet of Things," in *IEEE International Conference on Communications (ICC)*, Sydney, Australia, 2014.

[23] A. Darwish and A. E. Hassanien, "Wearable and Implantable Wireless Sensor Network Solutions for Healthcare Monitoring," *Sensors*, vol. 12, pp. 12375–12376, 2012.

[24] H. Alemdar and C. Ersoy, "Wireless Sensor Networks for Healthcare: A Survey," *Computer Networks*, vol. 54, pp. 2688–2710, 2010.

[25] M. H. Behringer, "End-to-End Security," *The Internet Protocol Journal*, vol. 12, p. 20, 2009.

[26] G. Summers, "Data and Databases," in *Developing Databases With Access*, Nelson Australia Pry Limited, 2004, pp. 4–5.

[27] J. Mirkovic and P. Reiher, "A Taxonomy of DDoS Attack and DDoS Defence Mechanisms," *ACM SIGCOMM Computer Communication Review*, vol. 34, pp. 39–53, 2004.

[28] S. Misra, P. V. Krishna, H. Agarwal, A. Saxena and M. S. Obaidat, "A Learning Automata-Based Solution for Preventing Distributed Denial of Service in the Internet of Things," in *2011 International Conference on and 4th International Conference on Cyber, Physical and Social Computing*, 2011.

[29] T. Heer, O. Garcia-Morchon, R. Hummen, S. L. Keoh, S. S. Kumar and K. Wehrle, "Security Challenges in the IP-Based Internet of Things," *Wireless Personal Communications*, vol. 61, pp. 527–542, 2011.

[30] D. Mansouri, L. Mokdad, J. Ben-Othman and M. Ioualalen, "Detecting DoS Attacks in WSN Based on Clustering Technique," in *Wireless Communications and Networking Conference (WCNC)*, 2013.

[31] D. Martynov, J. Roman, S. Vaidya and H. Fu, "Design and Implementation of an Intrusion Detection System for Wireless Sensor Networks," in *IEEE International Conference on Electro/Information Technology*, 2007.

[32] R. Roman, P. Najera and J. Lopez, "Securing the Internet of Things," *Computer*, vol. 44, pp. 51–58, 2011.

[33] M. Elkhodr, S. Shahrestani and H. Cheung, "The Internet of Things: Vision & Challenges," in *IEEE Tencon Spring 2013*, Sydney, Australia, 2013.

[34] B. Hoh, M. Gruteser, H. Xiong and A. Alrabady, "Enhancing Security and Privacy in Traffic Monitoring," *IEEE Pervasive Computing*, vol. 5, pp. 38–46, 2006.

[35] P. Beatty, I. Reay, S. Dick and J. Miller, "P3P Adoption on e-Commerce Web Sites: A Survey and Analysis," *IEEE Internet Computing*, vol. 11, no. 2, pp. 65–71, 2007.

[36] S. Sicari, R. Alessandra, A. G. Luigi and C.-P. Alberto, "Security, Privacy and Trust in the Internet of Things: The Road Ahead," *Computer Networks*, vol. 76, pp. 146–164, 2015.

[37] J. H. Ziegeldorf, O. G. M. Morchon and K. Wehrle, "Privacy in the Internet of Things: Threats and Challenges," *Security and Communication Networks*, vol. 7, no. 12, pp. 2728–2742, 2014.

[38] D. Gessner, A. Oliveira, A. S. Segura and A. Serbanati, "Trustworthy Infrastructure Services for a Secure and Privacy-Respecting Internet of Things," in *IEEE 11th International Conference on Trust, Security and Privacy in Computing and Communications (TrustCom)*, Liverpool, England, 2012.

[39] R. Roman, P. Najera and J. Lopez, "Securing the Internet of Things (IoT)," *IEEE Computer*, vol. 44, pp. 51–58, 2011.

[40] Z. Yan, P. Zhang and A. V. Vasilakos, "A Survey on Trust Management for Internet of Things," *Journal of Network and Computer Applications*, vol. 42, pp. 120–134, 2014.

[41] M. Taddeo and L. Floridi, "The Case for E-Trust," *Ethics and Information Technology*, vol. 13, pp. 1–3, 2011.
[42] I. W. Foundation, "Maximize Insight, Ensure Trust and Improve IT Economics – United States," 2015.
[43] Z. Yan and S. Holtmanns, "Trust Modeling and Management: From Social Trust to Digital Trust," in *Computer Security, Privacy and Politics: Current Issues, Challenges and Solutions*, Hershey, PA, IGI Global, 2008.
[44] S. B. Barnes, "A Privacy Paradox: Social Networking in the United States," *First Monday*, vol. 11, no. 9, 2006.
[45] G. Blank, G. Bolsover and E. Dubois, "A New Privacy Paradox: Young People and Privacy on Social Network Sites," in *American Sociological Association Annual Meeting*, San Francisco, CA, 2014.
[46] L. Rainie, S. Kiesler, R. Kang, *et al.*, *Anonymity, Privacy, and Security Online*, Pew Research Center, Washington, DC, 2013.
[47] L. F. Cranor, S. Egelman, S. Sheng, A. M. McDonald and A. Chowdhury, "P3P Deployment on Websites," *Electronic Commerce Research and Applications*, vol. 7, no. 3, pp. 274–293, 2008.
[48] A. Jøsang, L. Fritsch and T. Mahler, "Privacy Policy Referencing," in *International Conference on Trust, Privacy and Security in Digital Business*, Bilbao, Spain, 2010.
[49] A.-R. Sadeghi, C. Wachsmann and M. Waidner, "Security and Privacy Challenges in Industrial Internet of Things," in *52nd ACM/EDAC/IEEE Design Automation Conference*, San Francisco, CA, 2015.
[50] L. Da Xu, W. He and S. Li, "Internet of Things in Industries: A Survey," *IEEE Transactions on Industrial Informatics*, vol. 10, no. 4, pp. 2233–2243, 2014.

Chapter 9
E-health natural language processing

Saman Hina[1], *Raheela Asif*[2] *and Pardeep Kumar*[3]

Abstract

In health-care domain, electronic health-care records (EHR) comprise different types of information that are critical for analysis. This analysis can be used for advance research in health-care domain or for decision-making process for several important aspects. Text is one of the most significant forms that exist in EHRs and contain voluminous facts that need to be analyzed and used in advanced applications. Analysis of this text is associated with one of the important categories of Artificial Intelligence that is "natural language processing—NLP." NLP researchers working using data extracted from EHRs have contributed remarkable research in this field. For a better understanding of this chapter, authors have classified and named this type of research as "E-health NLP."

E-health NLP applications range from keeping privacy of an individual in a health-care system to extract important findings from unstructured patient's data. Patient's information lies in structured (data entry forms) and unstructured format (e.g. discharge summaries, consultation notes, remarks in laboratory reports). In this chapter, unstructured datasets available for research and development in E-health NLP will be discussed. In addition to the details related to unstructured datasets, challenges to tackle this unstructured information and methods and applications that have been developed for the identification and classification of important information from unstructured medical narratives will be elaborated. Finally, this chapter will be summarized using key points and providing insights of future work in the same domain.

Keywords: Medical health analysis; Unstructured text; Information extraction; IoT; Semantics

[1]Department of Computer Science & Information Technology, NED University of Engineering & Technology, Karachi, Pakistan
[2]Department of Software Engineering, NED University of Engineering & Technology, Karachi, Pakistan
[3]Department of Software Engineering, Quaid-e-Awam University of Engineering, Science & Technology, Nawabshah, Pakistan

9.1 Unstructured datasets for E-health NLP research

Unstructured text in health-care domain can be extracted in the form of discharge summaries, consultation notes, remarks on laboratory reports, etc. Unstructured text is mostly narratives written by a clinician or staff as shown in Figure 9.1. These medical narratives need to be analyzed and consist of important medical concepts that can also be helpful in the diagnosis or prediction of critical diseases [1]. The other work includes the identification and classification of medical concepts in unstructured datasets [2], anonymization of medical narratives to use these datasets ethically for research [3] because of the concerns of individuals regarding data privacy [4] and identification of relation between the medical concepts [5]. The size of these unstructured datasets is growing rapidly and variation in the writing styles of the text create challenges for NLP researchers to work on these datasets.

One of the major challenges to work on unstructured medical narratives is to acquire appropriate dataset by fulfilling all the legal regulations devised by "The Health Insurance Portability and Accountability Act (HIPPA)" [6] for such sensitive datasets. According to HIPPA, if the 18 identifiers (shown in Figure 9.2) are associated with any individual's health information then will be considered "protected health information—PHIs" and must be anonymized/de-identified/removed from the dataset for any research purposes. These HIPPA identifiers are important to be de-identified specially when used with health-care datasets.

De-identified research datasets to work in health-care domain are distributed as part of global NLP challenge "n2c2: National NLP Clinical Challenges,*" previously distributed through "i2b2: Informatics for Integrating Biology and the Bedside." Organizers of these NLP challenges collect data from reliable health-care providers and carefully devise research questions to be solved by research community. These research investigations are in major numbers till date; some of the investigations are listed as follows:

PRESENT ILLNESS

Mrs. ABC, an 80-year-old lady walked in today with the complain of chest pain. She had history of diabetes, chronic kidney disease and asthma. She also complained about weakness and nausea for one week.

FAMILY HISTORY

Diabetes mellitus, coronary disorder.

DIAGNOSIS

Anemia, Diabetes Mellitus type II, chronic kidney disease.

She was discharged with next follow-up check up with cardiologist.

Figure 9.1 Sample discharge summary representing "Unstructured text"

*https://portal.dbmi.hms.harvard.edu/projects/n2c2-nlp/

1. Name
2. Address (all geographic subdivisions smaller than state, including street address, city county, and zip code)
3. All elements (except years) of dates related to an individual (including birth date, admission date, discharge date, date of death and exact age if over 89)
4. Telephone numbers
5. Fax numbers
6. Email addresses
7. Social security number
8. Medical record number
9. Health plan beneficiary number
10. Account number
11. Certificate or license number
12. Vehicle identifiers and serial numbers, including license plate numbers
13. Device identifiers and serial numbers
14. Web URL
15. Internet Protocol (IP) address
16. Finger or voice print
17. Photographic image—Photographic images are not limited to images of the face.
18. Any other characteristic that could uniquely identify the individual

Figure 9.2 HIPPA PHI categories

- "Identification of smoking status from medical record"
- "Extracting medication information from clinical text"
- "Annotating temporal information in clinical narratives"
- "Identification and classification of concepts, assertions and relations in clinical narratives"
- "Evaluating state-of-the-art in automatic de-identification"

The datasets for the mentioned investigations are already annotated for these tasks [7–9] and are ready to use for training new techniques. For instance, it might seem simple to identify and classify concepts in clinical narratives by looking into medical thesaurus, but unstructured clinical narratives involve a variety of language issues (paraphrasing, synonyms, abbreviations, etc.) that cannot be identified and classified using a medical dictionary [10].

The organizers distribute de-identified research datasets/corpora to the researchers by fulfilling ethical requirements for dealing such sensitive information. For the clarity of readers, term "corpus/corpora" and "dataset" is interchangeably used in this chapter. Researchers need to register and submit "data user and confidentiality agreement—DUA[†]" to access these datasets. If one wants to work on similar research questions then taking part into these challenges provide

[†]https://n2c2.dbmi.hms.harvard.edu/dua

the opportunity to contribute devised NLP frameworks/methods and results and compete with competent research teams.

Gold standard corpus*/ground truth

The gold standard corpus is a dataset that is annotated with the information (results) that is required to be identified in dataset. This dataset can be used for the final evaluation of the developed methods or may be used for training the dataset for prediction purposes.

* In the field of natural language processing (NLP), corpus is the collection of documents and the plural of corpus is known as corpora. In the E-health NLP, these documents can be consultation notes, discharge summaries, etc.

In this way, research teams may get gold standard annotated datasets/corpora that are ready for the application of variety of supervised NLP techniques. On the other hand, working on a different research question, one might need to develop his/her own gold standard/ground truth for supervised techniques or evaluation. Development of gold standard dataset for domain-specific corpus is a time-consuming, expensive and challenging task as it needs the involvement of a domain expert who can annotate or validate the gold standard dataset.

9.2 Annotation challenges dealing with health-care corpora

As discussed in Section 9.1, one of the challenging tasks is to develop gold standard corpus for the required research task. Manual annotation of such large datasets requires an extensive amount of time and effort from domain experts, which is practically not possible. One way of extracting required information is to use health-care thesaurus available for research but still it will not serve the purpose completely. This is because the gold standard corpus to be developed is written by a domain/medical expert and does not follow any specific format. Variation in writing styles involves an understanding of "semantics" that cannot be directly captured from globally available health-care terminologies such as "Systemized Nomenclature of Medicine-Clinical Terms—SNOMED CT" [11] that have been used for preprocessing or theoretical implementations, or using "Unified Medical Language System—UMLS" for the development of E-health resources [12]. Despite the fact that these terminologies contain semantic information, these still are not able to completely capture domain knowledge from unstructured datasets. Some of the language issues that are related to semantic information are listed as follows:

1. A different way of writing synonyms of a medical concept: for instance, medical concept "X-Ray" may be written as "xray or xRay."

2. Variation of writing abbreviations: for instance, a patient may be abbreviated "Pt or pt."
3. Paraphrasing of multiword concepts[‡]: for instance, "CT-Scan of the brain" may be written as "ct of brain or CT scan of brain or brain CT."
4. Spelling errors can be challenging if present in major numbers.

With the abovementioned language issues, it is problematic for the annotators to annotate gold standard corpus for domain-specific corpus manually by going through variation of writing style. These language issues cannot be ignored while working on health-care datasets as it contains contextual information that is critical for extracting the domain knowledge.

However, semiautomatic approach (discussed in Section 9.2.1) of developing gold standard datasets is helpful in minimizing efforts of annotators working on manual annotations.

9.2.1 Semiautomatic approach for the development of gold standard corpus of medical narratives

It is a fact that manual annotation that involves more than one annotator may produce reliable gold standard dataset. On the other hand, it cannot be denied that efforts involve in the manual annotation of domain-specific corpus (corpus of medical narratives) is time-consuming and expensive. Instead of annotating data from scratch, it is effective to adopt semiautomatic approach. This approach may involve lexicons/dictionaries/gazetteers (health-care terminologies in this case) of the required entities that can automatically identify and classify majority of concepts/medical entities. Remaining entities that are missed due to language issues may be tackled manually by developing specific annotation guidelines. Here, researchers must not reply completely on the entities/concepts identified and classified using dictionaries because contextual information must be considered in annotating health-care corpus. For this problem, annotation rule to get these entities verified by domain experts (annotators) must be included as part of annotation guidelines. This approach will minimize efforts, will save time in overall annotation process and will also help in the identification of language issues that exist in unstructured health-care dataset.

Although automatic annotation framework has also been reported for limited scope that is specific lung cancer concepts in clinical narratives [13]; however, it is challenging to develop a generic annotation framework for automatic annotation. This is also one of the limitations of the available research datasets that these datasets are annotated for specific problems and cannot be used for every research problem. The next section will cover NLP methods that have been adopted to tackle semantics in medical text analysis.

[‡]Multi-word concept means that one concept may contain more than one concepts, for instance "Chest X-Ray" contain two medical concepts "Chest (body structure)" and "X-Ray (Procedure/Test)."

9.3 NLP methods that can be adopted to tackle semantics for medical text analysis

In the analysis of unstructured medical text that is written by different medical professionals, the variation of writing styles and expressions leads toward inconsistency that cannot be directly extracted using health-care terminologies. Contextual knowledge is another challenging issue that needs strong semantic analysis in the identification of medical concepts in the corpus of medical narratives. In this section, important methods that have been used to tackle semantics are discussed.

9.3.1 Rule-based methods

Hand-crafted rules or observed regular expressions are used in the identification of medical concepts that are ignored by semantics included in medical dictionaries/gazetteers [10]. In the related research, it is evident that unstructured medical narratives contain a variety of patterns that may help in "information extraction—IE,[§]" but still the output is questionable when working on contextual analysis of the identified medical concepts [14].

Rule-based approach may perform well on the datasets that follow a similar format of writing styles but when applied on any different format may lose its efficiency. This is difficult to achieve generic rule-based system that extends gazetteers/dictionaries and work accurately on different corpora. For instance, Figure 9.3 shows concept "Cardiac CT" and its synonyms extracted from global health-care terminology SNOMED CT.

Synonyms presented in Figure 9.3 do not cover every possible variation of writing this concept. One clinician might write "CT of the heart" or "CT-Scan of the heart" or "Heart CT." Inconsistency in expression will not be captured by terminologies or dictionaries. One approach is to modify the available terminology as per requirement by adding variations of concepts. This needs a lot of meaningless effort as format and writing of one corpus will be different from the other corpus.

Preferred Name	Cardiac CT
Synonyms	Computed tomography of heart (procedure) Cardiac CT (procedure) Computed tomography of heart CT of heart

Figure 9.3 Example concept "Cardiac CT" extracted using SNOMED CT ontology from a BioPortal web annotator (https://bioportal.bioontology.org/annotator)

[§]IE means extracting relevant information from the text.

Rule#1: //Identification and classification of the category/class 'Procedure'

(Procedure) (SP) (Body structure) |

(Procedure) (SP) (IN) (SP) (DT) (Body structure) |

(Procedure) (SP) (IN) (Body structure)

Where,

SP = Space Token excluding newlines and tab spaces. IN = Preposition, DT = Determiner, | = Or

Figure 9.4 Example rule applied after the identification of concepts using dictionaries/gazetteers

As the matter of fact, corpus of medical narratives in UK English will have different expression than corpus of medical narratives written in US English. When dealing with medical corpus of other countries (such as Pakistan, Australia), it will be more challenging to capture the variation of writing styles relying only on terminologies/dictionaries.

However, if corpus from similar source is used then generic rules may work as the extension of concepts identified using dictionaries as presented in Figure 9.4. Here, (Procedure) and (Body structure) refer to the dictionaries/gazetteers of medical concepts extracted using "SNOMED CT health-care terminology" under these categories.

Rule 1 in Figure 9.4 shows that it will extract all possible concepts present in the corpus of medical narratives. This rule has been developed by the analysis of "Corpus A" and tested on "Corpus B" that was of similar nature. Different concepts following variation in formats ("GI Prophylaxis," "pelvic lymphadenectomy," "abdomen X-ray," "Prostate biopsy," "X-Ray of abdomen" and so on) will be captured using Rule 1. However, if the scope of the system is to capture more details then the developed rules will not be enough to capture the required contextual information. For instance, another corpus containing multiple concepts "Ct-scan of head and neck" or "CT of head, neck" will not adopt these rules accurately.

Another example for the identification of multiword medical concept in the corpus of medical narratives is as follows:

Example text:

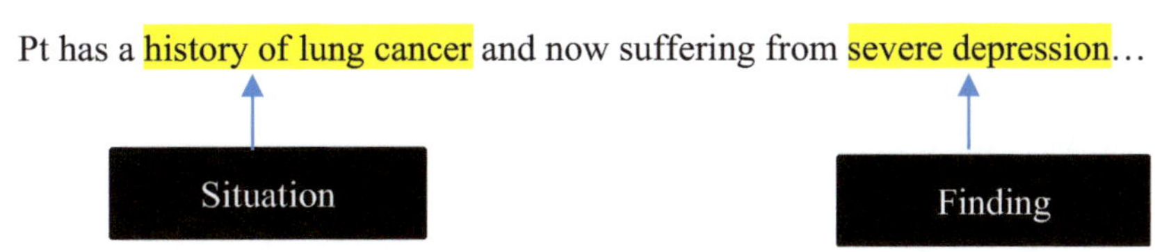

In this example text, the "history of lung cancer" is classified as situation and "severe depression" is classified as finding. The same case may be expressed as "lung cancer history" or "History: lung cancer"; hence there are a variety of expressions for the identification of multiword concept. Generic rules/patterns can only be observed when the dataset is analyzed thoroughly and it has a variety of observations in large numbers.

Despite the fact that rule-based approach provides in-depth analysis of linguistics features involved in the contextual analysis, which still failed to achieve generic scalability in the case of analysis of unstructured medical text. Reasons clearly indicate the variation in the writing structures used by different clinicians and furthermore, it will also add complexity of structures in the case of clinicians from different regions/countries.

However, hand-crafted rules may add value in improving machine learning methods that may be used for the identification and classification of required medical concepts. Output of rule-based methods used as features in the machine learning methods will certainly improve the performance of classification tasks.

9.3.2 Machine learning methods

Machine learning techniques for the identification and classification of text have proven significant improvement in E-health NLP. In addition to this, hand-crafted rules are time-consuming and expensive (discussed in Section 9.3.1) but effective to start with in the case of the following constraints required for supervised machine learning classification techniques:

- Unavailability of domain experts for data annotation.
- Unavailability of gold standard required for any specific application.
- Insufficient gold standard dataset.

Apart from these constraints, data that is publicly available may not satisfy all the requirements of E-health NLP systems but still provides quality content in terms of training and testing E-health systems. For the identification and classification of required clinical information in the unstructured text, both supervised and supervised approaches may be used. Researchers with clear requirements (known classes/labels) prefer to use supervised machine learning methods such as support vector machine, random forest. Annotation of gold standard dataset is a real bottle neck in using supervised machine learning methods [15]. A sample flow diagram (shown in Figure 9.5) describes the process of classification of unstructured text using supervised machine learning approaches.

In supervised machine learning application, different medical dictionaries/ lexicons can be incorporated to match medical concepts (feature). In some cases, researchers have to modify the format of the medical dictionaries according to the requirement of the tool they want to use [16].

In the first step, the corpus of medical narratives needs to be analyzed for preprocessing purposes. Preprocessing of the data involves cleaning unnecessary

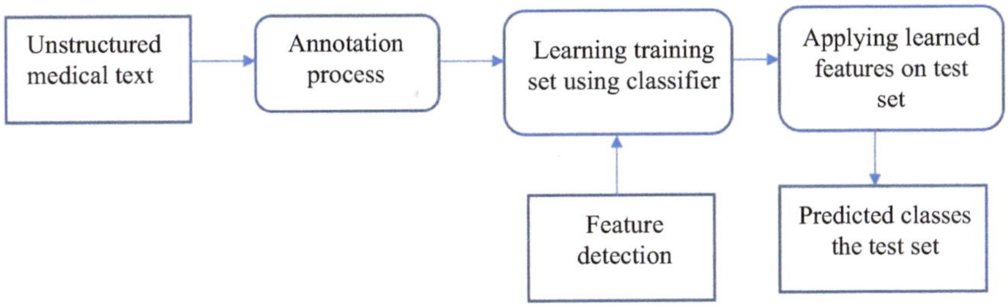

Figure 9.5 Process flow of supervised machine learning approach for medical narratives

information (date, removing stop words, headers, etc.) from the text or in some cases, de-identification of personal information from the text (for the ethical use of dataset). As mentioned earlier, data annotation is an important step in the application of supervised machine learning methods for the classification of required medical concepts. For this purpose, researchers also adopt semiautomatic approach to annotate datasets using medical terminologies/dictionaries such as UMLS or SNOMED CT [17]. These resources are available online at "National Library of Medicine"** and distributed by following registration process under terms and conditions. Different applications employ these terminologies as per requirements. Every medical concept is associated with codes and semantic categories; therefore, only concepts may be used with its category if any application did not require codes.

9.4 E-health and Internet of Things (IoT)

Other than research-based application as discussed in the previous sections, scalable and commercial applications are based on combining different areas such as NLP and Internet of Things (IoT). IoT is the future of E-health sector and will contribute in data exchange using different devices in E-health applications [18]. If commercial applications have been focused to facilitate multiple health-care users (clinicians, patients, other members), then only textual analysis will not serve the purpose. Patients need to be aware of required health-care information that is available to them via Internet, IoT sensors and mobile applications. Health-care assistance can be provided to the customers using automatic health-chatbots. Customer-centric applications are much more scalable in terms of usage where user can interact and get the required facilitation. This includes scheduling appointments through portals, awareness of procedures via websites/mobile and so on [19]. Smart health-care monitoring systems may help clinicians of developed countries to monitor health status of aging population. Smart devices may be used to record, analyze and predict health status and may help in the prediction of risk factors in special scenarios.

**www.nlm.nih.gov/research/umls/index.html

9.5 Contributions required from NLP researchers in health-care applications

Several research works have been published globally in the field of E-health NLP, still more valuable analysis and prediction can be done using real-time information growing every second [20]. Researchers and clinicians working in health-care sectors require an analysis of real-time information to deal with emergency scenarios such as COVID-19 pandemic. In addition to that, patients and people want to know the reliable facts regarding such sensitive information. In parallel, it is also a fact that real-time data is valuable and may not be shared with multiple users without following ethical requirements. One way is to design and implement multiple modules for different users that can share filtered information as per the requirement of type of users (doctors, researchers, patients) using cloud services. Data may be distributed via mechanism that is decided carefully considering ethical requirements for every user. An example architecture is presented in Figure 9.6 that

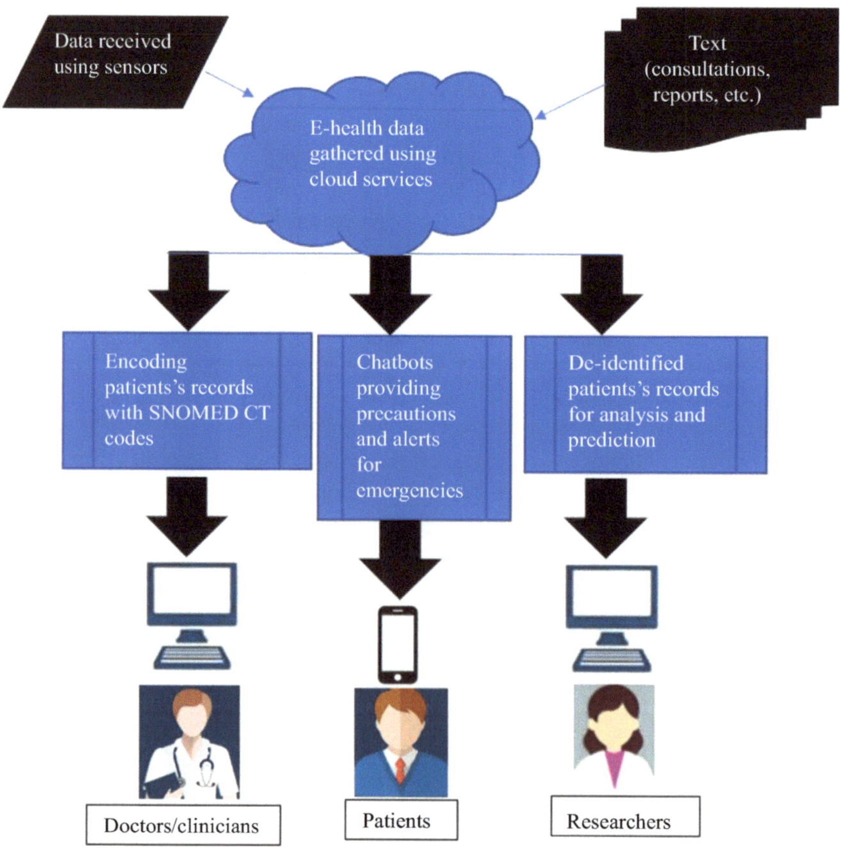

Figure 9.6 Potential architecture for sharing required data among potential users of E-health applications

shows the distribution of such information to multiple types of users after processing data using different modules.

In this architecture, data ethics have been designed keeping requirements of data for individual users. It can be observed that clinicians need to exchange consistent information of patients that is difficult in the case of textual format. A preprocessing encoding module may be implemented to convert all textual consultations in the form of medical codes that will ensure secure information exchange [21,22]. For patients, complete consultation records are insignificant; therefore required information such as "precautionary measures in emergency situations," "when to see doctors," "basic care advices based on symptoms," "support mental health issues" can be communicated to them via mobile alerts or chatbots [23,24]. Furthermore, researchers working in health-care domain need real-time information as well as information that resides in archived records. This information will ensure a reliable prediction of valuable information for health-care sector but may not be shared without the de-identification of personal information of individual. This information may be processed using anonymization system that will de-identify a patient (such as "patient name," "location," "address") and then be shared reliably for research purposes. State-of-the-art methods such as ensemble learning and neural networks [25] can be employed for securing the identities of patients in E-health applications [26].

Moreover, global pandemic has raised a variety of research questions that are related to different industry sectors. Different aspects were observed due to pandemic such as "social distancing" in workplaces, "decline in fuel rates" affected in aviation sectors, "hotels shut down" during lockdown situation in food industry [27]. These factors may be studied by NLP researchers using relevant datasets to improve alternate strategies that may be adopted in challenging situations like pandemic. Social media platforms can serve as open datasets that can be collected from the relevant community/group page with respect to pandemic and other risk factors that may affect these industries. "Aspect-based sentiment analysis" of these open datasets will highlight more aspects that can contribute in further analysis. Other than this, the mental health status of students as well as workers from different industry may be analyzed by extracting free text from social media platforms [28].

Another important research area that is critical in E-health NLP is related to "Fake news detection" and there is little contribution in this domain [29,30]. People of different age groups have access to social media platforms, news articles blogs and have been exposed to real and fake news related to health-care domain. This research also needs contribution from NLP researchers so that research community can create impact on this society in positive manner.

9.6 Conclusion and future work

Chapter summarizes the contributions of E-health NLP in the following multiple aspects:

- Challenges related to data have been explained and details of available datasets have been discussed.

- Data preparation and preprocessing of health-care datasets with respect to required research objective have been explained in detail. Semiautomatic approaches for the annotation of gold standard dataset of health-care data are effective than manual annotation.
- Different health-care terminologies ("UMLS," "SNOMED CT") may be employed for the initial annotation of the health-care datasets.
- Methods that can be explored to start initial research in E-health NLP have been explained using rule-based and machine learning method application pipeline.
- E-health NLP applications can be effective when used in combination with other domains such as "IoT" and "Cloud Computing."
- This chapter has been compiled by including important contributions that are required from NLP research community and have been discussed to benefit young researchers working in this area.

References

[1] H. M. A. A. Wahab, W. Mansoor, S. Hina, and S. M. Uzair, "Prioritization of diseases in patient's consultation notes using SNOMED CT," *International Journal of Computer Science and Network Security*, vol. 17, no. 7, 2017.

[2] G. R. Venkataraman, A. L. Pineda, O. J. Walk IV, *et al.*, "FasTag: Automatic text classification of unstructured medical narratives," *PLoS One*, vol. 15, no. 6, p. e0234647, 2020.

[3] S. Hina, R. Asif, and S. A. Ali, "Anonymization framework for securing protected health information in a complex dataset of medical narratives," *Mehran University Research Journal of Engineering & Technology*, vol. 39, no. 3, 2017.

[4] S. Kalkman, J. van Delden, A. Banerjee, B. Tyl, M. Mostert, and G. van Thiel, "Patients' and public views and attitudes towards the sharing of health data for research: A narrative review of the empirical evidence," *Journal of Medical Ethics*, 2019, doi: 10.1136/medethics-2019-105651.

[5] A. Mondal, E. Cambria, D. Das, A. Hussain, and S. Bandyopadhyay, "Relation extraction of medical concepts using categorization and sentiment analysis," *Cognitive Computation*, vol. 10, no. 4, pp. 670–685, 2018.

[6] W. Moore and S. Frye, "Review of HIPAA, Part 1: History, protected health information, and privacy and security rules," *Journal of Nuclear Medicine Technology*, vol. 47, no. 4, p. 269, 2019.

[7] A. Stubbs and Ö. Uzuner, "Annotating longitudinal clinical narratives for de-identification: The 2014 i2b2/UTHealth corpus," *Journal of Biomedical Informatics*, vol. 58, pp. S20–S29, 2015/12/01/ 2015.

[8] W. Sun, A. Rumshisky, and Ö. Uzuner, "Annotating temporal information in clinical narratives," *Journal of Biomedical Informatics*, vol. 46, pp. S5–S12, 2013.

[9] A. Stubbs, M. Filannino, E. Soysal, S. Henry, and Ö. Uzuner, "Cohort selection for clinical trials: n2c2 2018 shared task track 1," *Journal of the*

American Medical Informatics Association, vol. 26, no. 11, pp. 1163–1171, 2019.

[10] S. Hina, E. Atwell, and O. Johnson, "SnoMedTagger: A semantic tagger for medical narratives," *International Journal of Computational Linguistics and Applications*, vol. 4, no. 2, pp. 81–99, 2013.

[11] D. Lee, N. de Keizer, F. Lau, and R. Cornet, "Literature review of SNOMED CT use," *Journal of the American Medical Informatics Association*, vol. 21, no. e1, pp. e11–e19, 2013.

[12] L. Amos, D. Anderson, S. Brody, A. Ripple, and B. L. Humphreys, "UMLS users and uses: A current overview," *Journal of the American Medical Informatics Association*, vol. 27, no. 10, pp. 1606–1611, 2020.

[13] M. Najafabadipour, J. M. Tuñas, A. Rodríguez-González, and E. Menasalvas, "Lung Cancer Concept Annotation from Spanish Clinical Narratives," In: *Data Integration in the Life Sciences. DILS 2018. Lecture Notes in Computer Science*, Springer, Cham, vol. 11371, 2019.

[14] Ö. Uzuner, B. R. South, S. Shen, and S. L. DuVall, "2010 i2b2/VA challenge on concepts, assertions, and relations in clinical text," *Journal of the American Medical Informatics Association*, vol. 18, no. 5, pp. 552–556, 2011.

[15] I. Spasic and G. Nenadic, "Clinical text data in machine learning: Systematic review," (in English) *JMIR Medical Informatics*, vol. 8, no. 3, p. e17984, 2020.

[16] S. Hina, "Semantic tagging of medical narratives using SNOMED CT," PhD, School of Computing, University of Leeds, eThesis Online uk.bl.ethos.595145, 2013. [Online]. Available: https://etheses.whiterose.ac.uk/5289/1/HINA_S_COMPUTING_PhD_2013.pdf [Accessed 10 Jan 2021].

[17] A. T. McCray, O. Bodenreider, J. D. Malley, and A. C. Browne, "Evaluating UMLS strings for natural language processing," (in English), *Proc AMIA Symp*, pp. 448–452, 2001.

[18] M. Javaid and I. H. Khan, "Internet of Things (IoT) enabled healthcare helps to take the challenges of COVID-19 Pandemic," *Journal of Oral Biology and Craniofacial Research*, vol. 11, no. 2, pp. 209–214, 2021.

[19] S. Jarzabe, K. Cheong, Y. W. Lim, J. C. M. Wong, R. K. Kayanoth, and J. Y. Teng, "CBT Assistant Platform: Web/mobile co-design solution for cognitive behavioural therapy," *Journal of Hospital Management and Health Policy*, vol. 2, 2018.

[20] K. J. Hong, N. L. Park, S. Y. Heo, S. H. Jung, Y. B. Lee, and J. H. Hwang, "Effect of e-health literacy on COVID-19 infection-preventive behaviors of undergraduate students majoring in healthcare," *Healthcare*, vol. 9, no. 5, p. 573, 2021. [Online]. Available: www.mdpi.com/2227-9032/9/5/573.

[21] C. Gaudet-Blavignac, V. Foufi, M. Bjelogrlic, and C. Lovis, "Use of the systematized nomenclature of medicine clinical terms (SNOMED CT) for processing free text in health care: Systematic scoping review," *Journal of Medical Internet Research*, vol. 23, no. 1, 2021.

[22] A. N. Nguyen, D. Truran, M. Kemp, *et al.*, "Computer-assisted diagnostic coding: Effectiveness of an NLP-based approach using SNOMED CT to ICD-10 mappings," (in English), *AMIA Annual Symposium Proceedings*, vol. 2018, pp. 807–816, 2018.

[23] M. Bates, "Health care chatbots are here to help," *IEEE Pulse*, vol. 10, no. 3, pp. 12–14, 2019.

[24] Z. Safi, A. Abd-Alrazaq, M. Khalifa, and M. Househ, "Technical aspects of developing chatbots for medical applications: Scoping review," (in English) *Journal of Medical Internet Research*, vol. 22, no. 12, p. e19127, 2020.

[25] Y.-S. Zhao, K.-L. Zhang, H.-C. Ma, and K. Li, "Leveraging text skeleton for de-identification of electronic medical records," *BMC Medical Informatics and Decision Making*, vol. 18, no. 1, p. 18, 2018.

[26] K. Murugadoss, A. Rajasekharan, B. Malin, *et al.*, "Building a best-in-class automated de-identification tool for electronic health records through ensemble learning," *Patterns*, vol. 2, no. 6, p. 100255, 2021.

[27] A. Ayesha, B. Prabadevi, and S. Sudhagara Rajan, "Artificial intelligence for the novel corona virus (COVID-19) pandemic: Opportunities, challenges, and future directions," *International Journal of E-Health and Medical Communications (IJEHMC)*, vol. 13, no. 2, pp. 1–21, doi: 10.4018/IJEHMC.20220701.oa5.

[28] R. Skaik and D. Inkpen, "Using social media for mental health surveillance: A review," *ACM Computing Surveys*, vol. 53, no. 6, Article 129, 2020.

[29] P. Mookdarsanit and L. Mookdarsanit, "The COVID-19 fake news detection in Thai social texts," *Bulletin of Electrical Engineering and Informatics*, vol. 10, no. 2, p. 11, 2021.

[30] T. J. Banerjee, "A system of content analysis of social media using AI and NLP," *International Journal of Research in Engineering, Science and Management*, vol. 4, no. 6, pp. 132–136, 2021.

Chapter 10

Blockchain of things for healthcare asset management

Sajid Nazir[1], *Mohammad Kaleem*[2], *Hassan Hamdoun*[3], *Jafar Alzubi*[4] *and Hua Tianfield*[1]

Abstract

The healthcare sector has a large deployment of critical assets, which must be available at the right place at the right time. This necessitates not only the location of the assets being monitored in real time but also the serviceability being ensured through predictive maintenance. The Internet of Things (IoT) has transformed real-time data acquisition, which can be aggregated and analysed for meaningful inferences about the monitored process and assets. The information can be collected and exchanged through radio, Bluetooth or other communications technologies but raises privacy and security concerns as the critical asset information is susceptible to interception and tampering both in transit and at rest.

The asset information is critical both for privacy preservation and tamper proofing. Combining the use of blockchain technology with IoT can provide a high degree of trust and security. The data can thereby be securely shared within the private blockchain only with the authorised parties.

This chapter discusses the application of combining IoT and blockchain technologies into a solution to address challenges in the healthcare sector. In particular, we present an architecture for integrating IoT, edge artificial intelligence and blockchain technologies for asset management in the healthcare sector.

Keywords: Artificial intelligence; Blockchain; Healthcare; Cryptography; Real-time data acquisition; Data privacy; Asset management; Permissioned blockchain; Ethereum; Medical records; Distributed computing; Edge computing; Amazon Web Services (AWS); Hyperledger Fabric; Raspberry Pi; Polkadot; Asset tracking; Predictive maintenance; Hashing; Internet of Things

[1]Department of Computing, Glasgow Caledonian University, Glasgow, UK
[2]Department of Electrical and Computer Engineering, COMSATS University, Islamabad, Pakistan
[3]Mobile Architecture and Solutions, Service Platforms, British Telecommunications (BT), London, UK
[4]Faculty of Engineering, Al-Balqa Applied University, Al-Salt, Jordan

10.1 Introduction

The Internet of Things (IoT) has transformed many application domains through enabling real-time collection and processing of data. This is facilitated by the ever-decreasing cost of sensors and sensor platforms, miniaturisation, efficient communications protocols and low-power devices.

The blockchain concept has been popularised by cryptocurrencies such as BitCoin but has since then found applicability in many other application domains. The blockchain concept has been successfully applied in smart manufacturing, smart grid, food industry, supply chain management, unmanned aerial vehicles and healthcare [1]. An edge-of-things and blockchain-based system for autonomous and safe vehicle intersection management is described by Buzachis [2]. The large volume of data generated by the smart vehicles and its storage can be shared securely using blockchain [3]. The use of blockchain in the field of transport and logistics can bring a seamless mobility of goods and services across borders [4]. A blockchain of things architecture is proposed for manufacturing to combine Industrial IoT with permissioned blockchain to overcome the challenges of the centralised architecture of IoT [5]. A blockchain-based secure authentication and data-sharing scheme for IoT is described by Fan [6] providing a trade-off between security and efficiency.

A major project is the Web 3.0 foundation [7] which utilised some blockchain technologies as well as open-source web technologies to design and build development networks, cross-chain message passing (XCMP) methods and protocols providing secure environment for cross-chain composability of data, for example, Polkadot. Other applications of blockchains in sensor technologies are the HNT (Helium) [8] and MXC [9] projects. Helium is a wireless network powered by blockchain and MXC is a smart city IoT network built on blockchain. PharmaLedger project provides blockchain-based healthcare [10]. It is a consortium of 28 institutions with eight use cases and participation by major pharmaceutical companies. The project also offers interoperability with multiple blockchains [10].

Blockchain economy was expected to reach $1 trillion by 2020 [11]. Increase in blockchain-based asset management will be propelled by large enterprises in banking and healthcare [11]. It is predicted that blockchain will provide $3.1 trillion of value addition by 2030 [12]. Scalability and latency are the two major barriers for the adoption of blockchain healthcare applications [13].

In an increasingly connected society, the integration of blockchain with IoT, edge artificial intelligence (AI), cloud computing and 5G technologies is of paramount importance [4]. The combination of IoT, blockchain, edge AI and big data can produce significant impacts [14]. There is a need for IoT-based healthcare systems to evolve and adopt technologies such as AI, big data for processing the large data, while providing privacy and security [15]. The combined use of these cutting edge technologies can provide innovative solutions for critical areas such as healthcare asset management.

The remainder of this chapter is organised as follows. Section 10.2 describes the healthcare asset management. The challenges and opportunities in healthcare are presented in Section 10.3. Blockchain concepts and frameworks are covered in

Section 10.4. Section 10.5 describes the proposed healthcare asset management architecture. The major healthcare application areas that can benefit from blockchain and edge AI are presented in Section 10.6. Finally, Section 10.7 provides the conclusion and future work.

10.2 Healthcare asset management

Healthcare asset management is critical as it can have profound effects on the health and lives of both in- and out-patients that require the consumables, or a machine or data collection, consent and verification at various points in time/locations. The placement of medical assets improves the treatment of patients and can also have an effect on the outcomes in emergency situations [16].

Asset tracking represents an existing challenge in the healthcare sector [17]. It is estimated that an average hospital loses around 15 per cent of its assets every year, requiring unnecessary staff time to search for the equipment, and in some cases purchasing or renting the equipment, that the hospital already holds [18]. Thus, significant and otherwise useful staff time is lost in searching for supplies such as infusion pumps [18].

An asset management system for tracking and managing healthcare assets in a hospital setting with radio-frequency identification (RFID) technology is described in [19]. The collected information gets stored in a database from where it can be accessed over mobile phones to determine the position of the tracked asset [19]. The RFID tagging of the assets was used for tracking the assets. Within 2 years of an RFID solution, National Health Service Forth Valley saved over £343,000 through avoiding unnecessary purchases of additional equipment, and timely decommissioning of the equipment [18].

IoT devices can capture the real-time data of a patient, determine an accurate location for a physical asset such as infusion pumps and can also predict any fault or failure. Thus, at any time, an accurate location aids the utilisation of the medical devices which can then be redeployed readily whenever a change in location is required to serve another patient or operation.

It is important that the assets are located quickly once required. The use of IoT can be especially beneficial for mobile medical devices or assets by incorporating equipment-borne sensors and data collection which can provide real-time location information to the staff [20]. This can lead to an efficient utilisation of equipment and saves time in locating and transporting it across a medical facility [20]. This concept taken a step further can provide useful insights into the need for periodic and predictive maintenance based on equipment's usage pattern or any anomalous readings.

Blockchain is a distributed ledger with its data shared amongst the network peers [21]. Integration of distributed ledger technology (DLT) with the IoT technologies can provide improvements in health-related data sharing [22]. The study showed that a fully decentralised system for health data sharing is possible through edge computing devices that replace the local server [22].

Various communications technologies are being used in the healthcare sector. The commonly used communications technologies are barcodes, RFID, Bluetooth and Wi-Fi [16]. The choice of the technology can be governed by the required characteristics of the technology and constraints in the asset tracking application.

Smart healthcare systems require reliable and secure communications links, and good quality of service support at low power [15]. A good comparison of the technologies can be found in [15]. Low-power wireless technologies are essential for healthcare systems exploiting IoT; however, there are associated challenges in security and privacy [15].

The movement and utilisation of hospital resources through IoT tracking devices is possible due to the technology advancements [23]. A real-time system for asset tracking using Bluetooth low energy (BLE) and Wi-Fi for improving nursing workflow and hospital efficiency is described in [16]. The developed tags were attached to the assets which together with BLE beacons established the asset tracking system [16]. The authors suggest the sensor type, users, asset type and the area of operation as the important factors to be considered for asset tracking [16]. The system used the Wi-Fi for an approximate location within the hospital, whereas positioning with a higher degree of accuracy was determined through BLE beacons [16].

An IoT-based healthcare management system is proposed by Lee [23] that utilised Wi-Fi and RFID to track the location and also to monitor the condition of the assets by measuring temperature, acceleration, etc. [23]. The system is integrated with artificial neural network and Fuzzy logic module to provide additional features such as preventive maintenance and remaining shelf life [23]. All assets were fitted with RFID tags and the collected data through a back-end device was sent to cloud storage [23]. The system was capable of not only providing an asset location but also monitoring any asset with high deterioration value, such as blood bags for timely alerts [23]. The study tracked infusion pumps in a trial implementation [23].

AI can be used with IoT for collecting data, and a blockchain to improve security and avoid a centralised architecture [12]. The combined use of these technologies has immense potential for complex problems [12].

10.3 Challenges and opportunities in healthcare

10.3.1 Health and safety

The health and safety of the patient is of paramount importance. The data collection, transmission and storage should in no way compromise the health and safety of a patient. Given that the connections with a centralised server or the cloud platform may become unavailable due to Internet or hardware issues, this at no time should compromise the safety of the patient and any equipment that is in operation.

The edge or gateway devices with local storage can provide an interim storage of the data which can be uploaded and analysed at the cloud once the connection is restored.

10.3.2 Regulatory requirements

The regulations require use of certain communications bands to avoid interference with other medical equipment utilising it. In other cases the tracking system may experience interference from existing equipment [16]. Similarly, there may be constraints on the use of wired connections for the sensing and tracking equipment that brings its own challenges of the battery operation and replacement [16].

10.3.3 Data privacy

The data privacy for the patients is utmost important during acquisition, transmission, storage and analysis. The location, inventory and state of the medical equipment are also required to be shared only with the authorised parties.

The privacy concerns have resulted in the data protection regulations becoming stricter, such as General Data Protection Regulation [22]. The healthcare data can be communicated and analysed by preserving its privacy through blockchain technologies [20].

10.3.4 Data security

The health data stored in centralised databases is susceptible to data tampering and other types of malicious attacks [22]. Use of blockchain overcomes many of the associated problems with a centralised architecture [14]. The only single point of failure in blockchain is the clock required for timestamp [14].

The healthcare data is extremely valuable and patients need increasingly more and more control over their personal data captured through on-person devices such as smart watches [20].

Data security is important during data collection, transmission and analysis of healthcare records in cloud environments [24]. A secure and robust healthcare-based blockchain is proposed using encryption to transfer the data securely [24].

10.3.5 Device security

The security of IoT devices is still an open issue. There are a lot of devices provided by numerous manufacturers and as yet there is no consensus on the type of messaging protocols some of which are proprietary. Most protocols are simple with not so much security built into those. Some standardisation efforts have been seen in the development of communications protocols such as ISO/IEC 62443 [25] which can help strengthening security.

The gateway device for connecting to the cloud, such as Amazon Web Services platform, will need to have all the security credentials set-up on the device before a secure connection can be established. However, no such guarantees can be provided for other low-power devices which might be susceptible to eavesdropping and malicious attacks.

The security of IoT devices is also likely to be addressed through blockchain in the future [14,21], such as replacing a centralised server or cloud-based solution with a decentralised architecture.

10.3.6 Equipment interoperability

There are different medical equipment manufacturers, and most provide a proprietary system. This is a challenge for healthcare providers and clinicians as this could lead to vendor lock-in where the equipment from a particular manufacturer dominates the inventory and it is difficult to switch to better and cheaper alternatives due to the associated cost of switching and adjustment.

The vendors have to reach a consensus and agreement on the communications protocols and messaging protocols for equipment interoperability to happen. Medical device manufacturers' standards, such as ISO 13485, are used to harmonise regulatory requirements to achieve traceability, process validation and international compliance across healthcare products worldwide. Some aspects of interoperability also relate to usability by users. This is defined in IEC 62366-1:2015, Medical devices – Part 1: Application of usability engineering to medical devices and its equivalent standards in United States, EU and Canada, for a summary see [26].

10.3.7 Resource constraints

The low-power IoT devices do not have the necessary storage and computation facilities on board to store the entire blockchain or carry out the data processing. As a reference, BitCoin blockchain reached around 185 GB in September 2018 [1]. The standardised system for energy management for medical devices is specified in ISO 50001 [27].

10.3.8 Sustainability

Sustainability is an important concern for device manufacturers. This is usually implemented via adopting an environmental management system compliant with ISO 14001 [28] that helps to cut down waste and reduce overall carbon footprint. Blockchain can be used for creating measurements of CO_2 and waste points across the healthcare supply chain.

10.4 Blockchain: concepts and frameworks

The blockchain concept since its inception and popularity due to cryptocurrencies has increasingly been employed in other areas due to its advantage of privacy and security. The basic functioning of a blockchain is provided by Fernández-Caramés [21].

10.4.1 Block structure

The block structure and its relationship to the blockchain are shown in Figure 10.1. Each block comprises a block header and the block data. Each block contains the hash of the previous block's header. The first block in the blockchain is termed the Genesis block, and as it does not have a previous block, the value of previous block's hash in the first block will be zero. The field timestamp contains the time of block's addition to the blockchain. Nonce is an integer that provides additional

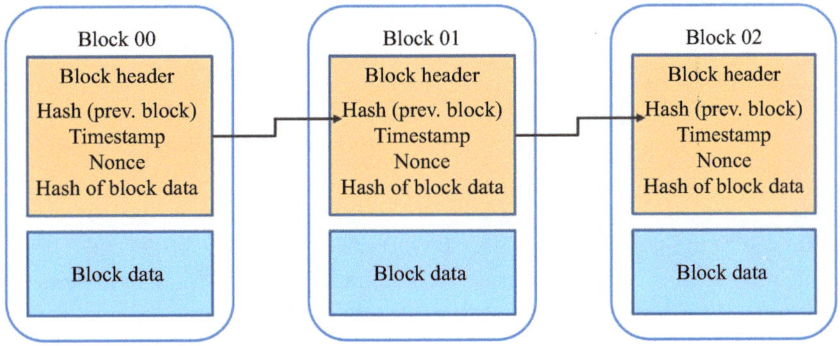

Figure 10.1 Structure of a block in a blockchain

security. As shown in Figure 10.1, each block also contains the hash of its own block data. Any tampering with the block data will result in the hashes to be invalid, and thus any tampering will be evident.

10.4.2 Smart contracts

Smart contract is defined as 'a self-executing programme in a blockchain environment, meant to implement automated transactions agreed by the parties' [4]. Smart contracts provide an automated mechanism for decentralised agreements and enable regulated resource exchanges between peers [29]. Ethereum is the most popular platform for running smart contracts [21]. Ethereum provides a programming language that can be used to encode complex interactions between the parties involved [29].

These smart contracts are analogous to paper contracts and thus can be used to meet regulatory requirements for the standards such as the Health Insurance Portability and Accountability Act of 1996 (HIPAA) [17].

10.4.3 Cryptography and distributed ledger technology

Every node in a blockchain peer-to-peer network has private and public cryptographic keys [21]. Transactions in a blockchain have to be signed and timestamped [21]. The technology uses public key cryptography for digitally signing the transactions between parties [14]. The private key is used to encrypt the information for providing a digital signature that is authentication, whereas the public key is used for decrypting the information sent by the corresponding private key holder. Blockchain makes possible the transactions between two or more parties without the requirement of a trust or validating authority between them [30].

Traceability can be achieved in blockchains through a series of blockchains with the timestamps [4]. A key development triggered by blockchain technology is the concept of DLT that allows the information to be exchanged across different endpoints while ensuring its integrity, security and privacy. Blockchain provides a tamper-proof ledger of transactions that can be shared. Blockchain architecture preserves privacy, provides security and decentralises architecture providing data integrity [3].

10.4.4 Consensus protocols

Consensus in a blockchain refers to the process used by the nodes to verify a transaction and to agree to its existence on the ledger [20]. A block can only be added to a blockchain after the majority of nodes agree that the block is valid. A discussion of consensus algorithms for healthcare is described in [31,32].

The transactions or blocks are linked together forming a blockchain [14]. These blocks require a consensus before being added to the chain and therefore it is extremely difficult or impossible to modify or remove a block [14]. A malicious attacker must have at least 51 per cent of the computational resources, thus making blockchain block corruption nearly impossible [33].

10.4.5 Blockchain classification

Blockchains can be classified according to the nature of access required as follows:

- private blockchain
- public blockchain
- consortium blockchain

The public blockchain can be joined by anyone as a simple node or as a validator/miner without requiring an approval [21]. On the other hand, the private blockchain has restricted access [21]. Consortium blockchain may be controlled by a single or multiple groups [1]. In addition, blockchains can also be further classified as permissioned and permissionless. The permissionless blockchains are open and public, whereas permissioned blockchains are closed and private.

10.4.6 Blockchain frameworks

Blockchain frameworks make it easier to implement a blockchain solution. Rather than developing a complete end-to-end blockchain solution from scratch, the process is simplified through the use of a framework.

The major cloud providers are also providing blockchain as a service and making it easier to use. Microsoft has released a framework, named CoCo, that helps one to create blockchain agnostic consortiums based on groups of trusted parties, such as multiple hospitals, device suppliers and manufacturers [17].

There are many blockchain platforms that suit healthcare applications. The details are provided in [31]. Besides, there are blockchain frameworks, such as Ethereum and Hyperledger Fabric which can be used to develop healthcare applications. The recent trend is towards open-source frameworks and two of the most favoured and popular blockchain frameworks are Hyperledger Fabric [34] and Ethereum [35].

10.4.6.1 Hyperledger Fabric

Hyperledger Fabric is an open-source permissioned DLT for enterprise use. Hyperledger supports smart contracts using general purpose programming languages which means that it is easy to be adopted by organisations. It is a permissioned blockchain, that is, the participants can trust each other as they are already known to each other. Another advantage is that different consensus algorithms can be used with it. Considering the previously mentioned advantages, Hyperledger Fabric is regarded as one of the popular platforms and enables privacy and confidentiality of the transactions [34].

10.4.6.2 Ethereum

Ethereum is also an open-source platform and has a large market capitalisation. It provides a blockchain with built-in Turing-complete programming language which means that any type of computation can be carried out. Smart contracts are written with Solidity programming language. Ethereum is a public permissionless blockchain and uses proof-of-stake as the consensus protocol [35,36].

10.5 Blockchain of things architecture for healthcare asset management

In this section, we present an architecture for healthcare asset management through the integration of the IoT, blockchain and edge AI technologies.

Assets in a blockchain are simply the items about which we intend to store records [20]. In this chapter, we use the term healthcare assets to include both the medical records and medical appliances. Moreover, some healthcare use cases involve information, such as databases, consent forms, which can benefit from distributed collection and verification in our proposed architecture.

In healthcare, opportunities exist for sharing of healthcare data, tracking of medical devices and tracking of the drug supply chain [17]. An IBM study has shown that 60 per cent of healthcare stakeholders believe that medical device asset management and integration has the greatest potential for disruption [17].

Healthcare assets are very critical, and it is of utmost importance for the authorised personnel to be aware of their location and serviceability so that these can be readily brought to use once required. Moreover, the status of the data collected/retained in those assets is of critical importance to better healthcare outcomes as well as important for patient privacy and confidentiality considerations.

There has been an increase in the number of devices per bed and the cost of mobile clinical assets is also on an increase [37]. Healthcare establishments have an opportunity to make enormous savings through accurate identification of their underutilised assets [37].

We provide a holistic solution for asset management by integrating blockchain, IoT and AI at the edge devices. Blockchain provides the required security of the critical and sensitive healthcare information whereas edge AI helps to take decisions closer to the source of the data on the edge device itself. Thus, AI can take decisions closer to the point of use [38].

We propose to use a round robin consensus algorithm [32]. The edge nodes will thus be selected in a predetermined order. This ideally suits the permissioned blockchain where there is a degree of trust between nodes and results in energy saving. The hospital facility or consortium can use a permissioned private blockchain where an entity will be allowed to join in only on being accorded permission. The entities involved here could be the hospital staff, medical suppliers, etc.

The proposed architecture for healthcare asset management is shown in Figure 10.2. The architecture could be visualised as layers. At the bottom layer, we have the medical assets whose location needs to be tracked and managed. The assets will have BLE tags attached so that their positions can be determined through strategically placed gateway devices. We anticipate communications and processing at the edge node and therefore consider a Raspberry Pi to be a suitable device to be used as a gateway. The Raspberry Pi has both Wi-Fi and Bluetooth interfaces and can also be used to communicate over the cellular network. The complete blockchain will be stored in the cloud where AI and analysis can be carried out. Based on the smart contracts, the cloud application can determine any anomalous behaviour to trigger an automated alert. The location of the asset can be made available through a mobile application.

The BLE standard facilitates better accuracy in determining the proximity compared to other technologies [39]. The latest standard in BLE technology has a reduced latency, and reduced airtime, facilitating a longer battery life for use with low-power devices [39].

The devices comprise sensor nodes which for larger and moveable assets can be placed with the device and can communicate over BLE in order to accurately locate the device. The architecture is communications technology agnostic and depending on the application, constraints could also use RFID tags or another technology that can be used to scan an asset as it moves from one healthcare zone

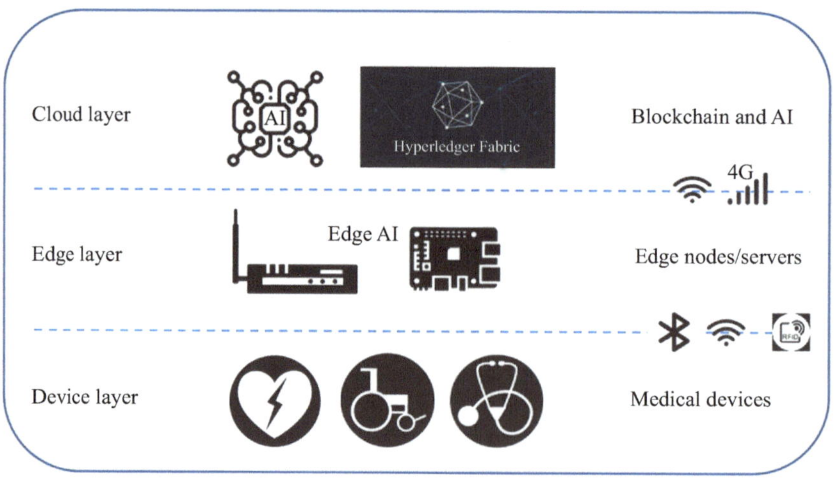

Figure 10.2 Proposed architecture for an integrated framework for IoT, edge computing, AI and blockchain

to another. However, BLE provides an automated way to track the assets as they move within the healthcare facility or are taken out of it.

In Figure 10.2, the edge nodes (i.e., edge servers/nodes) form a peer-to-peer network and participate in a blockchain that is managed by access control of the blockchain platform. Edge servers execute their smart contract policies and may initiate a new transaction on the blockchain platform. One original/root chain is grown based on the blockchain's consensus protocol to which all edge nodes subscribe themselves, and each edge server may maintain a local copy of the up-to-dated root blockchain. Also blockchain allows all verification to occur in the network – reducing the device complexity and data-processing requirements [40].

The healthcare blockchain for asset management can be shared between hospitals, maintenance and service providers, and other stakeholders. This ensures that all the authorised stakeholders can have access and independently verify each transaction [14].

With the recent uptake of blockchain technology by the healthcare establishments and large suppliers of medical equipment, it has also become important to consider communications mechanisms between blockchains.

We propose to use Polkadot [41] XCMP protocol. It defines how messages can be passed among parachains with no additional trust assumptions beyond the economic security of the relay chain. Such protocol will add value and simplifications to patient data record exchange across location boundaries – a typical challenge for current cloud providers.

Another protocol that can be used among different blockchains is inter-blockchain communication. This ensures authentication, statefulness of data, reliability and order of the patient records [42].

The combination of blockchain and IoT was described as blockchain of things [1]. Blockchain is a perfect way to overcome the challenges of decentralisation, diversity, heterogeneity and network complexity of IoT devices [1]. The authors describe the challenges of storing a blockchain at an IoT device and propose a full node, which stores the entire blockchain, and a lightweight node storing only a partial blockchain [1]. More details on types of blockchain nodes are provided in [31].

IoT devices can acquire real-time patient data, but generally this is processed and stored centrally, where the centralisation could become a single point of failure, subject to tampering and privacy exploits [31]. The IoT and blockchain integration can avoid such problems through decentralised processing and storage of IoT data [31]. Blockchain of things will be implemented in an edge computing environment, in which the edge nodes are equipped with the capabilities of information processing and computation necessary for the blockchain.

Nowadays, AI systems have seen a wide deployment in many areas. Major providers of the AI research are often the big cloud service providers. AI is also being deployed to the edge devices [12]. Edge devices such as Raspberry Pi devices are now quite powerful and can be equipped with enough storage to store data and processing locally in case the connection with the cloud is disrupted. Edge computing can support distributed and low-latency applications that can help to decrease the network traffic [21].

The big data generated by the IoT devices can be difficult to be managed by the centralised cloud model, and hence there is more emphasis on a decentralised model with edge devices storing and processing the information locally and sending only the required information to the cloud [2]. Decentralising the AI can result in more equitable development and use of AI compared to a centralised mechanism such as those based on cloud infrastructures [43]. The edge computing makes it possible to run AI algorithms on edge devices [38]. This not only ensures a close to source computation that safeguards sending the raw data all the way back to the cloud but also makes it possible to generate a quicker response.

Moreover, edge AI can be leveraged to accelerate certain processing requirements, verify healthcare data assets in time or make decisions faster, for example, in a healthcare decision support system use case.

Edge AI does not require the complex AI models to be trained on the edge device itself but rather pre-trained models can also be used [38]. Bringing computation to the edge of the network improves energy efficiency, latency and load optimisation [44].

10.6 Major healthcare application areas

This section describes the major application areas for blockchain of things in a healthcare setting. Use of blockchain technologies to solve the real-world problems in healthcare and biomedical sciences such as for research, supply chain, and for securing health data are described in [45].

Healthcare is a prime domain for the application of blockchain technologies as it provides fraud prevention, tamper-proofing and a trustless sharing of data [17]. A lot of potential for the application of blockchain exists in the healthcare sector, and there are not many examples that have gone into production [46]. The use of blockchain with smart contracts for Internet of Medical Things is provided in [30]. A healthcare data sharing system is proposed using IoT and DLT for a secure and tamper-resistant system [22].

10.6.1 Healthcare records

The medical data is increasing and requires being stored securely [20]. A blockchain-based solution for healthcare record storage can enable a trusted AI ecosystem [43]. A cloud-based secure storage of healthcare data is proposed in [24] where the clinical data can be shared and accessed by doctors, insurance agents, etc.

Data sharing has many opportunities for healthcare improvements but also involves many privacy challenges [17,46,47]. The data may need to be shared among the healthcare providers, insurance companies and patients [17]. Blockchain solves this by providing a secure record that is unalterable and can be shared in a decentralised setting [20].

A discussion of the various architectures for blockchain-based data sharing is provided in [47]. A data sharing scheme is proposed for sharing of IoT healthcare data, combining peer-to-peer network, blockchain and a digest chain [13]. An architecture termed IoB Health, by combining IoT and blockchain, is proposed for healthcare data management [31].

10.6.2 Device location management

The location management can include all activities relating to device tracking, knowing its current state and position at any given time, and removal on decommissioning [17]. This aids in the timely retrieval of devices and safeguards against unnecessary purchases [17]. The accurate and timely information about the medical assets is important to ensure that all the required supplies are available at the required location. The use of blockchain technology can not only help establish where a device currently is, but it can also trace its journey through its lifecycle aiding regulatory compliance [17]. Device tracking can assist with loss, theft and tampering due to the immutable nature of blockchain [17].

10.6.3 Preventive and predictive analysis

The maintenance can be planned both on a periodic basis based on the maintenance cycle of medical equipment and also the conditions of any imminent failure or malfunction can be predicted based on data analysis. For instance, an automated measurement of machine temperature or vibration on a periodic basis can determine if these are beyond normal range and hence indicate the need for an inspection or repair.

Similar to these applications, machine learning techniques can be applied to patients' data for predicting the onset of a particular medical condition even before the symptoms appear. Blockchain can be very useful for such sharing of data across hospitals in a secure manner [46].

10.6.4 Data visualisation

It is important that the information about healthcare assets is made available such that it makes it easy to determine the assets' location at any given time. The data visualisation would normally present the data after all the processing for a summarised depiction and may be presented through a desktop, web or mobile application [15]. This must take the user interface design principles into account for wide user adoption and benefit [15]. The data visualisation for the tracking information could also be provided through mobile phones to track the asset location [19].

10.6.5 Forecasting

In addition to the inventory management, the use of demand forecasting is also on the rise in healthcare applications [23]. This is helped by the advances in IoT technologies used in conjunction with inventory and forecast management [23]. The relevant data to make the right decisions at times is collected but stored in different information systems making its visibility and utilisation a challenge [23]. The improvements in forecasting can be achieved by using deep learning and fuzzy logic techniques [23].

10.6.6 Assisted living and patient monitoring

The use of on-person sensors can be very helpful to the healthcare professionals for remotely monitoring the health status of a person for any anomalies or deviations from the normal state. The assisted living makes it possible for the elderly persons to continue to live in their homes with or without the family support.

Senior citizens through wearable devices can provide a stream of monitored data such as blood pressure and heartbeat rate [1,15,48]. However, the degree of attention and monitoring similar to an in-patient in a medical facility can be provided through the latest digital technologies.

Blockchain can improve the security of the monitoring devices by protecting the patients' data [47]. A blockchain and IoT-based remote patient monitoring system is reported in [49], which can alert the healthcare providers in the case of need.

A system is proposed for ambient-assisted living using IoT sensors, healthcare devices and automated decision-making through AI at the edge [38]. A remote health monitoring architecture and the use case of ECG feature extraction with an IoT-based system with blockchain and edge computing is provided in [44]. The system utilised a Raspberry Pi as a sensor node, Wi-Fi and Bluetooth as communications technology, and a private Ethereum network [44].

10.6.7 Healthcare supply chain management

Supply chain management is important for any sector that has to track goods from an originating source to its destination [50]. It is important to ensure that the medication is authentic in order to safeguard patients' health and safety [50]. Drug counterfeiting is a major global problem and has its adverse effects on the health, and finances of the patient, together with making it less attractive for companies to invest in research and development [45]. The counterfeit medication is a prevailing issue in developing countries but is also present in developed countries [50].

10.6.8 Acquiring/processing patient's clinical data

The patients control over their personal medical data is on an increase. Blockchain can make it possible for personal medical data sharing where the control remains with the person sharing the data and they may also be compensated for this. Similarly, the medical images can also be shared with the consent of the patient [47]. This gives control to the patient as to who can access and use their data [50]. Using blockchain, various healthcare systems and providers can interoperate and share patients' data through the decentralised ledger [17]. A blockchain-based patient-centric architecture for sharing of medical records where the patient decides the shared information granularity is described in [43].

10.7 Conclusion and future work

Despite the advantages of blockchain, its full potential has not yet been realised in healthcare [46] and this will change in the very near future due to its recent uptake.

This chapter presents a blockchain based architecture for edge AI for healthcare asset management. The combined use of the latest technological advances in the fields of IoT, blockchain, AI and their availability on edge and also on the cloud platforms can provide insights and solutions to complex problems. This can provide enhanced security and privacy of the data. The proposed permissioned private blockchain architecture on edge and cloud platforms provides an appropriately secure framework for supporting healthcare applications such as asset management.

In our future work, we will implement the proposed architecture using the identified technologies for asset management in a healthcare facility. The data analysis on the cloud platform will be explored for providing data visualisation of the managed assets.

References

[1] Dai H.N., Zheng Z., and Zhang Y. 'Blockchain for Internet of Things: a survey'. *IEEE Internet of Things Journal*. 2019; 6(5): 8076–94.

[2] Buzachis A., Celesti A., Galletta A., Fazio M., Fortino G., and Villari M. 'A multi-agent autonomous intersection management (MA-AIM) system for smart cities leveraging edge-of-things and Blockchain'. *Information Sciences*. 2020; 522: 148–63.

[3] Javed M.U., Rehman M., Javaid N., Aldegheishem A., Alrajeh N., and Tahir M. 'Blockchain-based secure data storage for distributed vehicular networks'. *Applied Sciences*. 2020; 10(6): 2011.

[4] Koh L., Dolgui A., and Sarkis J. 'Blockchain in transport and logistics–paradigms and transitions'. *International Journal of Production Research*. 2020; 58(7): 2054–2062.

[5] Zhang C., Zhou G., Li H., and Cao Y. 'Manufacturing blockchain of things for the configuration of a data-and knowledge-driven digital twin manufacturing cell'. *IEEE Internet of Things Journal*. 2020; 7(12): 11884–94.

[6] Fan Q., Chen J., Deborah L.J., and Luo M. 'A secure and efficient authentication and data sharing scheme for Internet of Things based on blockchain'. *Journal of Systems Architecture*. 2021; 117: 102112.

[7] Web3 Foundation. [online]. Available from https://web3.foundation/projects/ [Accessed Jul 2021].

[8] People-Powered Networks. [online]. Available from https://helium.com/ [Accessed Jul 2021].

[9] Your Free Smart City IoT Network on Blockchain. [online]. Available from https://mxc.org/ [Accessed Jul 2021].

[10] PharmaLedger. The Project [online]. Available from https://pharmaledger.eu/about-us/the-project/ [Accessed Jul 2021].

[11] Swanson R. *TwoGap, the World's First Blockchain-Based Asset Management Platform, Expects Blockchain Economy to Reach $1 Trillion by 2020*. Financial Services Monitor Worldwide. Amman. 23 Sep 2017. [online]. Available from https://institutionalassetmanager.co.uk/2017/09/25/256392/twogap-expects-blockchain-economy-reach-usd1tn-2020 [Accessed Jul 2021].

[12] Daniels J., Sargolzaei S., Sargolzaei A., Ahram T., Laplante P.A., and Amaba B. 'The internet of things, artificial intelligence, blockchain, and professionalism'. *IT Professional*. 2018; 20(6): 15–9.

[13] Shen B., Guo J., and Yang Y. 'MedChain: efficient healthcare data sharing via blockchain'. *Applied Sciences*. 2019; 9(6): 1207.

[14] Kshetri N. 'Can blockchain strengthen the internet of things?'. *IT Professional*. 2017; 19(4): 68–72.

[15] Gardašević G., Katzis K., Bajić D., and Berbakov L. 'Emerging wireless sensor networks and Internet of Things technologies—foundations of smart healthcare'. *Sensors*. 2020; 20(13): 3619.

[16] Yoo S., Kim S., Kim E., Jung E., Lee K.H., and Hwang H. 'Real-time location system-based asset tracking in the healthcare field: lessons learned from a feasibility study'. *BMC Medical Informatics and Decision Making*. 2018; 18(1): 1–0.

[17] Bell L., Buchanan W.J., Cameron J., and Lo O. 'Applications of blockchain within healthcare'. *Blockchain in Healthcare Today*. 2018.

[18] Anstee C. *Tracking Medical Devices: The Role of Active and Passive RFID as Part of an Effective Medical Device Management System*. White Paper, Feb 2017. [online]. Available from https://gs1ie.org/download_files/solution-provider-files/paragonid/paragon-id-white-paper-medical-device-management-with-active-and-passive-rfid-july-2019.pdf [Accessed Jul 2021].

[19] Álvarez López Y., Franssen J., Álvarez Narciandi G., Pagnozzi J., González-Pinto Arrillaga I., and Las-Heras Andrés F. 'RFID technology for management and tracking: E-health applications'. *Sensors*. 2018; 18(8): 2663.

[20] Farouk A., Alahmadi A., Ghose S., and Mashatan A. 'Blockchain platform for industrial healthcare: vision and future opportunities'. *Computer Communications*. 2020; 154: 223–35.

[21] Fernández-Caramés T.M., and Fraga-Lamas P. 'A Review on the use of blockchain for the Internet of Things'. *IEEE Access*. 2018; 6: 32979–3001.

[22] Zheng X., Sun S., Mukkamala R.R., Vatrapu R., and Ordieres-Meré J. 'Accelerating health data sharing: a solution based on the internet of things and distributed ledger technologies'. *Journal of Medical Internet Research*. 2019; 21(6): e13583.

[23] Lee C.K., Cheng M.N., and Ng C.K. 'IoT-based asset management system for healthcare-related industries'. *International Journal of Engineering Business Management*. 2015; 7: 7–19.

[24] Mubarakali A. 'Healthcare services monitoring in cloud using secure and robust healthcare-based Blockchain (SRHB) approach'. *Mobile Networks and Applications*. 2020; 25(4): 1330–7.

[25] ISA-62443-4-2, Security for Industrial Automation and Control Systems: Technical Security Requirements for IACS Components. [online]. Available from https://isa.org/intech-home/2018/september-october/departments/new-standard-specifies-security-capabilities-for-c [Accessed Jul 2021].

[26] O'Leary D. *An Introduction to International Medical Device Standards*. May 2015. [online]. Available from https://meddeviceonline.com/doc/an-introduction-to-international-medical-device-standards-0001 [Accessed Jul 2021].

[27] ISO-50001:2018 Energy management systems—Requirements with guidance for use. [online]. Available from https://iso.org/standard/69426.html [Accessed Jul 2021].

[28] ISO 14001:2015 Environmental management systems—Requirements with guidance for use. [online]. Available from https://iso.org/standard/60857.html [Accessed Jul 2021].

[29] Mizzi A., Ellul J., and Pace G.J. 'Macroprogramming the blockchain of things'. In *2018 IEEE International Conference on Internet of Things (iThings) and IEEE Green Computing and Communications (GreenCom) and IEEE Cyber, Physical and Social Computing (CPSCom) and IEEE Smart Data (SmartData)*, 2018. pp. 1673–1678. IEEE.

[30] Sharma A., Tomar R., Chilamkurti N., and Kim B.G. 'Blockchain based smart contracts for internet of medical things in e-healthcare'. *Electronics*. 2020; 9(10): 1609.

[31] Ray P.P., Dash D., Salah K., and Kumar N. 'Blockchain for IoT-based healthcare: background, consensus, platforms, and use cases'. *IEEE Systems Journal*. 2020; 15(1): 85–94.

[32] Nguyen G.T., and Kim K. 'A survey about consensus algorithms used in blockchain'. *Journal of Information Processing Systems*. 2018; 14(1): 101–28.

[33] Almagrabi A.O., Ali R., Alghazzawi D., AlBarakati A., and Khurshaid T. 'Blockchain-as-a-utility for next-generation healthcare Internet of Things'. *CMC—Computers, Materials & Continua*. 2021; 68(1): 359–76.

[34] Hyperledger-Fabricdocs Documentation, 16 Jun 2021. [online]. Available from https://hyperledger-fabric.readthedocs.io/_/downloads/en/release-2.0/pdf/ [Accessed Jul 2021].

[35] Buterin V. *A Next-Generation Smart Contract and Decentralized Application Platform*. White Paper. 2014; 3(37). [online]. Available from https://translatewhitepaper.com/wp-content/uploads/2021/04/EthereumOrijinal-ETH-English.pdf [Accessed Jul 2021].

[36] Agrawal, R., Chatterjee, J.M., Kumar, A., and Rathore, P.S. (Eds.). (2020). *Blockchain Technology and the Internet of Things: Challenges and Applications in Bitcoin and Security*. Apple Academic Press, Palm Bay, FL.

[37] Horblyuk R., Kaneta K., McMillen G.L., Mullins C., O'Brien T.M., and Roy A., 'Out of control. How clinical asset proliferation and low utilization are draining healthcare budgets'. *Healthcare Financial Management*. 2012; 66(7): 64–8.

[38] Pazienza A., Mallardi G., Fasciano C., *et al.* 'Artificial intelligence on edge computing: a healthcare scenario in ambient assisted living'. In *Proceedings of the 5th Italian Workshop on Artificial Intelligence for Ambient Assisted Living 2019, co-located with 18th International Conference of the Italian Association for Artificial Intelligence, AI*AAL@AI*IA 2019*, Italy, Nov 2019. pp. 22–37.

[39] Di Marco P., Park P., Pratesi M., and Santucci F. 'A Bluetooth-based architecture for contact tracing in healthcare facilities'. *Journal of Sensor and Actuator Networks*. 2021; 10(1): 2.
[40] Qu C., Tao M., Zhang J., Hong X., and Yuan R. 'Blockchain based credibility verification method for IoT entities'. *Security and Communication Networks*. 2018.
[41] Burdges J., Cevallos A., Czaban P., *et al.* 'Overview of Polkadot and its design considerations'. arXiv preprint arXiv:2005.13456. 2020 May 27.
[42] Goes C. 'The Interblockchain Communication Protocol: An Overview'. arXiv:2006.15918v1 [cs.DC]. Inter-blockchain Communication. [online]. Available from https://ibcprotocol.org/ [Accessed Jul 2021].
[43] Jennath H.S., Anoop V.S., and Asharaf S. 'Blockchain for healthcare: securing patient data and enabling trusted artificial intelligence'. *International Journal of Interactive Multimedia & Artificial Intelligence*. 2020; 6(3): 15–23.
[44] Gia T.N., Nawaz A., Querata J.P., Tenhunen H., and Westerlund T. 'Artificial intelligence at the edge in the blockchain of things'. In *International Conference on Wireless Mobile Communication and Healthcare*, Nov 14 2019. pp. 267–280. Springer, Cham.
[45] Justinia T. 'Blockchain technologies: opportunities for solving real-world problems in healthcare and biomedical sciences'. *Acta Informatica Medica*. 2019; 27(4): 284.
[46] Mackey T.K., Kuo T.T., Gummadi B., *et al.* ''Fit-for-purpose?'–challenges and opportunities for applications of blockchain technology in the future of healthcare'. *BMC Medicine*. 2019; 17(1): 1–7.
[47] De Aguiar E.J., Faiçal B.S., Krishnamachari B., and Ueyama J. 'A survey of blockchain-based strategies for healthcare'. *ACM Computing Surveys (CSUR)*. 2020; 53(2): 1–27.
[48] Dadhich P. 'Security of healthcare systems with smart health records using cloud technology'. In *Machine Learning with Health Care Perspective*. 2020 (pp. 183–198). Springer, Cham.
[49] Dwivedi A.D., Malina L., Dzurenda P., and Srivastava G. 'Optimized blockchain model for internet of things based healthcare applications'. In *2019 42nd International Conference on Telecommunications and Signal Processing (TSP)*, 2019. pp. 135–139. IEEE.
[50] Boulos M.N., Wilson J.T., and Clauson K.A. 'Geospatial blockchain: promises, challenges, and scenarios in health and healthcare'. *International Journal of Health Geographics*. 2018; 17(1): 25.

Chapter 11

Artificial intelligence: practical primer for clinical research in cardiovascular disease

Shivendra Dubey[1], Chetan Gupta[1] and Kalpana Rai[1]

Abstract

Nowadays very popular field of computer science is artificial intelligence (AI) that aims to mimic human learning capacity, thought processes, as well as information storage. AI methods have been useful in cardiac treatment to explore original phenotypes as well as genotypes to increase the patient care quality, existing diseases; reduce readmission, mortality rates; and allow cost-effectiveness. Previously, some machine learning methods were used for predicting and diagnosing cardiac illness. In addition, the use of machine learning involves approximate degree of problem understanding, in terms of cardiac treatment as well as statistics, to put on the optimum machine learning methods. In the adjacent forthcoming, AI will come out in a pattern shift to precision cardiac treatment. The AI latent in cardiac medication is wonderful, although the challenges of ignorance might be dominating their possible medical effect. This chapter provides a preview of AI's application in cardiac medical care as well as discusses its latent role in simplifying precision cardiac treatment.

Keywords: Cardiac; Artificial intelligence; Cardiac illness prediction; Machine-learning

11.1 Artificial intelligence

Presently, the phrase "artificial intelligence (AI)" in the health field is glamorous, although there are misunderstanding and confusion of the techniques and terms. AI is an ambiguous and broad term that illustrates some computational agenda that mimics and simulates human intellect such as problem learning and solving. AI can point to general AI, in which the structure possesses cognition and self-sufficient [1]. However, such general AI has not come out along with application-specific AI, for a dedicated and specialized purpose, which is the AI that is presently offered by

[1]Department of Computer Science and Engineering, Sagar Institute of Research and Technology, Bhopal, India

"machine learning" that is an applied AI subfield, which routinely discovers data patterns with no use of precise instructions. Inside the machine learning, the appliances (machine) learn from the data as well as perform tasks based on the learn model, while uncomplicated computer programs execute tasks as per the fixed rules that are found in human knowledge and experience [2].

Machine learning and applied AI have been used as exchangeable within the health investigating context, since machine learning provide accommodation using AI skill in the health investigational setting. It contains a variety of algorithms intended for classification as well as prediction tasks that execute fine on composite big data. In this, "deep learning" is a machine learning algorithms subfield that is utilized deeply in the following processes such as numerous layered neural networks initially stimulated through the human brain structure [3]. These neural networks are intended presently, although they work significantly unusual as of how the human being neuron works. In the earlier decade, it was shown that the deep learning was improving and was used to be the best additional machine learning algorithms in a variety of fields, such as voice recognition, game playing, and image recognition. In the context of the classification of images, the current deep learning emergence, the CNN (convolution neural network) in 2012 had large collision on the sight. Amongst conventional machine learning algorithms that show 26% error rates, which were sensibly superior at the time, the CNN shows an exceptional 15.3% error rate [4].

CNN cloud image classification has been enhancing and the 3% current error rate improves the human eye abilities [5]. Their accomplishments are recognized to its ability to take out significant features from huge data throughout the processing of iterative data. In the selection of conventional machine learning methods that need arbitration degree as of the analyst (e.g. feature engineering: the creating variables, or features, and selection process, feature selection, which formulate algorithms and execute as superior), deep learning is usually additional self-directed one that is timely executed. For instance, in order to examine the images of chest X-ray with conventional machine learning, an analyst should primarily gather the parameters and measurements such as the heart size and the congestion present in a worksheet [6]. This categorization process loses information as well as is time-intensive. As a substitute, deep learning could supply unrefined image information and take out images' key patterns through itself. There are supervised, unsupervised, along with reinforcement learning is another terms cluster that explain the method as a machine learning as of supervised or unsupervised (Figure 11.1).

Algorithms can be trained from the data through information lying on the result; otherwise, ground fact to build up a prediction model in supervised learning. Typical responsibilities handled through supervised learning are regression as well as classification. Regression forecasts the worth (e.g. forecast the graph of echo cardio in appropriately diastolic missing ventricular recreation rate worth as of ECG information) while classification is a job for forecasting a categorized result, such as disease diagnosis and 1-year humanity (yes or no) [7,8] by specified parameters. On the opposite, the unsupervised learning techniques do not need ground fact as well as learn the data toward discovers associations and hidden patterns [9].

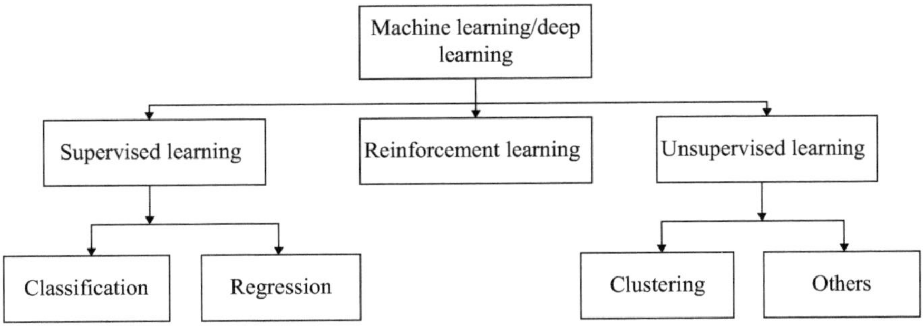

Figure 11.1 Machine learning

The main universal tasks within unsupervised learning are dimensionality reduction and clustering. Dimensionality reduction, which could be achieved within a supervised manner, is a job to decrease the dimensionality of data, i.e. the number of variables of data through observance primary variables that give details of the data. Clustering is an assignment to separate objects keen on groups by comparable characteristics. A method reinforcement learning in which an algorithm is trained toward an action gets highest reward in the position. This method is extensively used for decision-making within gaming plan. The initial plan that strikes on trained Go player is "AlphaGo;" moreover, it is used in reinforcement learning in the direction of learning the finest actions inside the Go game [10].

11.2 Traditional statistics versus AI

The standard method, namely statistics for health research is intended for the principle of viewing the new therapies benefit, identifying risk factors, predicting prognoses, and informative disease mechanisms. There are important overlaps in methodologies and techniques in the traditional statistics domain as well as AI. For illustration, linear and logistic regression replica, which are well known through nearly all health researchers, are also system in machine learning. Possibly, the primary dissimilarity is in their beliefs; statistics is an art that explains and estimates data, while machine learning or AI aims to attain realistic forecast from data by hand.

For instance, inside the linear regression models, the main significant interested parameters in statistics are the goodness-of-fit and weights or coefficients of every term, both of which explicate the data. On the other hand, AI focuses on unknown data prediction [11,12]. Therefore, the key concern of AI investigation is model concert in a test set, which is not used in the model training process, and it is offered with unusual terms as of statistics, such as confusion matrix (a cross-tabulation table category), F-measure (a harmony of positive predicted value and sensitivity), sensitivity, i.e. recall. In detail, the computation procedure is of fewer interests in AI, and various compound AI models do not yet offer other metrics and coefficients intended for interpretability.

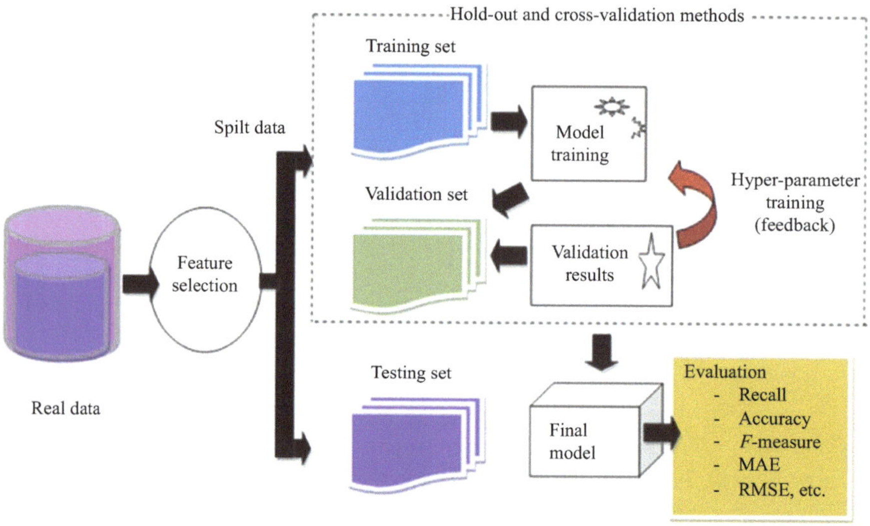

Figure 11.2 AI versus statistics

Therefore, typically AI requires a smaller amount of data assumptions and frequently uses extremely compound nonparametric models, in which it needs additional data than uncomplicated parametric models that are regularly used within conventional statistics, whereas conventional statistics execute well intended for a definite hypothesis through an appropriate sized data set, AI normally outperforms statistical methods designed for prediction within complex and large data. An additional significant consideration, particularly vital for medicine, is that AI techniques, distinct various complicated statistical investigations, have been recommended not to offer fundamental inferences.

In fact, there is changed interest in with machine learning intended for this incredible use. This developing model although should be established carefully by the offered domain information concerning disease mechanisms and pathophysiology to support the AI analysis results. Operational ability on different data structures is moreover a significant AI strength compared by conventional research [13]. Figure 11.2 sums up dissimilarity between statistics with traditional medical research and research by AI.

11.3 Representative algorithms of AI

Deep learning and machine learning consist of an algorithms multitude. Table 11.1 sums up the concise fundamental machine learning algorithms descriptions used within various tasks. Presently, deep learning and ensemble learning could be illustrated as the foundation of AI algorithms.

Deep learning is better than other conventional machine-learning algorithms in analyzing compound data such as texts, unstructured data, and images data. In universal, deep learning contained the output layer, hidden layers, and input layer, where output layers and input layers point to novel data and the algorithm output correspondingly [14]. Throughout many hidden layers, unprocessed input is steadily converted into supplementary essential features and abstract features that symbolize the novel data (Figure 11.3).

One of other machine learning methods is ensemble learning that merges several "weak" algorithms (learners) such as logistic regression and decision tree (Table 11.1) to get excellent prediction. Bagging, stacking, and boosting are the three major ensemble learning techniques [15]. Bagging is a technique in which several weak algorithms are qualified in comparable, and all algorithm results are collective to build a concluding result with minute variation. In boosting, several

Table 11.1 Description of ML algorithms

Algorithm	Uses	Description
Decision tree	Regression/ Classification	An algorithm like flowchart that separated data into different branches through allowing for information gain
Logistic regression	Classifications	A method that calculates the estimates of probability of outcome from different covariates through logistic functions
K nearest neighbor	Regression/ Classification	Methods that classify outcomes through comparing *k* instances that exist into the nearest location
Neural network	Regression/ Classification	A method that inspired through human brain architecture. Multiple layers consisting of multiple nodes are connected to one another with edges weighted as per training results
K means	Clustering	A clustering algorithm that makes a number of *k* clusters in which every outcome belongs to the cluster that has its mean in the nearby location from the outcome
SVM	Regression/ Classification	SVM draws a boundary line that increase margin from every class. New outcomes are classified through the line
PCA	Dimensionality reduction	A method that converts high-dimensional data into low-dimensional data with keeping important information as much as possible through transformation

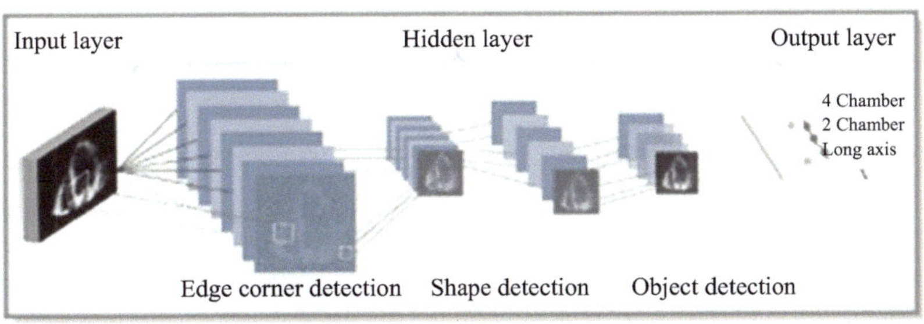

Figure 11.3 Detection system

weak algorithms are joined in series as well as qualified consequently with a consideration of preceding algorithm errors to compact bias.

The stacking method is another technique in which the weak algorithms results are used as other machine learning Meta learner (algorithm) inputs. This ensemble learning technique works extremely well through combining different types of generally outperformed and simple algorithms of any solitary machine-learning method [16,17].

11.4 Machine power along with big data

The methodologies and concept of AI methods themselves are not unused, though the unexpected wealth of AI in the earlier arises through the computing power evolution and big data emergence as well as the deep learning techniques development. Formerly, the data lacking that was a big challenge to train AI was one of the AI development's bottlenecks. Though this restriction vanished as big data happens to exist because of Internet popularization. The information in the form of digital is stored through smart devices by Internet link that could move data over a complex network with no requirement of human interface that additionally improved the functional data influx. Analyzing such big data by AI requires an enormous quantity of computational control. Graphic processing units were initially made up to execute specific tasks within gaming graphics, other than its parallel computing control fitted very well and fast also in deep learning tasks [3].

In the past decade, graphic processing units have turned reasonable whereas the computing control is continual toward developing exponentially. At present, researchers cloud also realizes services that are cloud based like infrastructure as a service, or else called machine learning as a service such as Google Cloud ML, Microsoft Azure ML, and Amazon Web Services. They offer graphic processing unit's power through a variety of AI applications along with unlimited data storage space on the cloud platform. Moreover, a number of machine learning services as a service offer automatic machine learning method, such as BigML and Google Cloud Auto ML, wherever different machine learning algorithms that are needed to minimum coding are offered [18,19]. This structure could be used through easy graphic user interfaces and might be an improved selection for researchers who are the learners of machine learning.

11.4.1 Image identification

The input layers point to the image raw pixels, and then primary layers recognize effortless image features such as lines and edges. The following layers recognize rather more compound characteristics such as tails, eyes, and ears. At last, final layers identify the features of dogs and cats. This deep learning method takes out main characteristics from unprocessed unstructured data and returns results as regression or classification. At present, most health research is completed with structured data effectively, which is organized and labeled properly into design field into a tabular shape [20].

11.4.2 Structured data

This data can be applied in unsupervised machine learning method efficiently and naturally. Recently, our group [21,22] applies a new data analytics [23] method to identify data analysis in a topological form to construct a patient–patient correspondence system that uses the mathematics foundation and a fundamentally unsupervised machine learning method. This data analysis is a structure intended for machine learning; it amalgamates and borrows different machine learning techniques to understand the essential property as well as the outline of the compound data. The learning is useful for the technique to realize the phenotypic illustration of left ventricular response pattern within the aortic stenosis progression.

11.4.3 Unstructured data

Whenever data stores up with unorganized collection called unstructured data that is applied on traditional statistical and tabular databases. Textual information in medical images, electronic health records, and visual clips and audio are the data examples that are considered unstructured data in the health field. The machine learning emergence has opened prospect to efficiently examine that data which is notion to have 80% toward 90% of every potentially method [17,24] as well as an enormous resource intended for medicinal research.

11.4.4 Medical images

Conventionally, it was hard to be used for a computer without human intervention dealing with medical images, while they have a huge range of illness patterns. The physician has had to completely analyze, interpret, and read medical images variety. These procedures could be one of the bottlenecks and time-consuming of medical practice. Deep learning, other derivative neural networks and particularly CNN are suitable for a game changer within the medical image analysis process by its ability to discover features to classify and segment objects and pixels in images [25,26].

A CNN to build up a pipeline for computerization of the following echocardiography tasks: (1) image segmentation, (2) view classification, (3) cardiac function and structure measurements, and (4) diseases discrimination. In the learning, this deep learning method was trained during a supervised approach to categorize images in 1 of 23 categories of views (remote parasternal long axis, normal parasternal long axis, etc.) by 70 000 preprocessed images produced of 277 echocardiograms. During a 5-fold cross-validation, that algorithm can wonderfully differentiate extensive subclasses from one other through a generally 84% classification accuracy. For the segmentation of images, the other method was trained to section cardiac chamber within five views (parasternal long, short-axis views, apical 2-chambers, 3-chambers, and 4-chambers), correspondingly. Subsequent to supervised learning method by 124 toward 214 images for each solo view, the methods were able to section areas of entity cardiac chambers through tremendous overlap toward human-annotated chambers areas. By these areas of auto-annotated chambers, they designed left ventricular mass, left ventricular expulsion portion, and chamber quantity, which was decided through physically calculated values as 15%–17% [27–29].

In this study, we have found out and disguised the direct diagnosis and auto-analysis possibility from echocardiography images by deep learning technique. Sign data including phonocardiogram's signal and ECG modalities contain sound, ECG, oscillometric devices, phonocardiogram, and several wearable approaches. One of the top-studied signals is ECG signal in cardiovascular medication. Deep learning methods have saturated this field as well. Recently, we have built up a deep learning method that classifies solitary lead ECG in different 12 rhythms classes, such as functional rhythm, sinus rhythm, atrial fibrillation, and atrioventricular block [30]. They used raw ECG signals 30 from solitary lead of 91232 ECGs ambulatory, which were marked via specialized ECG technicians, i.e. supervised learning toward trained or learned algorithm. Following training of that algorithm recognized arrhythmias within 328 test sets through enhanced accuracy, i.e. F-measure 0.84 other than cardiologists attains averaged F-measure 0.78. An additional signal of attention in cardiovascular medication is the heart sound information (i.e. phonocardiogram). PhysioNet Resources, an investigated source is recognized for the studies on physiologic signals and biomedical [31].

11.5 Challenges to implementation

The amount of clinical applications and research by AI [32] will additional augment paralleled through a constant evolution of customary AI platforms and computing power. Researchers and clinicians will be further probable to be concerned. Thus, learning and understanding terminologies and their limitations and possibilities will be additionally vital. This cardiovascular illness is one of the fields that cannot efficiently be diagnosed because of its multifactorial complex nature. Existing barriers to adoption occupy numerous issues concerning infrastructures slightly than AI techniques. Primary, by privacy concern, open data accessibility is incomplete compared with additional fields. Methodical companies and organizations will require setting up data infrastructure through adequate confidentiality policy. Regularization for ethical and legal issues is too significant. Since AI devices could change through learning as real-world data changes still after consumption, the conventional paradigm of health [33] tool regularization is not adequate.

As AI approach leads toward complicated medical results, current laws may not illuminate the accountability. However, systems and technologies are constantly enhancing. Furthermore, numerous rules are now individual recognized for the medical AI research standardization. Investigation data has exposed that there is a readiness to hold these changes, particularly in a younger surgeon.

A modern learning is that radiology residents approximately 95% would attend AI information courses if presented as well as 70% confirmed that they would be similar to sophisticated training into the field. Expectantly, in the approaching decades, a numeral of well-intended study on create big data will accompany in a novel model in medicine.

11.6 Conclusion and future work

AI has appeared as a promising apparatus within cardiovascular medicine. Through the popularization of machine power and big data, the healthcare fundamentals research and practice is a hurdle for change. Conventional statistics continues extremely effectual in an easy data set as well as in assessing fundamental relationship, although lots of areas in scientific research and practice will be led through powerful exploration and prediction of big data by AI. Mainly, the AI capabilities to examine unstructured data expand the cardiovascular research field. AI wills additional augment as its contribution toward synthetic data generation, computational modeling, and mobile health, with original regularizations intended for its ethical and legal issues. In this standard shift, disease mechanisms and physiology deep understanding remain primary to understand the AI results. Meanwhile, AI literacy will become necessary to appreciate the newest medical information and to utilize the new medical or health devices.

References

[1] Mozaffarian D, Benjamin EJ, Go AS, *et al.* Executive summary: heart disease and stroke statistics – 2016 update: a report from the American Heart Association. *Circulation*. 2016; 133: 447–454.

[2] Rajkomar A, Dean J, and Kohane I. Machine learning in medicine. *N Engl J Med*. 2019; 380: 1347–1358.

[3] LeCun Y, Bengio Y, and Hinton G. Deep learning. *Nature*. 2015; 521: 436.

[4] Krizhevsky A, Sutskever I, and Hinton GE. ImageNet classification with deep convolutional neural networks. *Adv Neural Inf Process Syst*. 2012:1097–1105. Available at: https://papers.nips.cc/paper/4824-imagenet-classification-withdeep-convolutional-neural-networks.pdf.

[5] Szegedy C, Ioffe S, Vanhoucke V, and Alemi AA. Inception-v4, inception-ResNet and the impact of residual connections on learning. *Thirty-First AAAI Conference on Artificial Intelligence*. 2017. Available at: www.cs.cmu.edu/~jeanoh/16-785/papers/szegedy-aaai2017-inception-v4.pdf. Accessed January 10, 2021.

[6] Mayr A, Binder H, Gefeller O, and Schmid M. The evolution of boosting algorithms. From machine learning to statistical modelling. *Methods Inf Med*. 2014; 53: 419–427.

[7] Narula S, Shameer K, Salem Omar AM, Dudley JT, and Sengupta PP. Machine learning algorithms to automate morphological and functional assessments in 2D echocardiography. *J Am Coll Cardiol*. 2016; 68: 2287–2295.

[8] Motwani M, Dey D, Berman DS, *et al.* Machine learning for prediction of all-cause multicentre prospective registry analysis. *Eur Heart J.* 2017; 38: 500–507.

[9] Lancaster MC, Salem Omar AM, Narula S, Kulkarni H, Narula J, and Sengupta PP. Phenotypic clustering of left ventricular diastolic function parameters: patterns and prognostic relevance. *JACC Cardiovasc Imaging.* 2019; 12: 1149–1161.

[10] Silver D, Huang A, Maddison CJ, *et al.* Mastering the game of go with deep neural networks and tree search. *Nature.* 2016; 529: 484.

[11] Shameer K, Johnson KW, Glicksberg BS, Dudley JT, and Sengupta PP. Machine learning in cardiovascular medicine: are we there yet? *Heart.* 2018; 104: 1156–1164.

[12] Sengupta PP, and Shrestha S. Machine learning for data-driven discovery: the rise and relevance. *JACC Cardiovasc Imaging.* 2019; 12: 690–692.

[13] Gandhi S, Mosleh W, Shen J, and Chow CM. Automation, machine learning, and artificial intelligence in echocardiography: a brave new world. *Echocardiography.* 2018; 35: 1402–1418.

[14] Seetharam K, Shrestha S, and Sengupta PP. Artificial intelligence in cardiovascular medicine. *Curr Treat Options Cardiovasc Med.* 2019; 21: 25.

[15] Wang G, Hao J, Ma J, and Jiang H. A comparative assessment of ensemble learning for credit scoring. *Expert Syst Appl.* 2011; 38: 223–230.

[16] U.S. Food and Drug Administration. FDA news release: FDA permits marketing of artificial intelligence-based device to detect certain diabetes-related eye problems. 2018. Available at: https://fda.gov/news-events/press-announcements/fda-permits-marketing-artificial-intelligence-based-devicedetect-certain-diabetes-related-eye. Accessed May 24, 2019.

[17] Gandomi A, and Haider M. Beyond the hype: big data concepts, methods, and analytics. *Int J Inf Manage.* 2015; 35: 137–144.

[18] Pilkerton CS, Singh SS, Bias TK, and Frisbee SJ. Changes in cardiovascular health in the United States, 2003–2011. *J Am Heart Assoc.* 2015; 4: e001650.

[19] Johnson KW, Shameer K, Glicksberg BS, *et al.* Enabling precision cardiology through multiscale biology and systems medicine. *JACC Basic Transl Sci.* 2017; 2: 311–327.

[20] Diller GP, Kempny A, Babu-Narayan SV, *et al.* Machine learning algorithms estimating prognosis and guiding therapy in adult congenital heart disease: data from a single tertiary centre including 10 019 patients. *Eur Heart J.* 2019; 40: 1069–1077.

[21] Casaclang-Verzosa G, Shrestha S, Khalil MJ, *et al.* Network tomography for understanding phenotypic presentations in aortic stenosis. *JACC Cardiovasc Imaging.* 2019; 12: 236–248.

[22] Frizzell JD, Liang L, Schulte PJ, *et al.* Prediction of 30-day all-cause readmissions in patients hospitalized for heart failure: comparison of machine learning and other statistical approaches. *JAMA Cardiol.* 2017; 2: 204–209.

[23] Sujatha R, Nathiya S, and Chatterjee JM. (2020). Clinical data analysis using IoT data analytics platforms. In Raj P, Chatterjee J, Kumar A, and Balamurugan B (Eds.) *Internet of Things Use Cases for the Healthcare Industry*. Cham: Springer, 271–293.

[24] Clifford GD, Liu C, Moody B, *et al.* Classification of normal/abnormal heart sound recordings: the PhysioNet/computing in cardiology challenge 2016. *2016 Comput Cardiol Conf (CinC)*. 2016; 43: 609–612.

[25] Zhang N, Yang G, Gao Z, *et al.* Deep learning for diagnosis of chronic myocardial infarction on nonenhanced cardiac cine MRI. *Radiology*. 2019; 291: 606–617.

[26] Wolterink JM, Leiner T, de Vos BD, van Hamersvelt RW, Viergever MA, and Isgum I. Automatic coronary artery calcium scoring in cardiac CT angiography using paired convolutional neural networks. *Med Image Anal.* 2016; 34: 123–136.

[27] Zhang J, Gajjala S, Agrawal P, *et al.* Fully automated echocardiogram interpretation in clinical practice. *Circulation*. 2018; 138: 1623–1635.

[28] Potes C, Parvaneh S, Rahman A, and Conroy B. Ensemble of feature-based and deep learning-based classifiers for detection of abnormal heart sounds. *2016 Comput Cardiol Conf (CinC)*. 2016; 2016: 621–624.

[29] Mallya S, Overhage M, Srivastava N, Arai T, and Erdman C. Effectiveness of LSTMs in predicting congestive heart failure onset. arXiv preprint arXiv:1902.02443. 2019. Available at: https://arxiv.org/abs/1902.02443. Accessed August 11, 2019.

[30] Hannun AY, Rajpurkar P, Haghpanahi M, *et al.* Cardiologist-level arrhythmia detection and classification in ambulatory electrocardiograms using a deep neural network. *Nat Med*. 2019; 25: 65–69.

[31] Molinaro AM, Simon R, and Pfeiffer RM. Prediction error estimation: a comparison of resampling methods. *Bioinformatics*. 2005; 21: 3301–3307; 135:e24–e44.

[32] Jain V, and Chatterjee JM. (2020). *Machine Learning with Health Care Perspective*. Cham: Springer.

[33] Agrawal R, Chatterjee JM., Kumar A, Rathore PS., and Le DN (Eds.). (2020). *Machine Learning for Healthcare: Handling and Managing Data*. Boca Raton, FL: CRC Press.

Chapter 12

Deep data analysis for COVID-19 outbreak

S.O. Owoeye[1], *O.J. Odeyemi*[1], *F.O. Durodola*[1] *and K.I. Adenuga*[2]

Abstract

The rampaging effects of the coronavirus disease in 2019 (COVID-19), which was pronounced a pandemic on 11 March 2020 by the World Health Organization (WHO), have become one of the biggest challenges of the twenty-first century in terms of general wellbeing and safety. The effects of COVID-19, with over 100 million positive cases and more than 3 million deaths, have caused great damage to the social, economic and family well-being of people around the world. Clinical studies of COVID-19 have shown that patients are mostly infected from the lungs as a result of the SARS-COV-2 virus (severe acute respiratory syndrome coronavirus 2), for which the data collected from various patients are huge for medical practitioners to analyse and capture the trends. To solve this problem, the concept of deep data analysis comes into play. Deep data analysis is a process used in deriving useful information, trends and analysing large-scale data. Making use of deep analytics processes will ensure that needed results are gotten from millions of COVID-19 data. This chapter discusses the various deep analytics applications and how they can be used specifically for COVID-19 data. One very useful deep analytics technique is the convolutional neural network (CNN) model. CNN has shown to be useful in analysing image data and this technique can be applied in COVID-19-related situations. A method of diagnosing positive COVID-19 patients involves chest X-ray, radiography. The captured X-rays can be fed to a trained CNN model that checks for differences between that of the positive patients and a healthy one. Thus, deep analytics through CNN can be useful in diagnosing COVID-19 patients. To carry out the deep analytics, the COVID-19 radiography database on Kaggle was used. This chest X-ray database consists of 3,615 COVID-19 positive images, 10,192 normal images, 1,345 viral pneumonia images and 6,012 lung opacity images. After cleaning the data, they were split into training, testing and validation sets. The trained CNN model was trained to distinguish between the four different groups of images. Eventually, the proposed system was synchronized with Internet of Things–based

[1]Department of Mechatronics Engineering, Federal University of Agriculture, Abeọkuta, Nigeria
[2]Farnborough College of Technology, University Center Farnborough, Farnborough, United Kingdom

health monitoring tools and provides results to doctors and health workers, in general, to adequately diagnose and assist in the treatment of COVID-19.

Keywords: Chest scan; Convolutional neural network; COVID-19; Deep data analysis; Diseases; Diagnosis; Internet of Things; X-ray

12.1 Introduction to deep data analysis

We live in a data-driven world where the success of businesses lies in how well the enterprise can derive maximum satisfaction for its clients. To ensure that customers are satisfied with one's product, businesses will have to collect, collate and analyse data. Data can be collected in the form of feedback from customers that can be obtained by questionnaires and other methods. Another means of collecting data could be by trying to understanding the specific needs of such customers. For instance, an online business can collect data by measuring customers' clicks on their websites; this will enable the business to understand the specific needs of their customers [1].

To understand what deep data analysis entails, we need to know what data is in the first place. Data is simply a means to represent information required for a particular purpose. In the technical sense, data is a set of values of quantitative or qualitative variables describing at least one person or object [2] while a datum (singular of data) is a single value of a single variable [3]. Data is useful only when it becomes information for making decisions after it has been properly analysed.

Deep learning can be defined as a group of learning procedures that are used to model data having various architectures, by utilizing multiple non-linear transformations. The basic element of deep learning is the neural networks that come together to produce the deep neural networks (DNNs).

The methodologies for analysing deep data include [4] the following sections.

12.1.1 Data visualization

Data visualization (Figure 12.1) involves drawing out a graphic representation of the data that makes it easier to locate trends and patterns in the data. This is an efficient and quick way of deriving conclusions from a dataset. Various visualization techniques can be employed such as bar graphs, histograms, scatterplots and heatmap.

12.1.2 Descriptive statistics

Descriptive statistics is the process of making quantitative descriptions or summarizing features from a collection of information [6]. Descriptive statistics simply helps to understand specific features of data by producing simple summaries about the dataset. It uses both analytical and graphical methods that provide the statistics needed to model and predict variations as well as to make numbers visible for communication purposes.

12.1.3 Predictive modelling

Predictive modelling is very important in data analytics as it gives accurate insights into the data and allows users to create forecasts of the available data. This method of modelling is very common in building artificial intelligent systems through the assistant of machine learning and data mining method, and the system can accurately predict what might happen next. Predictive modelling has several applications such as in HR analytics, whereby the model can identify employees who are high retention risks [7].

12.1.4 Machine learning

Machine learning (Figure 12.2) is a common method employed in data analysis. It is a branch of artificial intelligence with the working principle of a system learning from available data, by recognizing patterns and making decisions with little or no human interference [8]. Machine learning makes it possible to apply complex mathematical calculations to deep data very quickly and efficient.

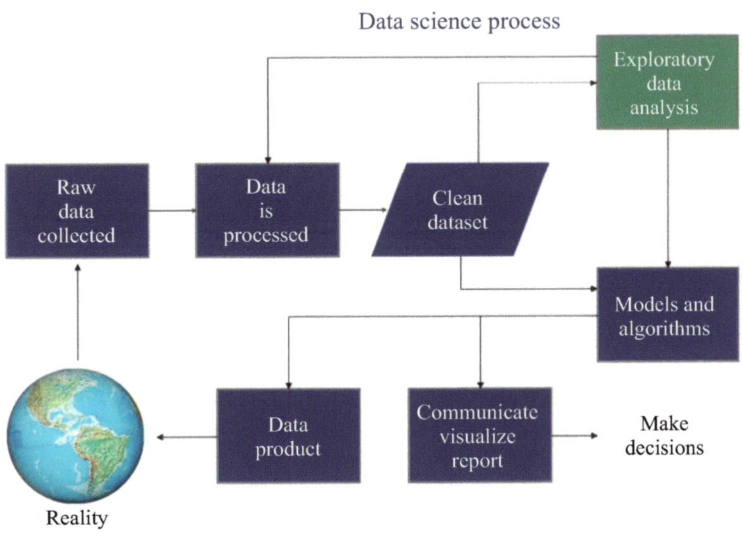

Figure 12.1 Data visualization in analysing data [5]

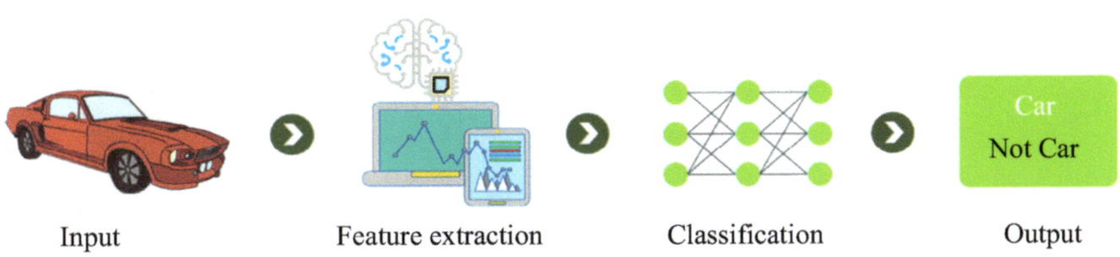

Figure 12.2 Machine learning [9]

Machine learning is of three broad categories as follows.

12.1.4.1 Supervised learning

This is one of the approaches used in machine learning in which a function or mapping is inferred from trained data, in supervised learning, each of the training examples (data) contains a pair of vectors (input vector and output vectors). The input vector is always explained by their respective supervisory signal that is known as the output vector, thereby creating an inferred function that can be used in mapping new examples [6]. The various stages involved in supervised learning are shown in Figure 12.3.

The supervised learning algorithms can be classified into two, namely regression and classification:

1. Regression: Supervised learning techniques whose output variables are continuous and can be assigned any real value that is regression type. The examples are weight, size and amount.
2. Classification: This is a type of supervised learning in which the output vectors are usually discrete or non-continuous such as gender (male or female), colour (black, white, red, etc.).

12.1.4.2 Unsupervised learning

Unsupervised learning is made up of unlabelled data, that means, it does not require a supervisory signal or training data (see Figure 12.4). It involves the grouping of data variables with similar characteristics or attributes.

12.1.4.3 Semi-supervised learning

Unlike supervised learning where all the classes of input variables are well labelled, in semi-supervised learning, only a few out of large datasets are labelled. The unlabelled datasets are then classified about the labelled sets, i.e. the labelled sets are used as a guide for the unlabelled data as shown in Figure 12.5.

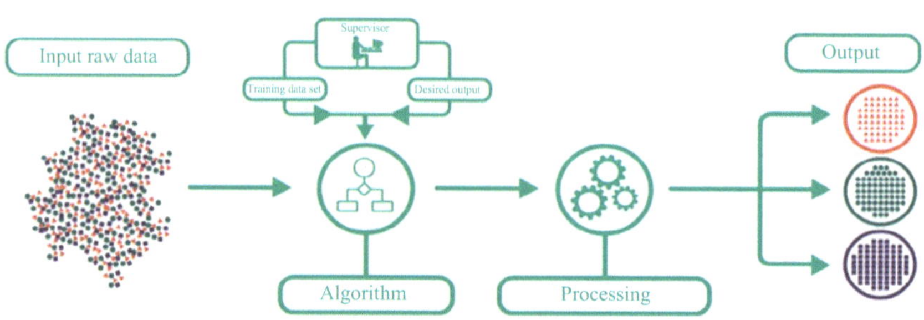

Figure 12.3 Supervised learning [10]

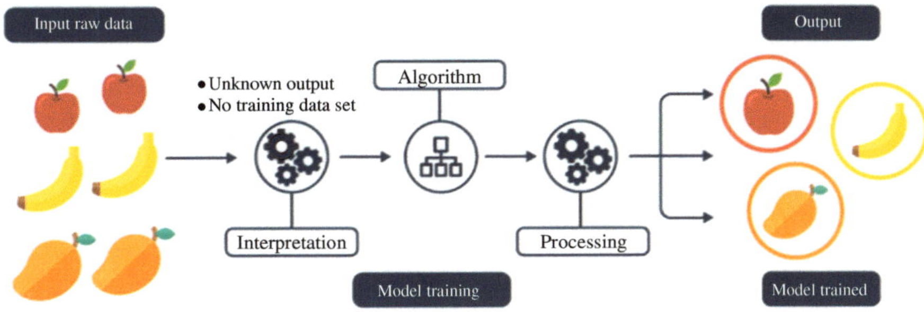

Figure 12.4 Unsupervised learning [11]

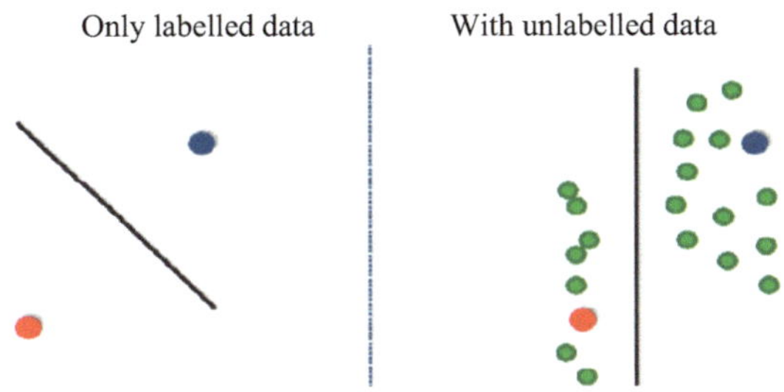

Figure 12.5 Semi-supervised learning [7]

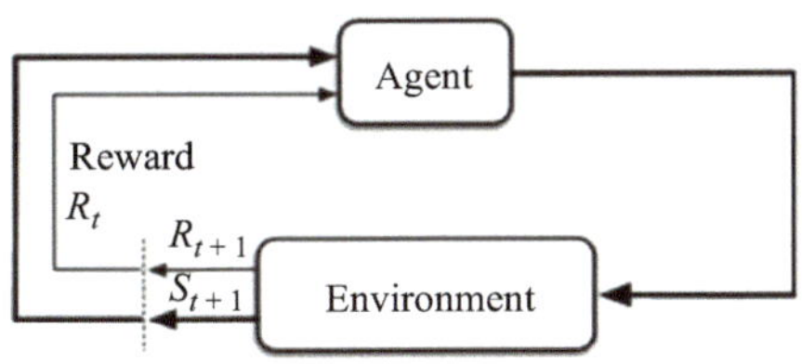

Figure 12.6 Reinforcement learning [12]

12.1.4.4 Reinforcement learning

This is also another method of machine learning in which output vectors are solely dependent on the inputs, and the next input vector is dependent on the output of the previous input. As shown in Figure 12.6, this chain continues until the processing is stopped. A typical example is a game of chess.

Machine learning has vast applications in various fields like financial market analysis, handwriting recognition, credit card fraud detection, image classification, disease diagnosis, natural language processing, speech recognition, recommender systems.

12.1.5 Data reduction

Data reduction simply means the reduction of certain parts of data. Data reduction is a method of data analysis that allows you to remove the information that is not needed from the data, thereby making it easier to draw meaning from the dataset. One way of achieving this is by a technique called dimensionality reduction. This involves transforming high dimensionally spaced data into data with a low dimensionally spaced such that the low-dimensional representation does not undergo any loss in the useful properties of the original data [13].

12.1.6 Multivariate analysis

Multivariate analysis is used in situations where several measurements are carried out for all the experimental units with special emphasis on the determination of the relationship between these quantities and their structures are of paramount importance [14]. It also involves the observation and analysis of more than one outcome of the statistical variable at a time.

12.1.7 Regression analysis

Regression analysis methods are employed to investigate the relationship between dependent variables and independent variables. There are various forms of regression analysis such as linear regression that makes use of a linear model by trying to fit a straight line through the data, and logistic regression is used to estimate the probability of an existing binary class.

12.1.8 Data wrangling

This is another method of analysing deep data which involves the gathering, selection and transforming data to answer various analytical questions [10]. It is a process that transforms and maps raw data from one form into a different format with the sole aim of making it more appropriate and useful for various purposes.

12.2 Deep data analysis for COVID-19

The virus causing COVID-19 is known as the severe acute respiratory syndrome coronavirus 2 (SARS-COV-2) [15]. This virus is known to be causing diseases ranging from the common cold to more serious types like the SARS. It is a highly communicable disease and it is contacted from person to person through infected air droplets, during coughing or sneezing by an infected person. It is also transmittable through hands contact or contact with an infected surface. There are several ways to diagnose COVID-19 such as viral tests in nose swab, CT scans and X-rays, while chest X-rays are a good means of diagnosing COVID-19 infections, it is not always easy for medical personnel to visually distinguish between the X-ray scans of a normal person and that of a COVID-19 positive patient. To solve this problem, the idea of deep data analytics for COVID-19 comes into play.

Deep data analytics for COVID-19 aims at finding an accurate and efficient means of diagnosing COVID-19 infections. Its models have proven to be very useful in image classification tasks and as such, they can be employed in tackling the problem of COVID-19 diagnosis. The method used in this chapter aims at building a deep data model capable of classifying X-ray image data into two groups of either the chest scan is that of a normal person or it belongs to an infected person. The question then arises on what deep data analytics algorithm is to employ in solving the problem at hand.

Artificial neural networks (ANNs) are systems that are designed using the mechanisms of neurons in the nervous system of the human brain as template, which could be either hardware or software. The deep learning technology utilizes this type of neural network that comes under the broad domain of artificial intelligence. Various categories of neural networks utilize different principles in defining their own rules. There are various types of ANNs and each of these types has its unique strengths.

Some popular deep learning architecture are ANNs, generative adversarial networks (GANs), DNNs, recurrent neural networks (RNNs), convolutional neural networks (CNNs) and deep belief networks (DBNs).

12.2.1 Artificial neural networks

ANNs are systems built to mimic the biological functioning of the human brain. The human brain is composed of 86 billion nerve cells called neurons [16] that are connected by axons which act as synapses to carry out specific functions when activated. Through this looping process, a neuron can send messages to other neurons in the unit.

Like the biological neural circuit shown in Figure 12.7, an ANN is composed of multiple nodes, connected by links and capable of interacting with each other.

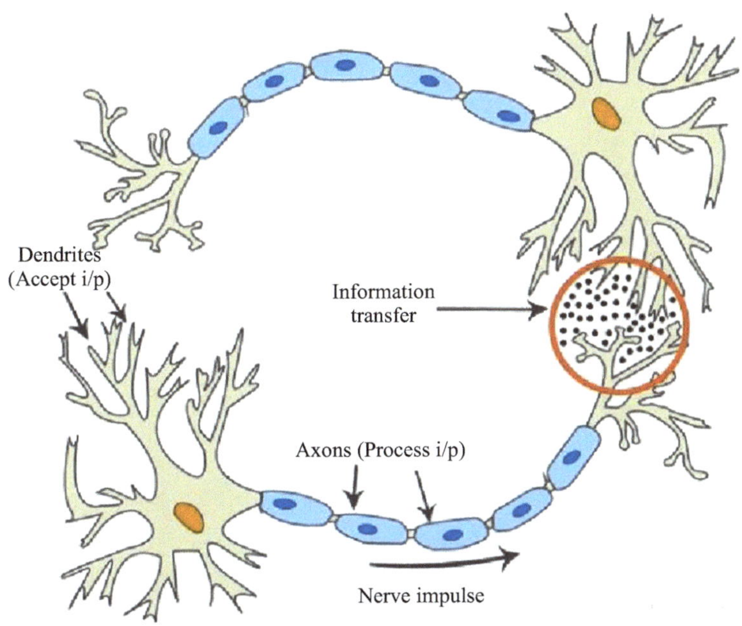

Figure 12.7 Biological neural circuit [16]

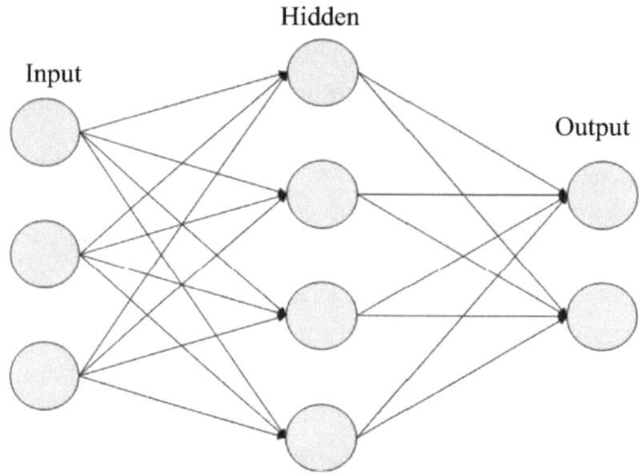

Figure 12.8 One-layer ANN [16]

Each link is a weight, and the ANN learns by continuously adjusting these weights according to a learning rule metric, till the error value is just small enough. Such systems learn to perform the task by analysing various examples. In image recognition, the system can learn to identify images of an animal according to the label name, such that, when the label is absent, the system will be able to make predictive inferences from the animal image.

Figure 12.8 shows a simple ANN model. It has three input neurons and produces two output neurons. As in every deep learning model, there are multiple hidden layers that have a particular task to perform. There are two types of ANN: feedforward ANN and feedback ANN.

Feedforward neural network is perhaps one of the easiest forms of ANNs. In a feedforward neural network, data is made to pass through various input nodes until the output node is reached. This implies that the movement of data is in a particular direction starting with the first level until it gets to the output point. This method, which can be achieved using the classifying activation function, is also referred to as a front propagated. Although in some complex forms of neural networks, backpropagation might not exist making the transfer of the data to be unidirectional only, in a feedforward ANN there might be only one layer or it might contain some other hidden layers.

Feedforward neural networks can be applied in different technological fields like face recognition, machine vision and computer vision. This is due to the difficulty in classifying the target classes in these applications. It has also the ability to deal with data that contains a lot of outliers. The relative simplicity in maintaining this type of neural network also contributed to its wide usage.

12.2.2 Deep neural networks

A DNN can be referred to as a complex form of the ANN. It is simply an ANN that has many hidden layers.

Figure 12.9 shows a DNN model. The major difference between the DNN and ANN is the number of hidden layers. The DNN and ANN both consist of the same components; neurons, synapses, weights, biases and functions. DNN are capable of modelling complex non-linear relationships by dedicating each hidden layer to perform a specific operation. For example, in an image recognition program, the first hidden layer can be used to train the system on facial features. The second hidden layer can be used to analyse other things like background, colour, etc.

12.2.3 Generative adversarial networks

GANs are DNNs that use two types of networks: the first is the generator that creates new data illustrations, and the other is the discriminator that assesses their level of authenticity, as shown in Figure 12.10. These networks are sited against each other, and they are in a constant battle till some form of equilibrium is reached. Equilibrium is achieved when the discriminator can no longer tell real images from fake ones created by the generator.

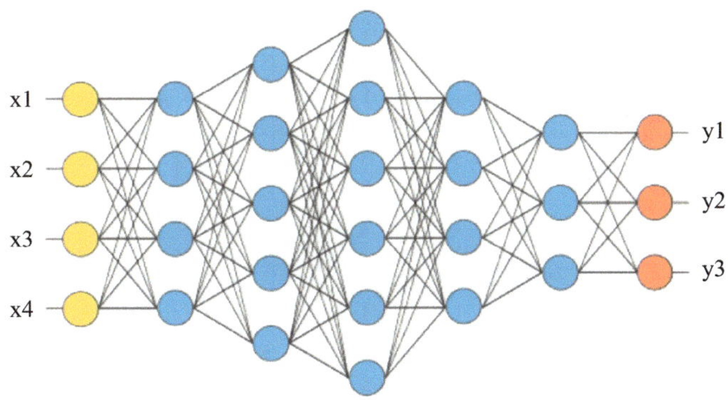

Figure 12.9 DNN with five hidden layers [17]

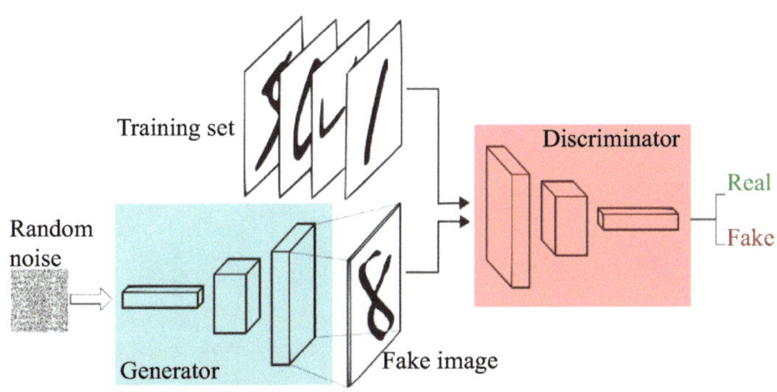

Figure 12.10 GANs [18]

12.2.4 Deep belief networks

In deep learning, a DBN is a form of DNN with several of its layer hidden, in which there is an interconnection among the layers, although no interconnection exists within units of individual layers [19]. A DBN could be visualized as a stack of restricted Boltzmann machines (RBM) where the visible layer of the RBM is the hidden layer of one RBM directly below it. DBNs have the ability to reconstruct their inputs then use them as feature detectors during training.

12.2.5 Convolutional neural network

This type of neural network is based on a variation of multilayer perceptions. A CNN comprises at least a convolutional layer. These layers are made to either have complete interconnectivity or pooled together. A convolutional operation is first performed on the layer, then the result is passed to the next layer. Because of this convolutional operation, the network becomes deeper though with lesser parameters, CNNs have also shown to be very effective in applications involving natural language processing, video and image recognition and recommender systems.

The CNN also shows great outcomes in semantic parsing and paraphrase detection. Their applications also extend to signal processing and image classification.

They are also being used in the analysis of images and recognition in agricultural sector to predict the growth of crops and yield of a farmland through the use of weather data obtained from satellites like LSAT. Figure 12.11 shows a representation of a CNN.

12.2.6 Recurrent neural network (RNN) – long short-term memory

This is a form of ANN in which the result obtained from a particular layer is feedback to the input, thereby making the prediction of the possible outcomes of the next layer.

The opening layer is achieved in the same way as it is in the feedforward network, that is, using the sum of the product of the weights and features. However, in subsequent layers, the RNN process begins.

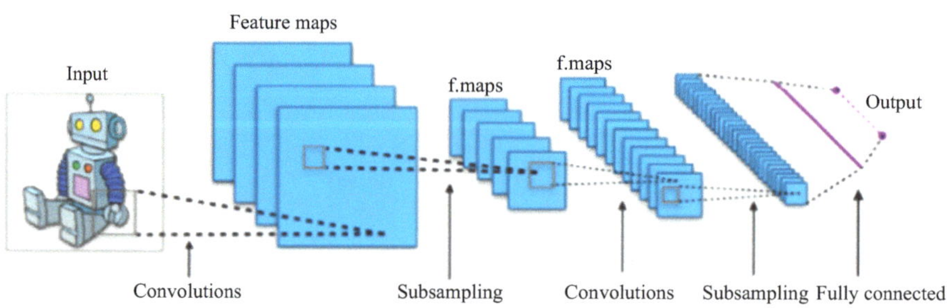

Figure 12.11 Image of convolutional neural network [20]

From each time step to the next, each node will recollect part of the information that it had in the previous time step. In other words, each of the nodes behaves like a memory cell during computations and when performing various operations. The front propagation is first carried out by the neural network but keeps the information it may need to use later.

The system self-learns, even if the initial prediction is not correct, and works at achieving the correct prediction during the backpropagation. This type of neural network is very useful in text-to-speech conversion technology. Figure 12.12 shows a representation of the RNN.

12.2.7 Modular neural network

Modular neural network has many networks that could function independently and perform sub-tasks. During the computation process, the various networks do not interrelate with or signal each other. They work independently towards achieving the output.

In this network, it is possible to carry out a large and complex computational process with great speed by breaking it down into independent components. The computation is significantly faster due to the fact that the networks are not either interacting with nor connected to one another. Figure 12.13 shows a modular neural network.

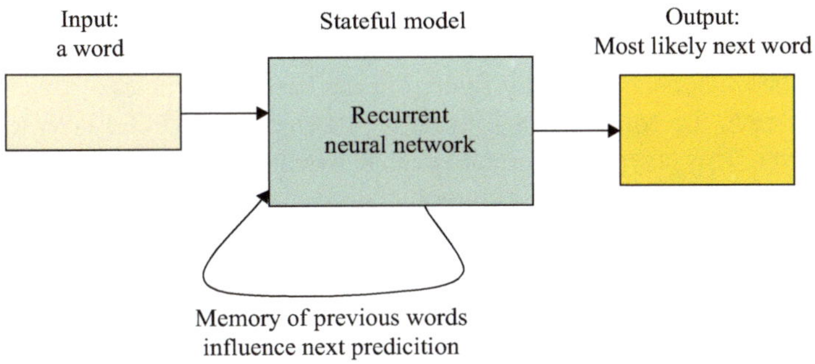

Figure 12.12 Recurrent neural network [20]

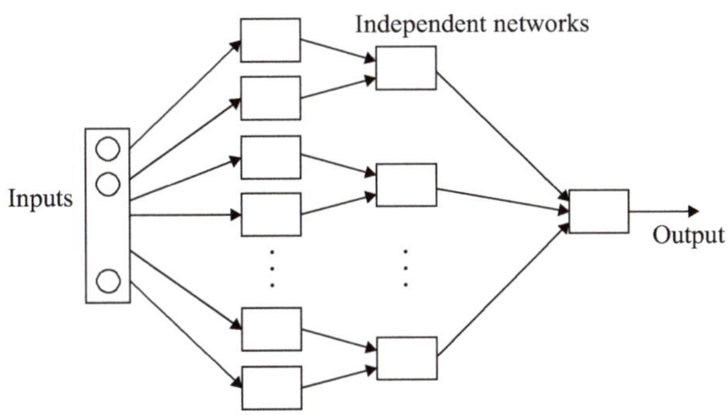

Figure 12.13 Modular neural network [21]

12.2.8 Sequence-to-sequence models

The sequence-to-sequence model is made up of two RNNs. It is made up of an encoder and a decoder that respectively processes the input and the output, the usage of the same or different limits is possible on the encoder and decoder. This type of model is suitable for application in cases where the input data length is not equal to the length of the output data. Sequence-to-sequence models can be used mainly in machine translation, chatbots, and question answering systems.

For deep data analytics in COVID-19 using chest scans, a neural network model that works effectively with visual data is needed to classify the X-rays into various groups. For this reason, a CNN model was used.

A CNN (Figure 12.14) can be referred to as an algorithm that is based on deep learning which can be modelled to accept images as input, and thereafter assigned learnable weights and biases to the different features or objects that exist in the image in order to distinguish them [16].

CNN is more efficient in dealing with visual imagery than other neural network models. For example, trying to feed an image to other neural networks can be very tasking for several reasons, one of which is the need for a large number of parameters (over 10,000 for very small images), which could lead to a loss of the 2D information due to flattening out of the image; therefore, the model will be far less accurate than if done with a CNN. In other to solve this, CNN makes a use of a convolution layer created when multiple image filters are applied to the input image. This convolution layer helps the model automatically figure out the best filter values.

In addition to the convolutional layers, CNN employs an extra layer known as a pooling layer. This layer is important because when dealing with coloured images and lots of filters, the number of parameters could be too much for the system to process. The pooling layer works by accepting an input, convolution layer then sub-sampling by picking maximum values with each stride. The pooling layer helps the

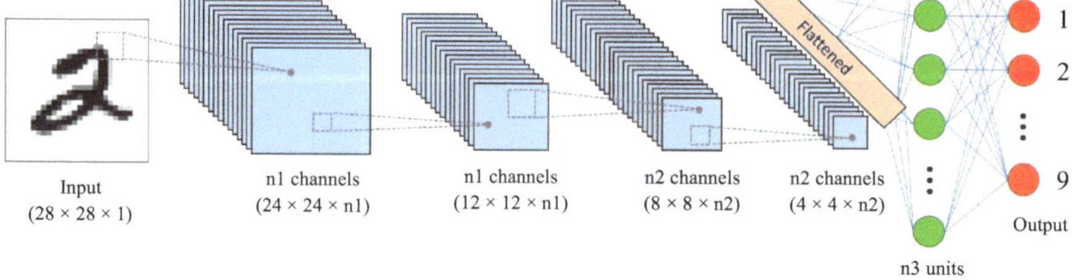

Figure 12.14 CNN algorithm to classify handwritten digits [16]

algorithm reduce the number of parameters by dropping lots of information. Another layer that works with CNN is the dropout layer. During training, units are randomly dropped to prevent the algorithm from gaining too much information, hence avoiding overfitting.

Aside from image and video recognition, CNN has various applications such as [17,18]

- Medical image analysis
- Natural language processing
- Financial time series
- Image segmentation
- Recommender systems

12.3 CNN architectures

12.3.1 LeNet

This is one of the most popular CNN architectures, and it is a digit recognition algorithm implemented in 1998 by a team of four [19]. The architecture (Figure 12.15) takes in an input image of 32 by 32 pixels and feeds it into a sequence of layers.

The first layer is convolutional and consists of six filters of size 5 by 5 pixels. A sub-sampling layer follows size 2 by 2 pixels and choosing 2 as the stride. Layer 3 is another convolutional layer having 16 filters and a size of 5 by 5 pixels, followed by the sub-sampling layer of size 2 by 2 pixels. The fifth layer connects the output of the fourth layer to the full connected layer, while the sixth layer is also a fully connected layer with 84 nodes and the final layer classifies the outputs into 10 layers representing the 10-digits.

However, the downside of this network is the inability to process large size images and classify data with a large number of classes.

12.3.2 AlexNet

AlexNet (Figure 12.16) is similar to the LeNet but has a larger number of filters, hence its ability to classify data into a large number of classes. It takes in a colour

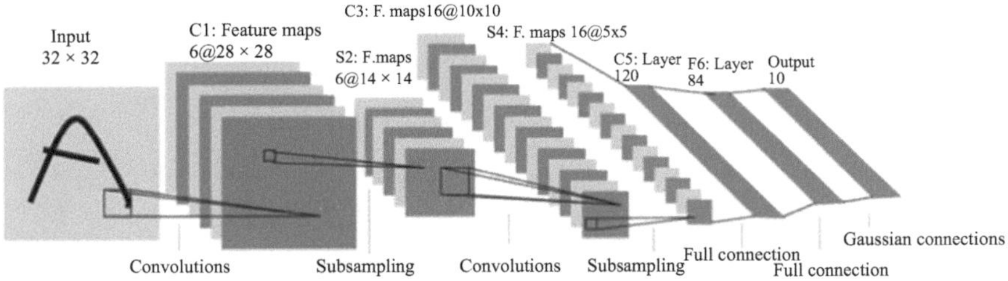

Figure 12.15 LeNet architecture [19]

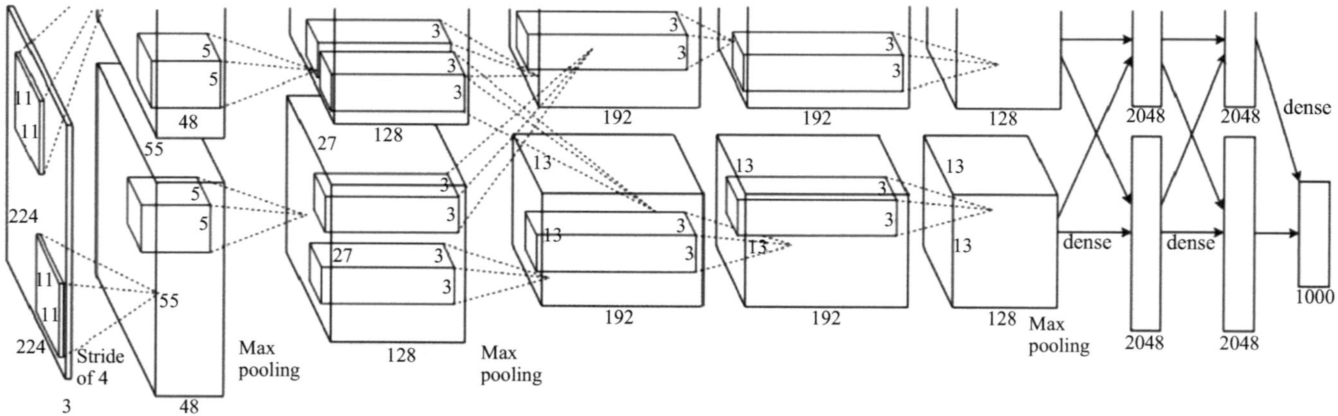

Figure 12.16 AlexNet architecture [20]

image with dimensions 224 by 224 pixels and feeds this input through 11 layers described in Table 12.1.

12.3.3 VGGNet 16

The VGGNet architecture (Figure 12.17) was designed by Simonyan and Zisserman and was able to achieve a top-5 error rate of 5.1%. It takes in a colour image with dimensions 224 by 224 and feeds this input through 21 layers described in Table 12.2.

12.3.4 Google Net/Inception

With a top-5 error rate of 6.67%, this network (Figure 12.18) won the ILSVRC 2014 competition [22]. The architecture was developed by Google and tries to implement the LeNet architecture more smartly. The Google Net architecture functions by concatenating the output of several convolution layers, thus producing a final output containing matrices from all filter operations together.

12.3.5 ResNets

This network was developed to tackle the problem of 'vanishing gradient'. Vanishing gradient problems occur when a large input space is mapped to a small one causing the derivatives to disappear. ResNet solves this problem by implementing a pre-activation variant of the residual block, to allow the gradient to flow through the connection to earlier layers [23].

Table 12.1 AlexNet features

S/N	Layer name	Features
1	Convolutional	96 filters, size = 11 by 11, stride = 4
2	Max-pooling	Size = 3 by 3, stride = 2
3	Convolutional	256 filters, size = 5 by 5, stride = 4
4	Max-pooling	Size = 3 by 3, stride = 2
5	Convolutional	384 filters, size = 3 by 3, stride = 4
6	Convolutional	384 filters, size = 3 by 3, stride = 4
7	Convolutional	256 filters, size = 3 by 3, stride = 4
8	Max-pooling	Size = 3 by 3, stride = 2
9	Connected to a hidden layer	4,096 nodes
10	Connected to a hidden layer	4,096 nodes
11	Connected to a hidden layer	SoftMax regression, 1,000 nodes

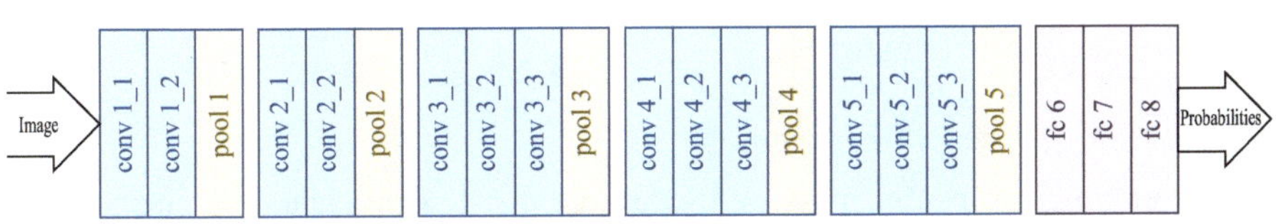

Figure 12.17 VGG16 network architecture [21]

Table 12.2 VGGNet features

S/N	Layer name	Features
1	Convolutional	64 filters
2	Convolutional	64 filters
3	Max-pooling	
4	Convolutional	128 filters
5	Convolutional	128 filters
6	Max-pooling	
7	Convolutional	256 filters
8	Convolutional	256 filters
9	Convolutional	256 filters
10	Max-pooling	
11	Convolutional	512 filters
12	Convolutional	512 filters
13	Convolutional	512 filters
14	Max-pooling	
15	Convolutional	512 filters
16	Convolutional	512 filters
17	Convolutional	512 filters
18	Max-pooling	
19	Connected to a hidden layer	4,096 nodes
20	Connected to a hidden layer	4,096 nodes
21	Connected to an output layer	SoftMax regression, 1,000 classes

12.4 Building the neural network

12.4.1 Dataset

To show how deep data analytics can be used in the diagnosis of COVID-19, we decided to build a neural network model capable of distinguishing between various chest scans images. This model does not claim 100% real-world effectiveness, but only researches about means by which deep data analytics can be employed efficiently in diagnosing COVID-19 from X-rays scans.

To aid our purpose, the dataset used for this research was culled from a Kaggle repository [24,25]. The dataset which was put together by a group of researchers from Qatar University, Doha, Qatar and the University of Dhaka includes several images of real chest X-rays. In the database, there are 10,192 normal chest X-ray images, a total of 3,615 images for COVID-19 positive cases, as well as chest X-ray images of other lung infections which include 1,345 viral pneumonia images and 6,012 lung opacity images. All images are provided with a resolution of 299 by 299 pixels in a PNG file format.

12.4.2 Data pre-processing

Before building the neural network model, the chest scans data was cleaned and processed to make it suitable for the network architecture. The data pre-processing was done over few steps:

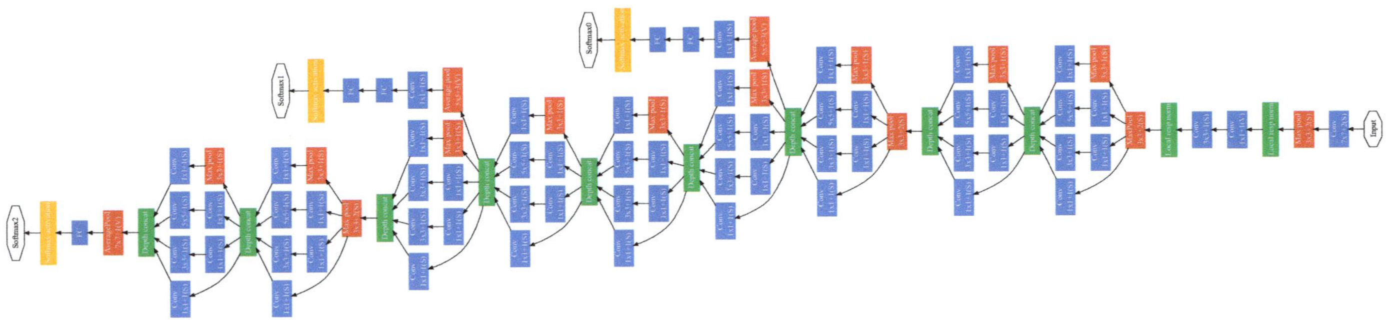

Figure 12.18 Google Net architecture [22]

1. Scaling down the data to a resolution of 100 by 100 pixels – This first step of data scaling was done to reduce the size of raw information to ensure fast training of our model.
2. Data splitting – This deep learning model involves splitting the raw data into training and testing sets. The purpose of splitting our data is to ensure that we do not make use of the same dataset for both training and prediction. This could bring about false accuracy scores and eventually lead to model overfitting. For this experiment, our data was split in the ratio 20–80 as shown in Table 12.3, where the test dataset contained 20% of the initial sample while the remaining 80% belonged to the training dataset which will be used to fit our model.

12.4.3 Train-test split

Table 12.3 Train-test split

	Total size (*t*)	Train (80%*t*)	Test (20%*t*)
Normal images	10,192	8,154	2,038
COVID-19 positive images	3,615	2,892	723
Viral pneumonia images	1,345	1,076	269
Lung opacity images	6,012	4,810	1,202

12.4.4 Data augmentation

To train the neural network sufficiently well, the learning models need a huge number of raw data to work with. Since large data is not always available, there is need for data augmentation. This is a technique in which the quantity of our raw data can be increased through the addition of some slightly modified copies to our already existing data. It generally helps to reduce model overfitting during training [26]. To augment the data, we employed several image transformation techniques such as rotating the images by 20 degrees, shifting image width and height by a maximum of 5%, image normalization, cutting away part of the image by a maximum of 10%, zooming into the image by 10%, flipping the images horizontally and filling the missing pixels with the nearest filled values.

12.5 Neural network architecture

Our proposed model as shown in Figure 12.19 involves feeding the pre-processed data into the neural network architecture. The neural network learns from it and makes predictions from which various metrics can be evaluated to determine model accuracy.

The neural network architecture (Figure 12.20) accepts an image of 150 by 150 pixels, runs it through 12 subsequent layers and produces an output of 4 classes.

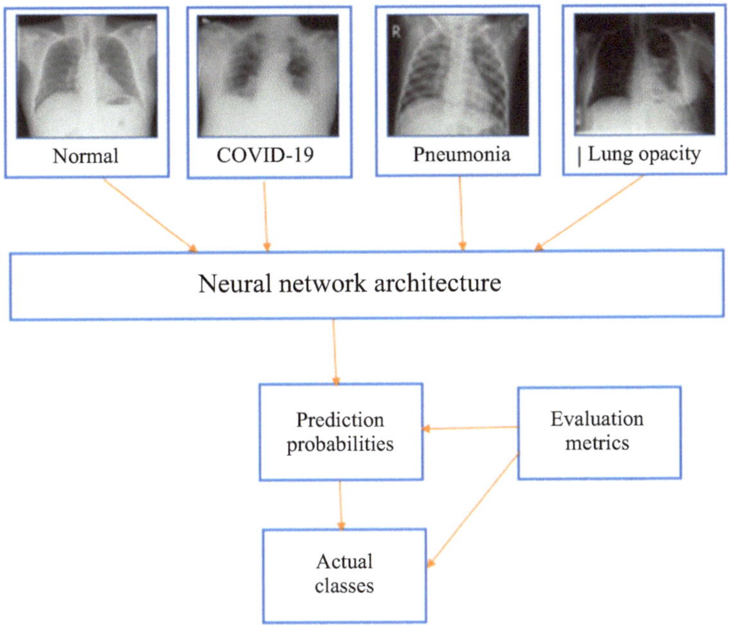

Figure 12.19 Proposed model

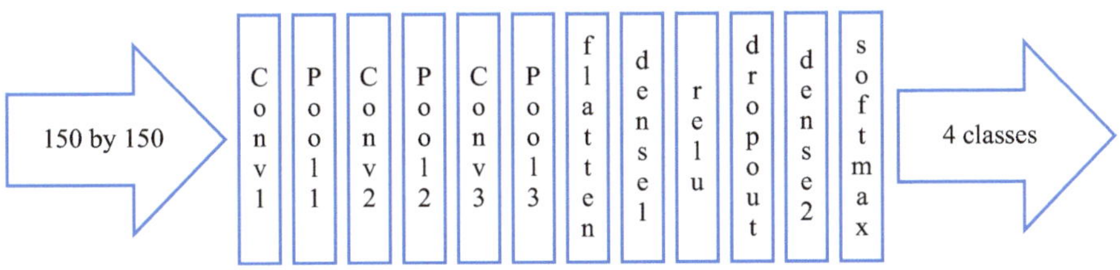

Figure 12.20 Neural network architecture

Our neural network architecture is described in Figures 12.20 and 12.21 and in the following list.

1. Layer 1 – The first layer is a 2D convolution layer that accepts images of shapes 150 by 150 pixels and converts each of these pixels in its receptive field into a single value. It has the following features:
   (i) 32 filters (represents the dimensionality of the output space)
   (ii) 3 by 3 kernel size (represents the height and width of the 2D convolution window)
   (iii) 150 by 150 input shape
   (iv) Figure 12.21 describes the rectified linear unit (ReLU) activation function. This function is governed by [27]
   $f(x) = \max\{0,x\}$ where $f(x) = 0$ if $x \leq 0$ or x if $x > 0$

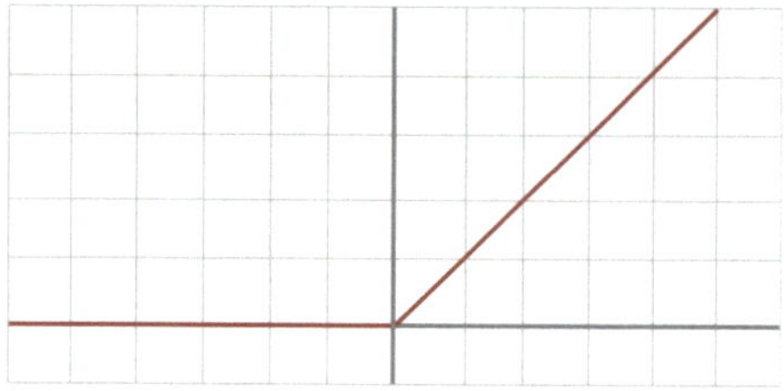

Figure 12.21 ReLU plot [27]

2. Layer 2 – This is the first max-pooling layer, it calculates the maximum values in each patch of each feature map. It also helps reduce overfitting by providing an abstracted form of representation. It was set with a 2 by 2 pool size which represents the window size over which to take the maximum.
3. Layer 3 – The second convolution layer. It has the following features:
   - 64 filters
   - 3 by 3 kernel size
   - 150 by 150 pixels input shape
   - ReLU activation
4. Layer 4 – The second pooling layer. It has a pool size of 2 by 2.
5. Layer 5 – The third convolution layer. It has the following features:
   (i) 64 filters
   (ii) 3 by 3 kernel size
   (iii) 150 by 150 pixels input shape
   (iv) ReLU activation
6. Layer 6 – The third pooling layer. It has a pool size of 2 by 2.
7. Layer 7 – The seventh layer is a Flatten layer which is used to fatten the input by converting the data into a one-dimensional array.
8. Layer 8 – This is a fully connected layer with 128 nodes. It connects the output to a hidden layer. It can be represented mathematically by

   $$Z = x \times w + b$$

   where w is the weights to the adjusted and b represents the biases.
9. Layer 9 – This layer applies a ReLU activation function to the dense layer, such that

   $$A = \mathrm{ReLU}(Z)$$

   where A is the activation function and Z is the output dense layer.
10. Layer 10 – This is a dropout layer. Dropout layers help to avoid overfitting by randomly turning neutrons off during training [28]. To configure our model, we set it to automatically turn off 50% of the neutrons.

11. Layer 11 – This is a fully connected layer with four nodes representing the four classes of predictions, i.e. normal cases, COVID-19 positive cases, viral pneumonia cases and lung opacity patients.
12. Layer 12 – This layer is an activation layer with a SoftMax activation function due to its multi-class classification task. It normalizes the final output of the network to a probability distribution over the predicted output class. This activation function is represented by the following equation [29]:

$$f(x) = \frac{e^x}{\sum_{j=1}^{J} e^x} \text{for } i = 1, J$$

12.6 Other parameters used to configure the neural network

1. Categorical cross-entropy loss function – This loss function as described in Figure 12.22 is used for multi-class classification tasks. It functions very similarly to the SoftMax activation function.
2. Adam optimizer – This is a very useful optimizer in neural network modelling. It simply optimizes the training algorithm so it can handle sparse gradients in the instance of noisy data.

12.7 Model summary

Our model was trained over the Keras framework which provides a way to summarize a model. This summary of our particular model is shown in Table 12.4 and simply describes information about:

- the layer types
- output shape of each layer
- the number of trainable and non-trainable parameters in each layer

12.8 Metrics used for evaluation

1. Confusion matrix – This is a popular metric used to evaluate the accuracy of a classification task. It computes a matrix on a test dataset for which the labels are known. The format of the matrix is described in Table 12.5.

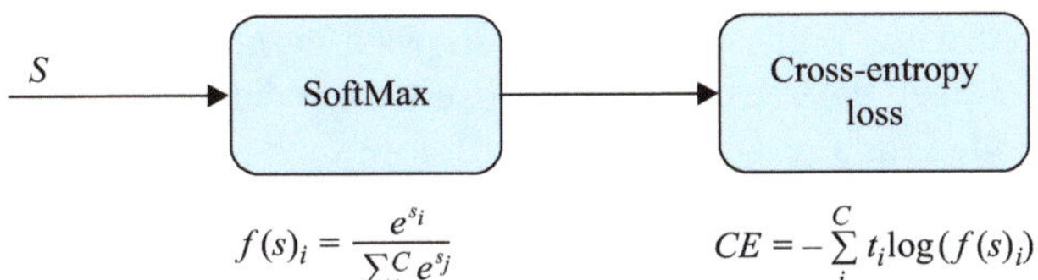

Figure 12.22 Cross-entropy loss function [30]

Table 12.4 Model summary

Layer (type)	Output shape	Parameter
2D Convolution_1	(297, 297, 32)	896
Max Pooling_1	(148, 148, 32)	0
2D Convolution_2	(146, 146, 64)	18,496
Max Pooling_2	(73, 73, 64)	0
2D Convolution_3	(71, 71, 64)	36,928
Max Pooling_3	(35, 35, 64)	0
Flatten	(78400)	0
Dense_1	(128)	10,035,328
Activation_1	(128)	0
Dropout	(128)	0
Dense_2	(4)	516
Activation_2	(4)	0

Trainable parameters – 10,092,164; non-trainable parameters – 0.

Table 12.5 Confusion matrix explained

	Predicted 'No'	Predicted 'Yes'
Actual 'No'	True negative values	False positive values
Actual 'Yes'	False negative values	True positive values

2. Confusion matrix explained.
3. Classification report – Classification report is another metric used to measure the accuracy of predictions for a classification problem. It evaluates three parameters which are as follows:

- Precision: Precision $= \frac{\text{true positives}}{\text{true positives}+\text{false positives}}$
- Recall: Recall $= \frac{\text{true positives}}{\text{true positives}+\text{false negatives}}$
- $F1$ score: $F1$ score $= 2\times \frac{\text{recall}\times\text{precision}}{\text{recall}+\text{precision}}$

12.9 Results and evaluation

After training the neural network, the prediction results showed a 70% accuracy which is rather impressive considering the few samples of image data we had to train the network with. While the network shows a high accuracy performance, it only depicts how deep data analysis can be used in the diagnosis of COVID-19 and is not recommended for a real-life situation. Before such a model can be considered for practical use, it needs to be retrained with a large number of data and the hyper-parameters duly optimized.

Figures 12.23 and 12.24 show the loss and accuracy analysis of the training and validation dataset.

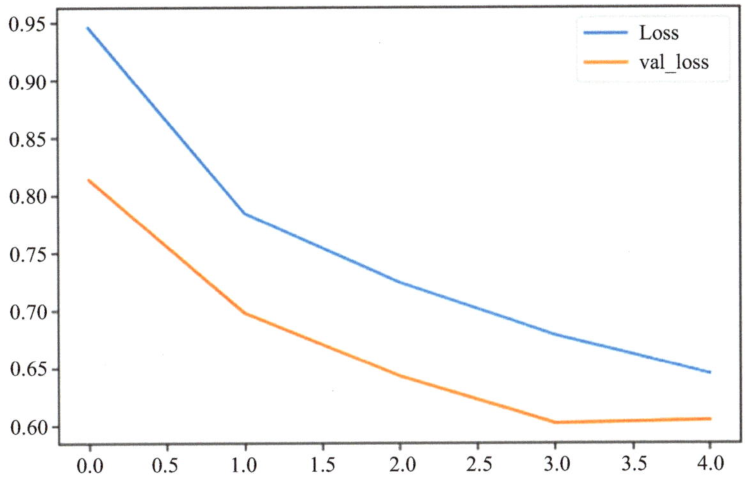

Figure 12.23 Training and validation loss

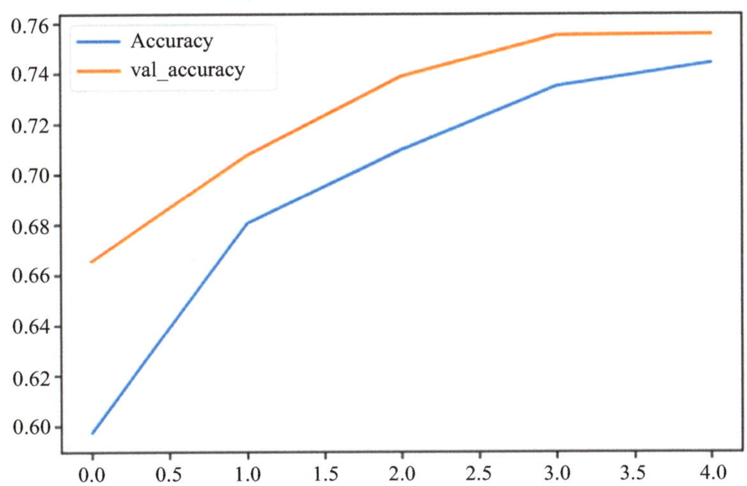

Figure 12.24 Training and validation accuracy

The following matrix and Table 12.6 discuss the results of the metrics used for evaluation which includes confusion matrix and classification report.

$$\begin{bmatrix} 287 & 155 & 279 & 2 \\ 43 & 829 & 320 & 0 \\ 60 & 222 & 1{,}743 & 13 \\ 6 & 18 & 133 & 112 \end{bmatrix}$$

Table 12.6 Classification report

	Precision	Recall	*F*1-score	Support
COVID-19	0.72	0.40	0.51	723
Lung opacity	0.68	0.70	0.69	1,202
Normal	0.70	0.86	0.77	2,038
Viral pneumonia	0.88	0.42	0.57	269
Accuracy			0.70	4,232
Macro average	0.75	0.59	0.63	4,232
Weighted average	0.71	0.70	0.69	4,232

12.10 Conclusion and future scope

The COVID-19 pandemic keeps growing by the day. Even with a breakthrough in vaccines development, it will take years before the world is completely vaccinated. Hence, a deep data analytics model that helps accurately detect positive COVID-19 cases will be very helpful during this period. In this chapter, we have experimented with a convolutional network and how it works well with image data. Here, we can classify chest X-ray scans into four different groups; normal scans and other lung infections which include COVID-19, lung opacity and pneumonia. Our neural network was basic with several convolutional and pooling layers but overall, we were able to achieve an accuracy of 70%.

Future scopes of this project should ensure that all hyper-parameters are well optimized for more accurate results as well as working with a larger database so the neural network has enough samples to train with.

References

[1] S. Otte, "What is Data Analysis?," Innoplexus, 7 December 2018. [Online]. Available: https://innoplexus.com/blog/what-is-data-analysis/. [Accessed 17 April 2021].

[2] OECD, "Glossary of Statistical Terms," Organization of Economic Co-operation and Development, p. 119, 2008.

[3] ABS, "Statistical Language – What Are Data?," Australian Bureau of Statistics, 13 July 2013.

[4] "Deep Data Analytics," Data Analytics Corp, n.d. [Online]. Available: https://dataanalyticscorp.com/consulting/deep-data-analysis/.

[5] C. O'Neil and R. Schutt, "*Doing Data Science*,", O'Reilly Media, Inc, Sebastopol, CA, October 2013.

[6] P. S. Mann, "*Introductory Statistics*," 2nd edn, Wiley, Hoboken, NJ, 1995.

[7] "What is Predictive Modelling?" MicroStrategy, n.d. [Online]. Available: https://microstrategy.com/en/resources/introductory-guides/predictive-modeling–the-only-guide-you-ll-need/. [Accessed 17 April 2021].

[8] SAS, "Machine Learning: What It Is and Why It Matters," Statistical Analysis System, n.d. [Online]. Available: https://sas.com/en_us/insights/analytics/machine-learning.html/. [Accessed 17 April 2021].

[9] DLT Labs, "Understanding Machine Learning & Deep Learning," 2 March 2020. [Online]. Available: https://dltlabs.io/.

[10] M. Thurber, "What Is Data Wrangling and Why Does It Take So Long?" Elder Research, 6 April 2018. [Online]. Available: https://elderresearch.com/blog/what-is-data-wrangling-and-why-does-it-take-so-long/.

[11] World Health Organization, "Statement on the Second Meeting of the International Health Regulations (2005) Emergency Committee Regarding the Outbreak of Novel Coronavirus (2019-nCoV)," WHO Press release, 30 January 2020.

[12] "COVID-19 Pandemic," Wikipedia, 2021 [Online]. Available: https://en.wikipedia.org/wiki/2019%E2%80%9320_coronavirus_pandemic/. [Accessed 17 April 2021].

[13] L. van der Maaten, E. Postma and J. van den Herik, "Dimensionality Reduction: A Comparative Review (PDF)," *Mach Learn Res*, vol. 10, pp. 66–71, 2009.

[14] I. Olkin and A. R. Sampson, "Multivariate Analysis: Overview," *International Encyclopedia of the Social & Behavioral Sciences*, Pergamon, Turkey, pp. 10240–10247, 2001.

[15] G. Hinton "Deep Belief Networks," *Scholarpedia*, vol. 4, no. 5, p. 5947, 2009.

[16] S. Saha, "A Comprehensive Guide to Convolutional Neural Networks – The ELI5 Way," Towards Data Science, 15 December 2018. [Online]. Available: https://towardsdatascience.com/a-comprehensive-guide-to-convolutional-neural-networks-the-eli5-way-3bd2b1164a53.

[17] R. Collobert and J. Weston, "A Unified Architecture for Natural Language Processing: Deep Neural Networks with Multitask Learning," *Proceedings of the 25th International Conference on Machine Learning*, pp. 160–167, 2008.

[18] A. van den Oord, S. Dieleman and B. Schrauwen, "*Deep Content-Based Music Recommendation*," Curran Associates, Red Hook, NY, pp. 2643–2651, 2013.

[19] Y. LeCun, L. Bottou, Y. Bengo and P. Haffner, "*Gradient-Based Learning Applied to Document Recognition*," IEEE, Manhattan. NY, 1998.

[20] A. Krizhevsky, I. Sutsekever and G. E. Hinton, "*ImageNet Classification with Deep Convolutional Neural Networks*," University of Toronto, Toronto, Ontario.

[21] K. Simonyan and A. Zisserman, "Very Deep Convolutional Networks for Large-Scale Image Recognition," *University of Oxford Conference Paper at ICLR*, 10 April 2015.

[22] C. Szegedy, W. Liu, Y. Jia, *et al.*, "Going Deeper With Convolutions," 17 September 2014.

[23] H. Kaiming, X. Zhang, S. Ren and J. Sun, "*Deep Residual Learning for Image Recognition*," Cornell University, 10 December 2015.

[24] M. Chowdhury, T. Rahman, A. Khandakar, *et al.*, "Can AI Help in Screening Viral and COVID-19 Pneumonia?" *IEEE*, vol. 8, pp. 132665–132676, 2020.

[25] T. Rahman, A. Khandakar, Y. Qiblawey, *et al.*, "Exploring the Effect of Image Enhancement Techniques on COVID-19 Detection using Chest X-ray Images," *Computers in Biology and Medicine*, vol. 132, 104319, 2021.

[26] C. Shorten and T. M. Khoshgoftaar, "*A Survey on Image Data Augmentation for Deep Learning*," Springer, New York City, vol. 6, p. 60, 2019.

[27] V. Nair and G. E. Hinton, "Rectified Linear Units Improve Restricted Boltzmann Machines," *International Conference on Machine Learning*, pp. 807–814, 2010.

[28] G. E. Hinton, N. Srivastava, A. Krizhevsky, I. Sutskever and R. R. Salakhutdinov, "Improving Neural Networks by Preventing Co-Adaptation of Feature Detectors," 2012.

[29] I. Goodfellow, Y. Bengio and A. Courville, "*6.2.2.3 Softmax Units for Multinoulli Output Distributions*," MIT Press, Cambridge, MA, pp. 180–184, 2016.

[30] R. G. Blog, "Understanding Categorical Cross-Entropy Loss, Binary Cross-Entropy Loss, Softmax Loss, Logistic Loss, Focal Loss and All Those Confusing Names," 23 May 2018. [Online]. Available: https://gombru.github.io/2018/05/23/cross_entropy_loss/. [Accessed 17 April 2021].

Chapter 13

Healthcare system using deep learning

J.B. Shajilin Loret[1] *and P.C. Sherimon*[2]

Abstract

The human healthcare system is entering a new era in which biomedical data will play a critical role. Deep learning (DL) is becoming more widely used in the healthcare system, and it benefits patients and clinicians in a variety of ways. DL allows the healthcare system to analyze data at a high rate while maintaining accuracy. DL is not machine learning or artificial intelligence (AI); rather, it is a sophisticated hybrid of the two that employs a layered algorithmic architecture for analyzing the data at breakneck speed. The basis of DL starts during 1943, once the two scientist Walter Pitts and Warren McCulloch generated a computer model that is according to human brain neural networks. The term “DL” is a made-up term. DL is a function of AI that plays the role of the human brain in the decision-making process in terms of data processing and pattern development. The names such as deep neural learning or deep neural network are the additional names of DL. This DL is quite useful when dealing with unstructured data, and to handle vast amounts of features. DL uses both organized and unstructured data for training. Some of the DL includes face recognition, vision for driverless cars, virtual assistants, and money laundering.

Generative adversarial networks, multilayer perceptron, radial basis network, recurrent neural networks, and convolutional neural networks are five key components of core neural networks in DL. DL has the potential to revolutionize the delivery of healthcare in the future. For computer vision, medical imaging and diagnosis can be more precise to DL. Classifications of images, object detection, image restoration, and image segmentation have all been achieved with superhuman accuracy. Digits written by hand can also be accepted. DL, which employs massive neural networks, teaches machines how to automate the tasks that human visual systems perform. DL approaches make use of data from EHR records to solve a variety of healthcare concerns, including lowering the rate of misdiagnosis and predicting operation outcomes.

We look at how these computational methods can influence a few key areas of medicine in this chapter, as well as how to construct end-to-end systems. Moreover, we discuss about the different kinds of algorithms in DL and the advantages. DL in

[1]Department of Information Technology, Francis Xavier Engineering College, Tirunelveli, India
[2]Faculty of Computer Studies, Arab Open University, Muscat, Sultanate of Oman

healthcare applications includes electronic health records, disease prediction and treatment, DL for cancer diagnosis, and DL for cancer diagnosis research.

Keywords: Deep learning; Healthcare; Recurrent neural networks; Multilayer perceptron; Convolutional neural networks

13.1 Introduction

Healthcare is entering a new era in which abundant biomedical data plays an important role. Recently, artificial intelligence (AI), semantic computing deep learning (DL), and machine learning (ML) have been steadily infiltrating the medical field, which brings technologies and solutions that are changing healthcare. Each of these innovations is interconnected, which conveys something new to the industry and changing the way in which doctors handle their duties and provides patient care. Despite the fact that AI is the most eminent technology principle, DL in healthcare is a subfield of AI that has the potential to transform healthcare and add a new level of sophistication to medical technology solutions.

The healthcare production has the capability to explore information at rapid speeds while maintaining high precision. It is not AI or ML; rather, it is a complex combination of the two that sifts through data at breakneck speed thanks to a layered algorithmic architecture. The advantages of DL in healthcare are numerous, including the ability to be fast, accurate, and precise, to name a few; however, it does not stop there. The neural networks created by various layers of AI and ML, as well as their capability to learn, provide further advantages. When it derives to DL, learning is just the name of the game.

In 1943, DL became a reality, after Walter Pitts and Warren McCulloch generated a model of computer that is as in neural networks of human brain [1]. This DL has allowed the healthcare industry to process data at high speeds while maintaining high precision. It is not ML or AI; rather, it is a complex hybrid of the two that sifts through data at breakneck speed thanks to a layered algorithmic architecture. The networks and technology allow unparalleled processing power and the capability to sort through huge amounts of data that might otherwise be lost, overlooked, or overlooked in the healthcare industry, and the complicated problems can be solved by DL networks and pull the strands of information from huge amounts of data.

According to IDC, by 2022, the global bazaar for cognitive and AI systems is anticipated to hit US$77.6 billion by 2025. IDC anticipated that by the end of 2019, it would have risen to US$97.9 billion, or a composite annual growth rate of 28.4 percent. Because of the technology's ubiquity and potential to transform different sectors, not just healthcare, the demand has been steadily increasing.

DL in healthcare, on the other hand, continues to be a field ripe with opportunity and cutting-edge innovation. Organizations have used the algorithm's power, as well as AI and ML capabilities, to generate results that are ideal for the healthcare industry's stringent requirements.

13.2 History of healthcare deep learning

DL has previously made an impact in the area of healthcare. Google has devoted a significant research to in what way the DL models might be used to forecast the patients who are hospitalized and assist physicians in monitoring patient data and outcomes. "DL for Electronic Health Records" explained in what way DL might be used to diminish administrative burden while improving a better understanding of patient care and needs. This application is considered the best application in healthcare because it diminishes the logistical overhead while enabling medical specialists to concentrate on what they do best.

The NHS in the United Kingdom has pledged to use DL, AI, and ML to become a pioneer in healthcare. The healthcare provider realizes the importance of this technology. The NHS, which is struggling with cost-cutting and continuing capability shortages, observes the potential to transform patient care through intelligent assessments and DL toolkits. Investing in DL technologies may help the association escape few of the legacy problems that have stifled efficiencies and improve patient attention. It could also support healthcare staff in a desperate need of assistance.

DL applications in healthcare include medical imaging solutions, chatbots that detect trends in patient complaints, the algorithms of DL discriminate various kinds of cancer, and imaging solutions that employ DL in order to discover erratic diseases or precise kinds of pathology. The ML will cover linear classifiers such as logistic regression and naïve Bayes, tree-based classifiers, support vector machine, as well as nearest neighbor, and neural networks [2]. DL has proved critical in providing medical personnel with insights that allow them to spot problems early on, allowing them to give even more individualized and effective patient care.

13.3 Deep learning benefits

A type of ML is referred to as "DL" that can solve problems that traditional ML cannot. In DL, neural networks are used to enhance computational work and produce reliable results. DL applications include natural language processing, speech recognition, and face recognition. When a picture is uploaded in the Facebook with a friend, for example, the Facebook tags your friend and suggests his name. DL approaches are used on the Facebook to recognize people's faces and the algorithms in DL also understand and convert human speech to text. In future, the combination of DL and IoT could pave the way for a slew of game-changing advances.

13.4 Components of deep learning

The five core neural networks used in DL include the following:

- Generative adversarial networks (GANs)
- Multilayer perceptron (MLP)
- Network with radial basis

- Recurrent neural networks (RNNs)
- Convolutional neural networks (CNN)

13.4.1 Generative adversarial networks

These networks are absorbing new ML innovation. GANs are generative models, which means that they use your training data to create new data instances. GANs, for example, may produce images that appear to be photographs of human faces despite the fact that the faces are not real.

Unsupervised learning is used in the process of developing generative models in ML that mechanically recognize and learning regularities or patterns in incoming data such that this model can be used to generate or output new instances from the original dataset.

By rephrasing, a generative model is a supervised learning problem with two sub models. GANs are an ingenious way to train the generator model, which we train to construct novel samples, and the discriminator model, which seeks to categorize these examples as true or false, based on whether they are from within or outside the domain. Both the models are trained in an adversarial zero-sum game until half of the time the discriminator model is misled, indicating that the generator model generates trustworthy examples.

GANs are an interesting as well as fast emerging field that demonstrates the power of generative models by giving genuine examples in a range of issue domains. Furthermost in particular, image-tagging, especially in image-to-image conversion jobs like turning summer to winter or night-to-day images, as well as in creating lifelike photos of items, settings, and even people, cannot tell incorrect.

GANs are a type of generative model that uses a model that is both generative and discriminative to train it automatically to treat an unsupervised problem as if it were supervised. GANs offer a way to improve domain-specific data that is sophisticated as well as a solution to problems that necessitate generative solutions, and image-to-image translation is an example of this.

GANs are computational structures that pit two neural networks against each other to create new, synthetic data that can pass for real data (thus the term "adversarial"). They are frequently employed in the creation of photographs, films, and audio recordings.

Generative modeling neural network architecture called a GAN is a type of generative adversarial network. After being practiced, this GM can be used to produce new plausible samples on demand. GANs have very unique use cases, which can be difficult to grasp while you are just getting started. GANs are a type of model architecture that is used to train generative models. In general, the most frequent one of which is DL models.

The GAN architecture mainly consists of dual submodels such as a discriminator model that is used in conjunction with a generator model to create new instances and to determine whether the created examples are true or false.

- Generator: A model for generating fresh credible instances from the area of the problem.

- Discriminator: A model for detecting whether or not instances are authentic (domain-specific).

13.4.1.1 The generator model

This model uses a fixed-length arbitrary vector as input to generate a sample in the domain [3]. A Gaussian distribution is employed to construct the vector, which is afterward utilized to kick-start the creative process. Following the instructions, the issue domain will correspond to points in this multidimensional vector space, resulting in a concise representation of the data distribution.

A latent space, also called vector space with latent variables, is a vector space with latent variables. Hidden variables, usually referred to as latent variables, are the variables that are significant to a field but are difficult to see. This generator model (Figure 13.1) is retained and utilized to produce fresh samples after it has been prepared [4].

13.4.2 Multilayer perceptron

MLP is the technical term for a feed-forward neural network [5]. An input layer, a hidden layer, and an output layer are the three layers as shown in Figure 13.2. The signal that will be processed is obtained by the input layer. The output layer is in charge of things like prediction and classification. The MLP's real computing engine has an endless amount of hidden layers among the input and output layers. Data flows from the input to the output layer of an MLP in a forward manner, similar to a feed-forward network. The neurons of the MLP have been conditioned using a back-propagation learning technique. MLPs can tackle issues that are not linearly separable and can estimate any continuous function [5]. The most common MLP applications include pattern classification, identification, prediction, and approximation.

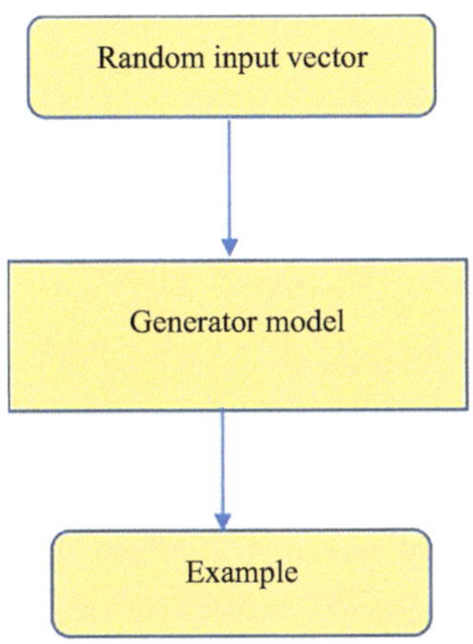

Figure 13.1 Generator model

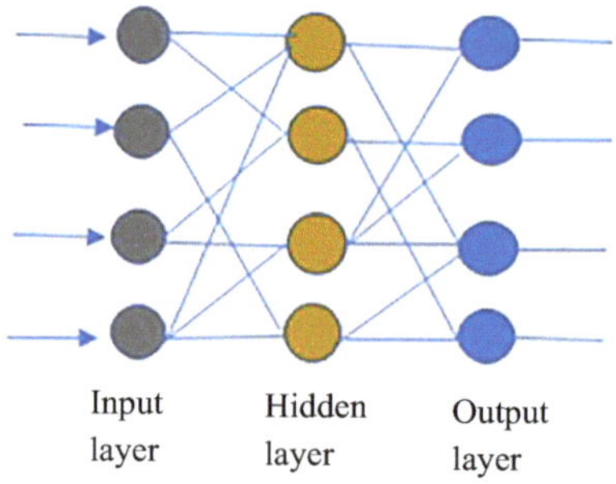

Figure 13.2 Multilayer perceptron

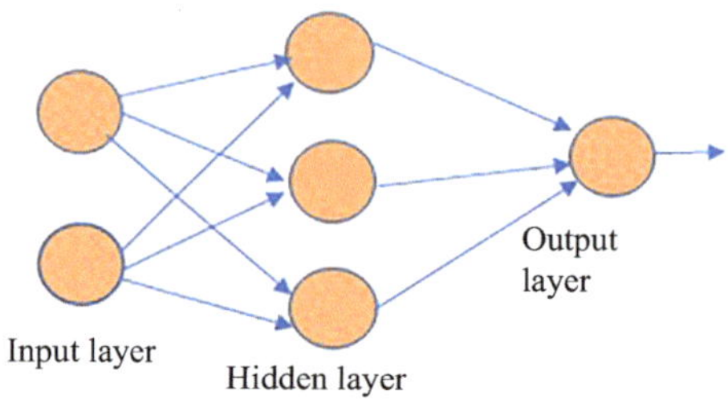

Figure 13.3 Three-layer MLP

This perceptron solves complex issues by collaborating with other perceptrons stacked in many layers [6]. Figure 13.3 illustrates a three-layer MLP. The input layer present in the left sends outputs to the entire hidden layer perceptrons and the output layer receives signals from this hidden layer. An MLP is a perceptron with many layers. Several signals were sent by each perceptron, one to each perceptron above it. The perceptron assigns different weights to each signal. Each line that connects a perceptron in one layer to the perceptron in the next layer in Figure 13.3 represents different outputs. The MLP will have a high amount of perceptrons in each layer, and there may be several levels; thus it might soon become a very complicated structure [7]. A neural network is another name for an MLP.

A three-layer MLP is a shallow or nondeep neural network. An MLP that includes four or more than four layers are known as a deep neural network. The decision function of a conventional perceptron is a phase function, and binary as output, which distinguishes an MLP from a neural network [6]. Activation functions that yield in outputs of real numbers, typically between 0 and 1 or −1 and 1, may be employed in neural networks derived from MLPs. This enables probabilistic forecasting or object classification with numerous labels.

13.4.2.1 Perceptron structure

In a neural network, the perceptron structure, or neuron, is simple but inventive. As in Figure 13.4, this perceptron is divided into four parts.

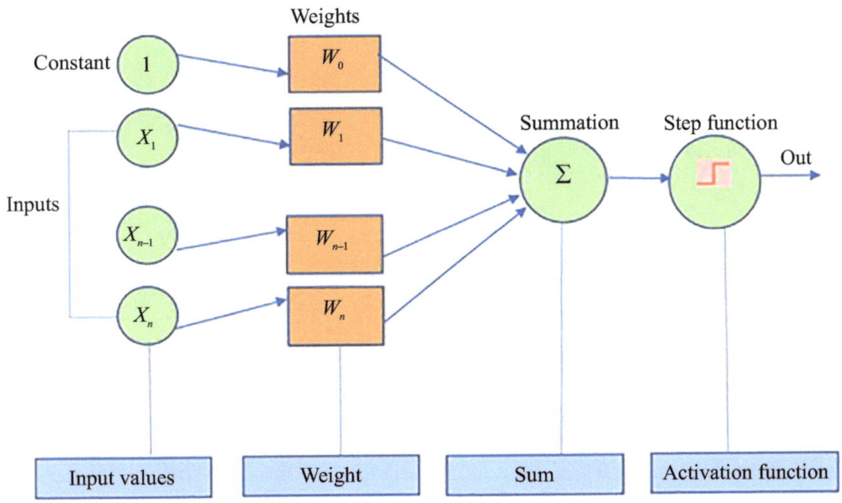

Figure 13.4 Perceptron structure

The perceptron learning process

A perceptron's steps are as follows:

1. A number of the inputs are computed after multiplying the inputs by their weights. In order to evaluate the relative value of each output, the weights are used by the perceptron. When new weights are discovered, the accuracy of neural network algorithms improves over time, which results in predictions that are more accurate. Varieties of techniques are employed in the fine-tuning of the weights, the most popular of which being back-propagation.
2. A bias variable is introduced where step 1 is multiplied by a weight. This technical step permits you to adjust the curve of activation function left and right as well as up and down on the number graph. It permits the numerical efficiency of the perceptron to be fine-tuned.
3. The activation function is used to feed the sum. The intended output values are transformed from the input values by means of the activation function. For instance, the range of the input values is from 1 to 100, which gives the outputs as 0 or 1. Learning is also aided by the activation role of a perceptron that is part of an MLP. Complex neural networks are trained thanks to the qualities of the activation function, particularly its nonlinearity.
4. The effect is the perceptron's production. A classification decision is the contribution of perceptron. The output of one layer's perceptrons is the input of the following layer in an MLP. The last perceptrons output in the "output layer" is the perceptron learning model's final prediction.

13.4.3 Radial basis network

The input layer, a hidden layer, and an output layer are the three layers present in a radial basis function (RBF) neural network as in Figure 13.5. The output of the

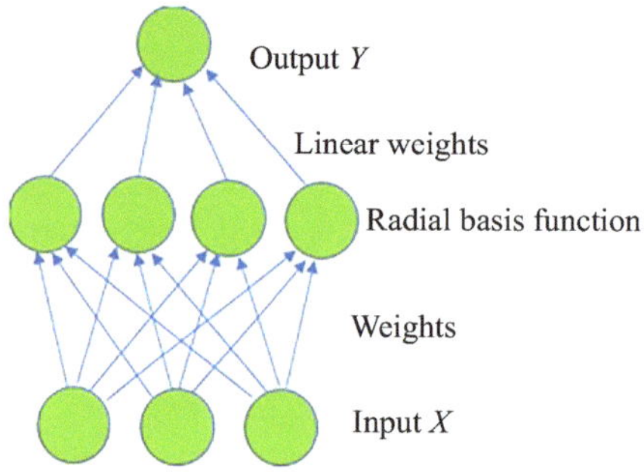

Figure 13.5 Radial basis network

hidden layer is inversely proportional to distance from the center of the neuron Gaussian transfer functions. *K*-Means clustering and probabilistic neural network/generalized regression neural network (PNN/GRNN) networks are the examples of RBF networks. Individual neurons exist for every point in the training file in PNN/GRNN networks, while the number of neurons in RBF networks is often substantially lower than the number of training points. When compared to RBF networks, PNN/GRNN networks are usually more dependable for small-to-medium-sized training sets problems, but they are impracticable in big training sets.

Since single perceptron/MLP are made up of input and output layers, they only have linear separability (some hidden layers in MLP). The AND and OR functions are linearly separable, while the XOR function is not.

One or more RBF neurons are inserted in the space of an RBF network, which are described by the predictor variables (e.g., *X*, *Y*). There are as several dimensions in this space as there are predictor variables. RBF is used to measure the Euclidean distance between the point being evaluated (in this case, the triangle) and the center of each neuron (also known as a kernel function). Due to the fact that the radius distance is the function's argument, it is called the RBF:

weight = RBF (distance)

RBF networks are made up of three layers as shown in Figure 13.6:

1. **Input layer:** Individual predictor variable is expressed by a single neuron in the input layer. $N-1$ neurons represent categorical variables, where N denotes the total number of categories. The value spectrum is normalized by subtracting the median and dividing by the interquartile range in the input neurons. The values are then supplied to each of the secret layer neurons by the input neurons.
2. **Hidden layer:** The number of neurons varies in this hidden. A radial base function centered on a point with the same number of dimensions as the predictor variables makes up each neuron. For each dimension, you can change the RBF's spread (radius). The training technique establishes the centers and spreads. A hidden neuron employs the RBF kernel function and the spread

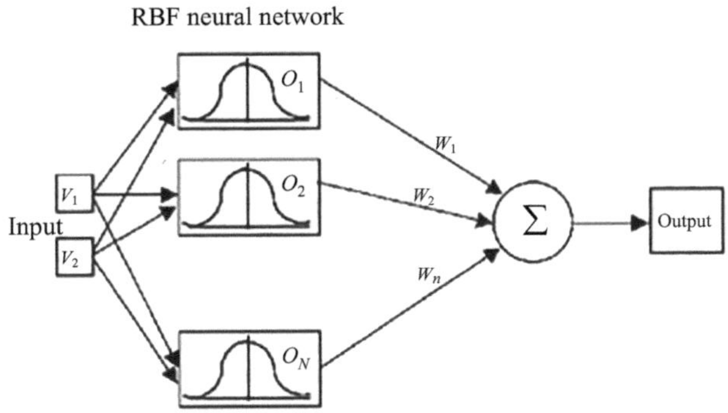

Figure 13.6 RBF network architecture

values to compute, when given, the x vector of input values from the input layer, the Euclidean distance of the test case from the neuron's center point [8]. The summation layer receives the result.

3. **Summation layer:** The weight of the neuron is multiplied by the hidden layer output (i.e. W_1, W_2, ..., W_n in this diagram) is sent to the next layer, which combines the weighted values together and displays the network's output as the sum of all weights. In the summation layer weight W_0 is multiplied by a bias value of 1.0. Every target category has its own performance in classification problems (along with its own set of weights as well as summation unit). The likelihood that the case being examined has that category is the value performance for that category.

13.4.3.1 RBF networks training

The training technique determines the following parameters [9]:

1. The hidden layer's total number of neurons.
2. The center coordinates of each RBF in the hidden layer.
3. The size of each RBF's radius in every dimension.
4. The RBF's outputs were given weights as they transit through the summing layer.

In order to train RBF networks, a variety of techniques have been used. K-Means clustering is one method for locating cluster centers, and RBF feature centers are then created from these. K-Means clustering, on the other hand, is a computationally costly algorithm that frequently fails to produce the best number of centers. Alternative possibility is to use the centers of an arbitrary selection of the training points.

Sheng Chen, Xia Hong, and Chris J. Harris created the DTREG training algorithm, and this algorithm decides the best core points and spread for individual neuron uses an evolutionary approach. It also identifies when it is to be stopped adding new neurons to the network by keeping an eye on the expected leave-one-out error and dismissing at what time it rises owing to overfitting.

Ridge regression is used in the hidden layer and the summation layer to determine the weights between neurons that are ideal. Mark Orr devised an iterative method for computing the optimal regularization, the lambda parameter is used to reduce generalized cross-validation error.

13.4.4 Recurrent neural networks

These RNNs vary from various feed-forward networks in that they can relay information in time steps. A leading researcher, Juergen Schmidhuber, offers a fascinating interpretation of RNNs.

In a sequence of input vectors, each vector is modeled individually by RNNs. As the network models each input vector through the input vector window, this allows it to maintain state. RNNs are well known for their ability to model the temporal dimension.

13.4.4.1 Time dimension modeling

RNNs with Turing completes are capable of simulating any program. RNNs can be thought of as "optimization over programs" if we think of this neural networks as an "optimization over functions." RNNs are suitable for modeling the functions with vector inputs and/or outputs that are time dependent. By forming cycles in the network, RNNs model the time dimension of data.

13.4.4.2 Lost in time

Without modeling the time dimension or assuming independence, many classification algorithms, including logistic regression, support vector machines, and conventional feed-forward networks, have been effectively developed. To capture the time dynamic, further variations of similar approaches model the input as a sliding window.

The assumption of time independence between model inputs prevents our model from capturing long-range time dependencies, which is one drawback of these methods. Sliding window approaches have a predefined window size; thus results that are larger will be missed. Modeling how conversation operates and teaching machines how to act in a meaningful manner as the discussion evolves over time are fantastic examples. For example, a well-trained RNN could participate in the famous Turing Test of Alan Turing's, in which a human is led to believe he is conversing with a real person.

13.4.4.3 Connections with temporal feedback and loops

RNN loops connections are possible. This enables them to accurately represent temporal behavior in areas like language, time series, audio, and text.

The data in this domain is intrinsically ordered and context-sensitive, with succeeding values relying on preceding ones. An RNN's wiring permits feedback in such a way that these temporal effects can be recorded. For applications, in time-series domains, the RNN architecture are most commonly used.

A feedback loop is used by an RNN to learn from sequences of various durations. To represent temporal relationships in data, RNNs use/train an additional parameter matrix for connections between time steps.

The formation of sequences is taught to RNNs in which the current input and the input from all past time steps determine the output at each time step. Back propagation through time is a gradient computation algorithm used by standard RNNs.

13.4.4.4 Time-series data and sequences

In this industry, we encounter sequential data in a variety of issue areas, and our model must output a series of vectors:

- Speech fusion
- Captions for images
- Music composition
- Participating in video games
- Language modeling
- Text-generation models at the character level

In additional a series of input vectors are needed:

- Prediction of time series
- Music information retrieval
- Audiovisual evaluation

There are also domains that necessitate the use of an input and an output vectors collection such as

- Translation into natural language
- Dialoguing with others
- Robotic control

Vector sequences, such as video frames, can be processed by this RNN [3]. It also has the capability to deal with the input and output in infrequent ways.

13.4.4.5 Understanding the input and output of the model

A single fixed-size input vector is used in traditional ML. We expect to observe a fixed input-to-output relationship with a fixed output scale in classic modeling practices. This is a typical modeling pattern for image categorization or columnar data classification classifiers.

Each time phase has its own input vector, with each vector containing a large number of columns that are used in RNNs to change the input dynamic. Some examples of how RNNs operate with input and output vector sequences are given in the following:

- **Sequence output (one-to-many):** Image captioning, for example, an image is taken and converts it into a series of words.
- **Sequence input (many-to-one):** Consider sentimentality analysis, which uses a single sentence as input.
- **Many-to-many:** For instance, each frame should be labeled in video classification.

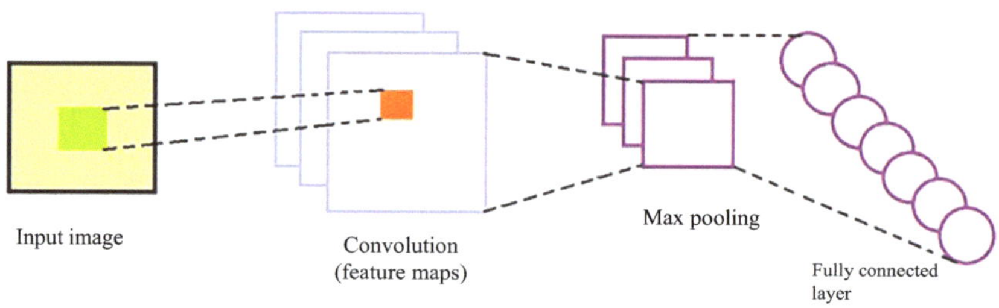

Figure 13.7 Convolutional neural network

The number of input records is mentioned to as the mini-batch size per batch that we want to model. The amount of columns in a standard input vector correlates to the number of function columns. The number of time steps describes the evolution of the input vector in time. This is the input data's time-series part. Any time step that counts greater than one in terms of input and output architecture is referred to as "many-to-many classification."

13.4.5 Convolutional neural networks

In order to acquire higher order features from information, using convolutions is the main aim of a CNN. They consistently place first in image classification competitions and excel at image object recognition [10]. Faces, people, street signs, and a number of other visual data are all recognized by them [11]. When looking at words as separate textual elements, CNNs come in handy, and they overlay with text analysis through the identification of optical characters. They can also perform sound analysis.

The effectiveness of CNNs in picture identification is one of the primary reasons why the world understands DL's potential. As shown in Figure 13.7, from raw visual data, CNNs excel at extracting location and (relatively) rotation invariant properties.

CNNs are accelerating machine vision developments, which have clear applications in self-driving vehicles, robots, drones, and blindness treatments. CNNs have also been used for sentiment analysis and natural language translation and generation. Convolution can be used to construct a more stable feature space from a signal.

13.4.5.1 CNN architecture

By transmitting data across all connected layers, CNNs convert data from the input layer to a collection of class scores provided by the output layer. Despite the fact that there are many different CNN architecture, they all follow the same layering structure, as in Figure 13.8.

The image's size (width×height) and depth (which indicates the color channels) are sent to the first layer as three-dimensional data (usually three for RGB color channels). The following layers for feature extraction are arranged in a sequence that repeats itself.

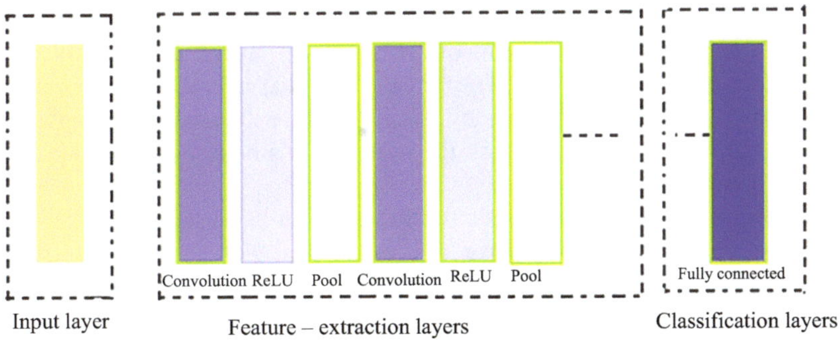

Figure 13.8 General CNN architecture

Convolution layer

To match up with other literature, a unit called the rectified linear unit is represented in the diagram, in which the activation function is depicted as a layer.

Pooling layer

These layers search the images for a variety of features and create higher order features as they go. This is consistent with a recurring subject in DL: the features are learned automatically rather than manually.

Finally, there are classification layers that are made up of one or more completely linked layers that use higher order characteristics to generate class probabilities or scores. As the name implies, the entire neurons in the previous layer are completely connected in these layers. The output of these layers is usually two dimensional, with dimensions $[b\ N]$, where N specifies the number of classes; we are interested in scoring and b is the number of instances in each class.

Neuron spatial arrangements

Traditional multilayer neural networks have fully connected layers, where each neuron in one layer is linked to the following layer's neuron. To fit the input volumes, the neurons in the layers of a CNN are constructed in three dimensions. Rather than the number of layers as in a multilayer neural network, depth refers to the third dimension of the activation volume.

Development of links between layers

The way layers in a convolutional architecture are related is another difference. CNNs have different kinds of layers than conventional multilayer networks, which have layer-oriented architecture. Each layer uses a differentiable function with or without parameters to transform the previous layer's neuron activations that are converted from a 3D input volume into a 3D output volume.

Input layers

For network processing, the image's raw input data is loaded and processed in input layers. The distance, height, and number of channels are specified by this input data. Three channels usually express each pixel's RGB values.

Convolutional layers

CNN architecture is built on the basis of convolutional layers. Convolutional layers convert incoming data using a patch of locally coupled neurons from the previous layer, as shown in Figure 13.9. This layer will compute the area of the input layer's dot product and the weights to which the input layer's neurons in the output layer are locally connected.

Despite the fact that the output's third dimension has a large number of components that may frequently increase, the resultant output often has the same (or fewer) spatial dimensions as the input. Let us look at convolution in more detail, as it is a critical concept in these layers.

Convolution

A mathematical procedure that explains how two sets of data are combined is called convolution. It uses Fourier transforms to link the frequency domain with the space/time domain, which is useful in both physics and mathematics. It takes data, runs it through a convolution kernel, and then outputs a feature map.

A CNN's function detector is the convolution operation. The input to a convolution can be either raw data or a function map built by another convolution. The kernel is sometimes misunderstood as a strainer, with the kernel data input filtering out specified data types.

The kernel is slid across the input data to produce the convoluted function (output) data that is explained. The supplied data values are multiplied by the kernel inside its constraints at each point, resulting in a single output function map entry. In reality, if desired function is discovered in the input, the output is immense.

A filter is the term used to describe the collection of weights in a kernel. A function map is the product of bringing this filter into alignment with the data or activation map. Based on the activations and parameters of the input volume, convolutional layers apply conversions on the volume of input data. To construct the 3D output volume, the activation maps for each filter are stacked along the depth axis.

Both layer parameters and hyper parameters are provided in convolutional layers. The parameters in this layer are trained using gradient descent so that the training set labels match the class scores. Convolutional layers are made up of the following main components:

- Parameter sharing
- Filters
- Activation maps
- Hyper parameters for certain layers

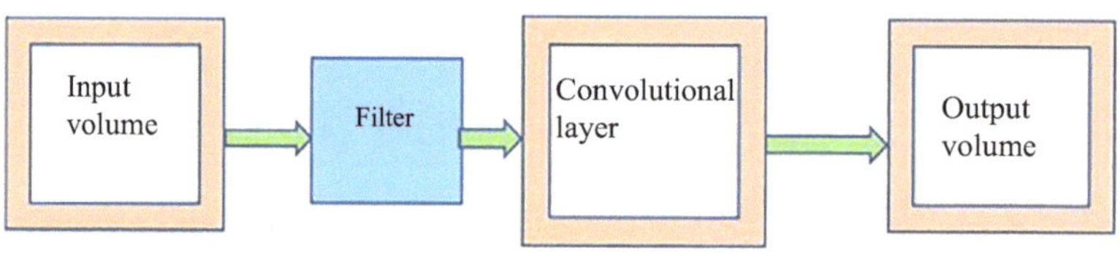

Figure 13.9 Convolution layer

Filters
A convolutional layer's filters are regulated by the layer's parameters. Filters are functions of width and height that are bigger than the input volume's height and width. In a sliding window, filters are applied around the width and height of the input volume. Each depth of the input volume receives a filter. The filter's output is determined.

Activation maps
When a neuron decides to allow information to pass through it, it is said to be activated. The activation function's inputs, as well as the weights on the connections, determine it. When we say the filter "activates," we mean that it allows data to flow from the input volume to the output volume.

During the forward transit of information through the CNN, we slide each filter across the spatial dimensions (width, height) of the input volume. For that particular filter, this results in a two-dimensional output known as an activation map.

Parameter sharing
This system can be used by CNN to keep the overall parameter count under control. Because of the usage of less resource to acquire the training dataset, the training time will be decreased. In CNNs in order to guarantee parameter sharing, we define a "depth slice" as a sole two-dimensional portion of depth. Each depth portion's neurons must then use the same weights and biases. As a result, a given convolutional layer has much less parameters.

If the input images used for training have a unique centered structure then it will not be able to use parameter sharing. This effect is experienced, when a precise feature to show up in a specific location on a face is expected. In this case, parameter sharing would not be used. The invariance of CNNs to translation/position is due to parameter sharing as well.

Learned filters and renders
There is a demonstration of the 96 filters of size $11 \times 11 \times 3$ that have been learned. Using the parameter-sharing scheme, due to the translationally invariant presence of images, a horizontal edge is recognized, which is advantageous in numerous spots in the image. This implies that all you have to do is to learn the horizontal edge once and do not have to recall it in all of the image's positions.

To further dissect this, consider a two-dimensional image and the neural network can learn the features of position-invariant images if the image is partitioned into four bits. These are location invariant due to the way the network divides the information into quadrants. It then learns small sections of the image at a time, eventually combining the results. This aids in learning of a global representation by the neural network that is independent of any particular set of features.

13.5 The role of deep learning in healthcare in the future

Healthcare's future has never been much bright. Not only because AI and ML enable developers to create solutions that address very specific industry demands, but also because DL in healthcare has the potential to be incredibly useful in assisting physicians and enhancing patient care. Dr. Eric Topol, a cardiologist and geneticist, recently published "Deep Medicine," in which he explains how DL can "restore the treatment in healthcare." He discussed in an interview, why DL is so important to the healthcare sector.

It is not intended to replace a doctor; rather, it is meant to support them. DL will not be able to replace people in the end, but it will give clinicians the resources they need to excel in their fields. Aidoc has developed algorithms that help radiologists to diagnose and treat patients more quickly. For its innovative algorithms, the company has received multiple accreditations and certifications from the Food and Drug Administration, the European Union CE, and the Australian Medicinal Products Administration (TGA). This AI and DL tool assists the busy radiologist by flagging areas of concern, allowing the healthcare professional to direct patients with more control and efficiency. It also eliminates paperwork by integrating into workflows and improves access to relevant patient data.

All of these point to DL, which is the direction of healthcare in the future. Finally, medical technology is evolving to include AI-based algorithms that can rationalize and simplify complex data analysis while also improving diagnosis. It is capable of being taught and educated. It has the ability to optimize workflows and reduce reporting times. It can also be used to adjust patient-care benchmarks in a certain time and a region with a limited budget.

DL will continue to gain traction in the healthcare industry, especially now that more doctors are recognizing the benefits. Close engagement with industry and specialist organizations is required to support this technology. In order to remain relevant to the profession at all times, it must remain versatile and adaptable.

Aidoc's DL radiology platform has already seen a number of successful implementations, which results in greater clinician support and workflow improvement. Radiologist workloads are more evenly dispersed, and abnormalities are more quickly reported and prioritized. In order to keep up with demanding workloads and industry expectations, radiologists often work 10–12-h days, making it one of the most difficult occupations. They will be able to spend more time with patients and other practitioners while also benefiting from Aidoc's in-depth review of medicinal images and data.

While DL in healthcare is still in its early phases, it has already made substantial progress. The benefits it provides have been recognized by leading institutions and medical agencies, and the solutions' popularity has surged. Compared to only one or two booths in 2017, AI and DL in healthcare applications now have their own platform, show space, and talk at the RSNA conference. Medical professionals still hold the future, but they are now aided by technology that recognizes their unique requirements and settings, as well as technology that helps them cope with the daily challenges they confront.

13.6 Deep learning applications in healthcare

In healthcare, DL will identify hidden opportunities and trends in clinical data, helping doctors to better treat their patients. For a long time, recently, AI, ML, and

DL have all received a lot of attention. These developments are transforming retail, banking, travel, manufacturing, healthcare, and other industries. DL algorithms use data from EHR documents to solve a number of critical healthcare problems, such as reducing misdiagnosis rates and predicting procedure outcomes. ANNs can assist clinicians in analyzing information and recognizing a range of diseases by processing vast volumes of data from numerous sources, such as medical imaging:

- Analyze blood samples.
- Monitor glucose levels in diabetic patients.
- Diagnose heart defects.
- Detect tumors using image analysis.
- Detecting cancerous cells and receiving a cancer diagnosis.
- An MRI scan can detect osteoarthritis before it causes any damage.

One of the sectors that makes the best use of these technologies is healthcare. Medical practitioners are constantly searching for new and creative ways to implement new technologies and deliver real outcomes because health is so critical. DL has game-changing implications in healthcare. DL uses neural networks to analyze a vast volume of data, such as patient records, medical reports, and insurance records, to generate the best results.

DL is being used by medical practitioners and researchers recently to discover any hidden possibilities in data and to better serve the healthcare industry. In healthcare, DL allows physicians to accurately identify and treat any disease, resulting in better medical decisions.

13.6.1 Drug discovery

In healthcare, DL assists in the discovery and creation of new medicines. The technology looks at the medical history of the patient's and makes suggestions for the finest course of treatment. Furthermore, this technology collects data from the symptoms and tests of patients.

13.6.2 Medical imaging

Heart disease, cancer, and brain tumors are diagnosed via the various techniques involved in medical imaging such as MRI scans, CT scans, and ECGs [4]. As a result, DL helps physicians in furthering disease research and delivering effective patient treatment.

13.6.3 Insurance fraud

To assess health insurance fraud claims, DL is applied. It has the ability to foresee potential fraud claims in the future using predictive analytics [4]. DL could potentially be used by the insurance business to deliver offers and promotions to their targeted patients.

13.6.4 Alzheimer's disease

This disease is one of the major diseases facing difficulties in the medical sector. Alzheimer's disease is diagnosed early using a DL technique.

13.6.5 Genome

To read a genome and assist patients in understanding illnesses that may affect them, DL technology is used. In genetics and the insurance sector, DL has a bright future. DL techniques are utilized to make doctors speedier and more precise [12]. Cellscope is a mobile app that allows parents to monitor their children's health in real time, avoiding the need for frequent doctor visits. DL in healthcare can help doctors make more informed medical decisions, which can benefit both doctors and patients.

13.7 Conclusion and future work

This chapter deliberates how computational approaches can affect a few major areas of medicine, as well as how to build end-to-end systems. Nowadays DL is being employed commonly in the healthcare system, and it has a number of advantages for both patients and professionals. DL enables the healthcare system to process data quickly while preserving accuracy. Furthermore, we have covered the various types of DL algorithms with their benefits. Also, this chapter considers some of the applications of DL such as DL for cancer diagnosis, disease prediction and treatment, electronic health records, and DL for cancer diagnosis research in healthcare.

References

[1] S. Asadianfam, M. Shamsi, and A. R. Kenari. "Hadoop Deep Neural Network for Offending Drivers", *Journal of Ambient Intelligence and Humanized Computing*, 2021. https://doi.org/10.1007/s12652-021-02924-4.

[2] H. Khan, A. Srivastav, and A. K. Mishra. "Use of Classification Algorithms in Health Care". In P. Tanwar, V. Jain, C.-M. Liu, and V. Goyal (Eds.) *Big Data Analytics and Intelligence: A Perspective for Health Care* (pp. 31–54), Emerald Publishing Limited, Bingley, 2020.

[3] L. Sehovac, and K. Grolinger. "Deep Learning for Load Forecasting: Sequence to Sequence Recurrent Neural Networks With Attention", *IEEE Access*, vol. 8, pp. 36411–36426, 2020.

[4] V. Silaparasetty. *Deep Learning Projects Using TensorFlow 2*, Springer Science and Business Media LLC, Berlin, 2020.

[5] S. Abirami, and P. Chitra. *Energy-Efficient Edge Based Real-Time Healthcare Support System*, Elsevier BV, Amsterdam, 2020.

[6] G. Saribas, E. A. Aydin, and A. R. Torun. "Multilayer Perceptron Approach to PLA, PLA/Copper and PLA/Carbon Substrate Bow-tie Antenna Production", *2020 4th International Symposium on Multidisciplinary Studies and Innovative Technologies (ISMSIT)*, 2020.

[7] Y. Geng, M. Liu, Q. Li, and R. He. *Introduction of Machine Learning*, Institution of Engineering and Technology (IET), London, 2019.

[8] A. Z. Al-Garni, W. G. Abdelrahman, and A. M. Abdallah. "Aircraft Turbines Time-to-failures Process Modeling Using RBF NN", *Journal of Quality in Maintenance Engineering*, vol. 26, no. 2, pp. 249–259, 2020.

[9] A. Bianconi, C. J. Von Zuben, A. B. de S. Serapião, and J. S. Govone. "Artificial Neural Networks: A Novel Approach to Analysing the Nutritional Ecology of a Blowfly Species, *Chrysomya megacephala*", *Journal of Insect Science*, vol. 10, no. 1, 2010.

[10] K. I. Lakhtaria, and D. Modi. "Deep Learning: Architectures and Applications". In A. Hassanien, A. Darwish, and C. Chowdhary (Eds.) *Handbook of Research on Deep Learning Innovations and Trends* (pp. 114–130), IGI Global, Hershey, PA, 2019.

[11] P. D. Hung, T. Minh, L. Hoang, and P. Minh. "Vietnamese Speech Command Recognition using Recurrent Neural Networks", *International Journal of Advanced Computer Science and Applications*, vol. 10, no. 7, 2019.

[12] A. Muniasamy, S. Tabassam, M. A. Hussain, H. Sultana, V. Muniasamy, and R. Bhatnagar. "Deep Learning for Predictive Analytics in Healthcare". In A. Hassanien, A. Azar, T. Gaber, R. Bhatnagar, and M. F. Tolba (Eds.) *The International Conference on Advanced Machine Learning Technologies and Applications (AMLTA2019). Advances in Intelligent Systems and Computing*, Vol. 921, Springer, Cham, 2020.

Chapter 14

Intelligent classification of ECG signals using machine learning techniques

Kuldeep Singh Kaswan[1], Anupam Baliyan[2], Jagjit Singh Dhatterwal[3], Vishal Jain[4] and Jyotir Moy Chatterjee[5]

Abstract

Bioengineering sign is responsible for processing biosignal acquisition preprocessing and evaluation. It is used so that physicians can decide on valuable information. New methods of image processing helped us to expose data, which was initially used to treat various diseases completely modified by this approach. Healthcare professionals use several types of face detection and machine learning (ML) techniques to examine physiological data. Using intelligent biomedical analytical techniques, software-based signals may be examined to allow physicians to make much better judgments in clinical trials. ML techniques in healthcare, biology and bioinformatics are becoming very effective. Biomedical signals processing and analysis progresses have been unbelievable in many fields, comprising biometrics, medical data management, etc. Biosignal monitoring and database technology that are applications- and data based not only get profit from learning machines but also promote the implementation of intelligent procedures. In this chapter, we will discuss new development and techniques in the interpretation of signals and ML for biological brain signals. In this, we will focus on the intelligent algorithms, covering novel theories, electrocardiography signals preparation and knowledge discovery analysis categorization, etc.

Keywords: Electrocardiography (ECG); Electroencephalogram (EEG); Electromagnetic (EMG); Machine learning; Arrhythmias; Feature extraction

[1]School of Computing Science and Engineering, Galgotias University, Greater Noida, India
[2]Chitkara University Institute of Engineering and Technology, Chitkara University, Rajpura, India
[3]Department of Computer Science and Applications, PDM University, Bahadurgarh, India
[4]School of Engineering and Technology, Sharda University, Greater Noida, India
[5]Department of IT, Lord Buddha Education Foundation, Kathmandu, Nepal

14.1 Introduction

Machine learning (ML) is a method used to obtain important information and optimize system performance from a certain dataset with high computing techniques. ML-based approaches are widely applied in a variety of fields, including video monitoring, voice identification, ML, news categorization, weather prediction, equity market analyzes and medical services [1]. ML has already been used by health experts for the precise and/or fast diagnosis of patients in the field of biomedical applications. ML may also be used to anticipate the severity of symptoms and to testing stations or treatments. Biomedical signals are mainly electrical signals produced because of particular cells' optoelectronic properties [2]. The medical information of a person may be gathered by monitoring these signals. Different forms of biomedical signals, including electrocardiography (ECG), electroencephalogram (EEG) Ming and EMG (electroretinogram), and electrooculogram can retrieve this data from a range of other sources. The valuable signal is tainted with several kinds of noise and undesired signals while recording these signals using an appropriate electrode.

Artifacts: In order to gain usable information, biomedical signal processing focuses with the evaluation of such measurement values. The filtration and collection of the signal and categorization by use of appropriate mathematical formulas, algorithms or technique tools are necessary in order to provide useful intelligence. In order to provide medical practitioners with real-time data, traditionally biological signals were recorded and calculated by software, therefore analyzing the safety of the population. The ML-based signal conditioning technology increases data quality and offers a correct choice. The conventional educated imagination of healthcare practitioners is eventually eliminated. In recent decades, the mortality rate owing to heart disease has risen dramatically. ECG is the most frequent cardiology diagnostic tool for monitoring and diagnosing a cardiac disease. The heartbeat has a particular electric system that expands and contracts its atrium and ventricles. ECG is the assessment of cardiac bioelectrical activities by inserting appropriate electrodes on the body of the patient. During the capture and transmission of ECG signals, it is damaged because of several types, including muscle noise (high confidence), foundation movements drift, 50 Hz base station interference, etc.

Electrode interference: These devices have to be eliminated using appropriate filters in order to get more accurate and useful information from ECG. In comparison with typical audio and video filters, the ML-adaptable filters for reprocessing the ECG signal produce excellent performance. The ML algorithms give precise and quicker solutions for the automation and decision-making of ECG functions, and cardiac abnormality classification [3]. Several ML techniques are described here to analyze biological data, especially ECG. The chapter is organized as follows.

14.2 Heart-generated ECG signal

The ECG measures the magnitude and timing of the bioelectric activity produced by the heart. The depolarization or repolarization of the heart cells located in atriums and ventricles is responsible for these vibrational signals. Proper electrodes enable to the monitoring of the electromagnetic field's rhythms of the person in different parts of the body [4]. The standard ECG signal is recorded with the bidirectional lime (three electrodes) criteria, and with working electrode on substrates. Bipolar norms are used to augment the typical ECG signal (six electrodes). A triangle called the Einthoven equilateral triangle is used in ECG [4]. Figure 14.1 shows three members of an electrode that are injected: the right arm (RA), the left arm (LA) and the left leg (LL). Considering the voltage differential between two limb leads, the conventional limb leads will be achieved, as described as plumb I, plumb II and plumb III are known. The summation of plumb I and plumb III is equal to plumb II according to Einthoven's law. The increased limb conduits are unipolar, and a null point called null reference prospective is produced, as illustrated in Figure 14.2. The differential here between zero point and the lead of each limb is shown in Figure 14.1 as aVR, aVL and aVF. The amplified limbs provide extra development in multiple distinct directions by capturing the characteristic impedance in the heart [4].

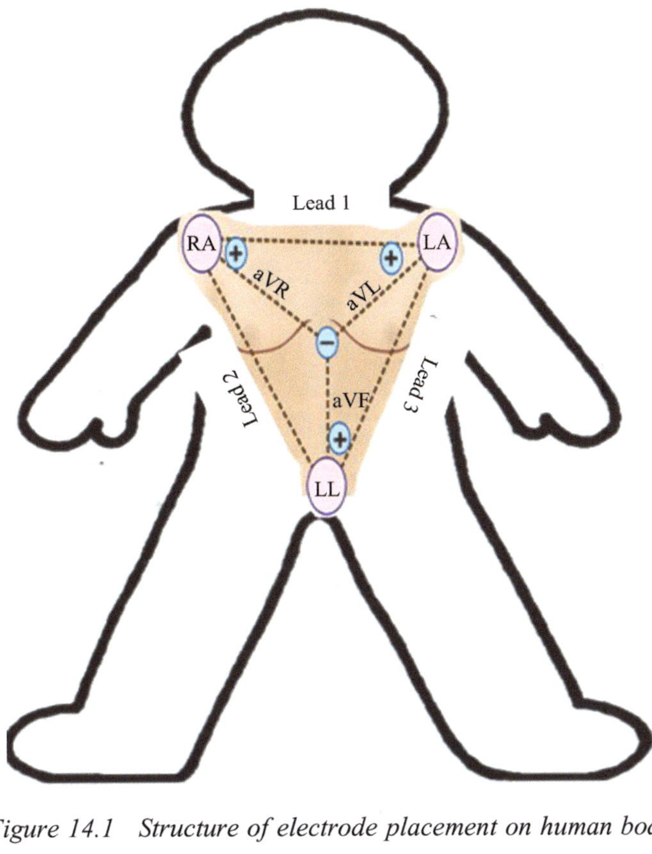

Figure 14.1 Structure of electrode placement on human body

The thoracic pathways designated as V1–V6 are also known as electrodes that are placed pathways. The aforementioned limb measures electrical impulses both in the left and the right directions, and in the rear and the front directions, compulsory in order and leads evaluate electrical impulses. The Middlesex Technology Institute Zigzag University Hospital [5] offers a variety of datasets of the ECG signal. As observed in Figure 14.3, the ECG waveform destabilization cycle consists of PQRST (U) impulses. The regular ECG signal, arrhythmias and QT interval and PR segmentation will examine P-wave observations, T-wave complication, PR interval and complicated QRS (whose endurance is also termed QRS). The ECG signal is recorded by electrodes which are sometimes skillfully contaminated by several

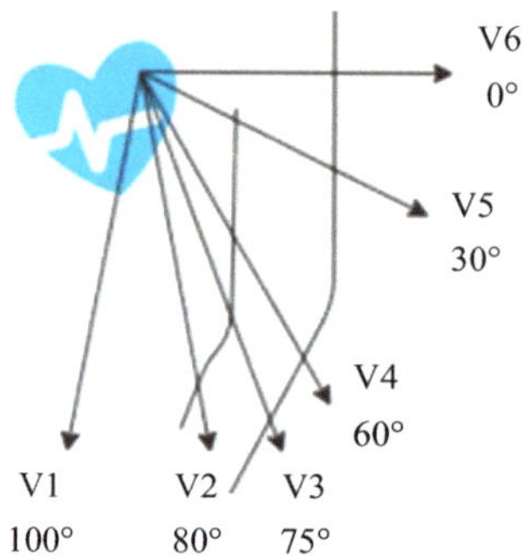

Figure 14.2 Structure of lead placement human chest

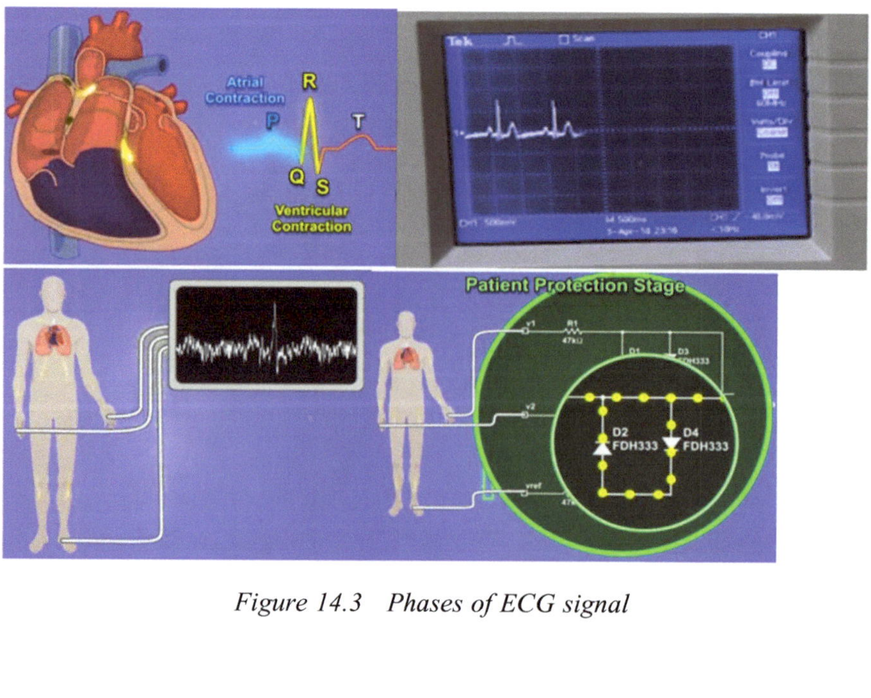

Figure 14.3 Phases of ECG signal

different sources systems. The ECG signal requires an image analysis of ECG data for the purpose of obtaining adequate understanding from the ECG signal. The different phases of ECG signal handling are shown in Figure 14.3. Various ML-based technologies utilized for ECG signal preparation and categorization will be explored in the following sections.

In Figure 14.3, ECG signal amplification utilizing algorithms based on the ML pretreatment of an ECG signal is necessary in order to remove undesired interfering portions and increase the beneficial feature of the biomedical signals. With the significant topics on cardiac electrical impulses concentrated between 5 and 35 Hz and the intensity of the ECG signal that is approximately 12 mV [6,7], it may be called a low-frequency physiological signal. The ECG signal is normally recorded after electrolytes gel is applied by inserting appropriate electrodes on the human body. Electrode or patient motion, inappropriate contact with the skin surface between some of the electrodes and other impulses may contribute to the addition of disturbance in the ECG signal. Due to improper channels transmission and data collection, and 50/60-Hz powerlines distortion and electromagnetic radiation pollution, the ECG signal may have a larger Stochastic filtering frequency. Depending on the voltage distribution of the complete modulating signal, the interference signals in the ECG may be categorized amongst four groups of abnormalities.

- Gaussian white sound: The ECG signal is damaged by this amplitude modulation particularly when the ECG signal is wirelessly transmitted.
- Noise from EMG: Electromagnetic signals, like skeletal muscles that are recorded in microelectrodes, are produced from other cells, culminating in ECG signal contaminated during signals of ECG. EMG noise reductions from ECG data are challenging as the frequency spectrum is the PQRST signals set in the ECG signal and, hence, the spectroscopic muscle activation frequencies are all the same.
- Hiking noise of baseline: This is a very low, gradually variable artifact, produced by variations in the impedance of the skin electrodes; skin contact, breathing, etc. movements in electrodes. Baseline roaming noise differs from its typical baseline from the whole signal.
- Noise interference with powerline (PLI): PLI noise is recognized as 50/60-Hz continuous powerline carrier disturbance with its electric field-generated harmonics. In view of the fact that the necessary characteristics need to be extracted from the ECG signal, the preparation methodology focuses largely on the elimination of undesired ECG signal sound elements. Background noise constituents can be eliminated with a preset coefficient by choosing the proper filter or filtering banking. The moment filters are adjusted with control parameters. ECG signals are timely signals with nonstatic environments. Fixed filter algorithms cannot significantly handle those signals when addressing these signals whose features differ over time. The ideal way to filter the ECG signals in an unset situation is to use an adaptive algorithm based on ML.

An instrumentation amplifier may update its correlation coefficient with environmental change continuously, such that optimal operational characteristics

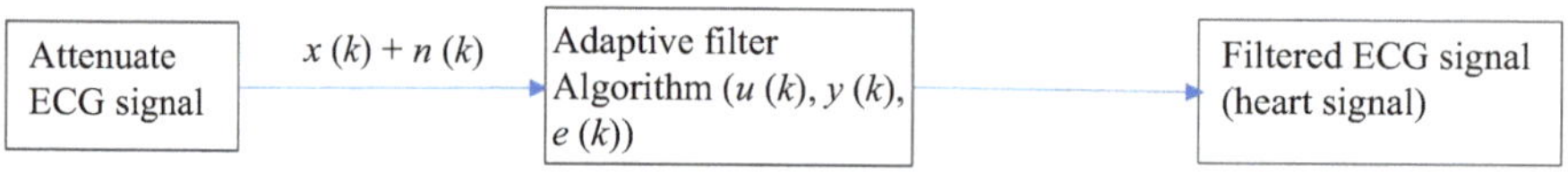

Figure 14.4 Enhance ECG signal

are achieved. Hamilton is playing a responsible role for maintaining national performance standards for removing PLI distortion by employing adaptive and non-adaptive filtering from the ECG waveform [8].

An instrumentation amplifier improves productivity with less complexity and improved ECG signal noise rejection. The iterative optimization architectures of Thakor and Zhu [9] have been created with the aim of removing noise in the ECG signal. They employed a recurring adaptable framework to identify heart rhythm. In Figure 14.4 for the treatment of the ECG data, there is an iterative optimization setup. Two signals are provided in Figure 14.4. The first is a perspective views comprising the requested signals. The $x(k)$ electrocardiogram and $n(k)$ signals that are noted in the ECG are not desired. The extra voltage level is a noisy signal $u(k)$ but is not related to the ECG signal $x(k)$. The signal $u(k)$ is delivered to the goal functional. The $e(k)$ activation function is specified as

$$e(k) = x(k) + n(k) - y(k) \tag{14.1}$$

The output of the adaptive filter is defined in equation (14.1) as

$$y(k) = \sum_{i=0}^{N} wn(k-1) \tag{14.2}$$

where wn is the coefficient of weight. The result (MSE) is then provided as

$$E\left[e^2(k)\right] = E\left[x^2(k)\right] + E\left\{[n(k) - y(k)]^2\right\} \tag{14.3}$$

The adaptive improvement adapts the parameters of the wl according to the predicted signal $e(k)$. When the modified signal generator value is achieved, the objective function modifies your equations to optimize MSE, as indicated in (14.3). The organizational strategy for coefficients alteration is based on the error signal minimization $e(k) = d(k) - y(k)$. Various alternative algorithms are also being suggested, based on their features, to remove the different kinds of interference. The following are addressed using the error propagation equations of Qureshi *et al.* [7], the most often used adaptive threshold methods for noise reduction present in the ECG signal.

14.3 Filtering parameters least-mean-square algorithm

In order to reduce the average standard errors in between filter output voltage and the expected exit signals, the least-mean-square (LMS) algorithm modifies the filter paramour. LMS consists of a strong algorithm of descent. The modified LMS technique filter parameter is provided as

$$w(k+1) = w(k) + 2\mu \times e(k) \times x(k) \tag{14.4}$$

where step sizes are μ. For analyzing the iterative refinement methodology, ECG data from both the MIT-BIH collections are used. This information is readily available for scholars. The ECG signal is directly collected in the central database, then warped and twisted by 50 Hz PLI and reference point undulating deformation in the MIT-BIH dataset. The simulations have been carried out using MATLAB® to examine the LMS-adaptive filter techniques' effectiveness. The input node of the objective function is used to provide PLI and baseline walking noise to polluted ECG, and at the required node the known ECG noise is used. The LMS-adaptive filter shows effectiveness with a medium error squared.

14.3.1 Updated filter coefficient in normalized least-mean-square (NLMS) algorithm

The normalized least-mean-square (NLMS) technique is utilized to resolve the problem of suitable step size selection. The choosing of stages is adaptable to result oriented and reliability. The modified NLMS algorithms filter coefficient is calculated as

$$w(k+1) = w(k) + \frac{2\mu}{x(n)xT(n)} e(k) \times x(k) \tag{14.5}$$

where $2\mu/x(n)xT(n)$ is all the sampling frequency standardized. ECG signals corrupted by PLI and foundation lines disturbance are used with the NLMS-adaptive method.·Effectiveness with square error of the NLMS adjustable filter is shown.

14.3.2 Improved performance LMS (DENLMS) algorithm delaying normalization inaccuracy

If high calculation performance with high computational is necessary, the DENLMS adaptation algorithm is chosen. The current DENLMS algorithm filtering frequency is specified as

$$w(k+1) = w(k) + \mu e(k - nD) \times x(k - nD) \tag{14.6}$$

where μ is the step and nD is the amount of delay normalization. In [10] a DENLMS-based adaptable filter technique removes Gaussian noise from the ECG data. Pipeline structures of the DENLMS algorithm improve the effectiveness and reduce the power consumption.

14.3.3 LMS is variant of sign data least-mean-square (SDLMS) algorithm

Sign data least-mean-square (SDLMS) algorithm is obtained by modifying the sgn(k) LMS input by making SDLMS far less difficult than LMS. Traditionally, this is consistently consistent, but subsequently accelerated with the crash of the MSE market. This strategy is often adopted when high-speed computation is required, for instance, in a particular component. The changed filtering coefficients for SDLMS algorithms is supplied as

$$w(k+1) = w(k) + 2\mu \times e(k) \times \text{sgn}(k) \tag{14.7}$$

Rather than the input signal, the quantification of the error sampling frequency is more required. The LLMS algorithm has an upgraded filter parameter:

$$w(k+1) = w(k) + 2\mu \times Qe(k) \times x(k) \tag{14.8}$$

The measurement function is $Qe(k)$, and logarithm functional Q is indicated as

$$Q(z) = 2^{\log_2(z)}\text{sgn}(z) \tag{14.9}$$

Main function of wavelet transform is the removal of various items that impair signal integrity and contribute to performance degradation. In this regard, the awareness of the impulse response and the attributes are essential for the maximum performance. The purpose of the adapting technique is to reduce MSE and increase the ECG signal for the retrieving of useful approach. NLMS offers improved MSE performance when compared to LMS, but at the expense of additional computation and storing. Due to its high-speed calculation, the SDLMS method is chosen for speedier results.

For the elimination of stationary and nonstationary disturbances from ECG, different iterative optimization techniques were compared [11]. Algorithm's effectiveness is checked by structural complexity, high computational and signal-to-noise ratio. EMG noise is eliminated using recurrent low-square adaptive algorithm from the ECG signal [12]. Parameters like filter order, signal-to-noise ratio, coefficient of remembering are used to verify the effectiveness of the classification method [13]. The motion devices are eliminated by employing an LMS based, iterative optimization method, a cosine transformer, from the ECG signal. Compared to conventional LMS algorithms developed, the suggested technique can eliminate higher frequencies noise relatively effectively. The ECG signal is polluted by several artifact kinds with varying frequency spectra. Distillation columns adaptable filtering may be designed for ECG filtration.

14.4 Retrieve and classify ECG signals utilizing ML-based techniques

The extraction of the ECG signal and the categorization of the signal present several obstacles. Due to the different aspects of EGC signals, the lack of defined characteristics and heterogeneity in ECG illness patterns/normal person by person [1], etc., the major issues in ECG signal categorization include many academics work on ML classification systems that can classify arrhythmias. The fundamental problem of the results of the ML-based classification is its reliance on heuristic knowledge. The learning process is essentially three types of ML-based algorithms: training data, unmonitored learning and enhanced learning. The monitored learning algorithm incorporates data from staff of expertise. This form of learning needs know-how and takes time. Uncontrolled learning detects new illnesses without human guidance from the query plan. However, this might lead to biased conclusions because other data groups do not verify it. Supervised and uncontrolled learning in combination is termed enhancement learning. But strengthening learning needs more time and unsupervised learning to get greater results. In general, measures such as sensitivity (*Se*), positive prediction (+*P*), specificity (*Sp*) and accuracy (*Ac*) [14] are validated for the efficacy of the classification method. The statistical metrics mentioned previously are as follows:

$$Se = \frac{TP}{TP + FN} \tag{14.10}$$

$$+P = \frac{TP}{TP + FP} \tag{14.11}$$

$$Sp = \frac{TN}{TN + FP} \tag{14.12}$$

$$Ac = \frac{TP + TN}{TP + TN + FN + FP} \tag{14.13}$$

where *TN* is genuine losses, *FP* is slightly inaccurate, and *FN* is false negatives, while *TP* is true positive. If the judgment of the doctor is accompanied by the identification of the arrhythmias of the classification, the *TP* decision will be taken. If both the physician's choice and the classifying arrhythmia are negative, the *TN* decision is made.

FP is decided when the classifier calls a healthy patient an arrhythmia. An *FN* decision is made if an arrhythmic patient is identified by the classification. The good *FN* and *FP* judgments are minimized by a strong classification method. As a component of *Se* and +*P*, another potential measurements *F*1 score is used. The *F*1 value is set to

$$F1 = \frac{2(Se + P)}{Se + P} \tag{14.14}$$

where the *F*1 score is used as a categorization indicator in the learning phase. Various techniques were developed for the categorization of ECG signals and collection of characteristics such as the methodology Pan and Tompkins, neural networks, wavelet based, mapping supports, personality mapping, fluid logic, related topic. In this part, innovative ML-based approaches are investigated.

14.5 Artificial neural network (ANN)-based ECG signals

Artificial neural network (ANN) is a scientific data categorization network based on biological activities. The usage of ML algorithms based on ANN offers several benefits, for example, their own flexibility, rapidity, accuracy and nonlinearity. Expandable and robust ANN also has irrelevant features. ANN applies to the ECG signal, given its major strengths: (1) the ECG signal is of a nonlinear character and the ANN uses different enabling functionalities to deal with nonlinearity; (2) the EG signals are less often used, and the ANN has an adaptable model to the shorter wavelengths. However, ANN has various problems surrounding its application, such as (1) ANN needs adequate information for training and testing objectives; (2) ANN may not be able to give an overall, ideal ECG electrocardiographic clinics approach; several ANN-based algorithms have been offered for the ECG classification. A square ANN is provided in [15] for the electrocardiogram classification. The proposal has been made in [16] for a robust and general ANN method to categorize the ECG data. In combination with an eigenvector-based approach, the recurrent neural network (RNN) is used for the classification of four ECG beats [17]. For this classification, the physiotherapy banking information is evaluated. The two classifier-based RNNs are suggested for heartbeat detection in [18]. Currently, numerous academics have begun using deep neural networks (DNNs) categorization. In [19], the active DNN categorization of ECG signals through training and interactions were suggested. In [20] the proposal for the identification of five kinds of cardiac beats in ECG readings is for a convolution neural network (CNN) of nine-layer models. In [21], a model DNN architecture including a CNN and a recurrent structure was designed. An ECG categorization approach was created, independent and interpatient. In the model described in [22], for cardiac arrhythmia identification of ECG data, a 1D-convolutional ANN model was presented. For technical identification of deep CNN-based arrhythmia, Reference [23] has been used. In [24], for myocardial infarction (MI) identification using ECG data, a CNN method is presented. The noise present on the signal obtains a precision of 93.53 percent. The ECG beat is searched by RNN in [25].

The ECG beat rating is global and updated based on morphological and temporal data from the RNN.

14.6 Classification of ECG signals based fuzzy logic (FL)

The ML based on fuzzy logic (FL) is an ECG signal technology and a classification of biological processes. The FL might provide more useful and intelligible linguistic knowledge estimations. In the ECG signal categorization, this specialty for the FL is significant as it entails knowledge-based decision-making. The FL employs smooth parameters with various membership functions. Instabilities may also be handled by the FL through the rules in expert systems. The ECG recordings presented a fuzzy rule-based set support system [26]. They have created an illness identification decision system. An ECG treatment of cancers-adaptable computational intelligence system with parameter sets has been proposed in [27]. The classification proposed was 88.2 percent on average right. The ECG signal also provides atherosclerosis parameters. A foggy endothelial dysfunction system has been established to predict blood vessel disease [28]. They highlight a membership function for searching regulations architecture, which accurately predicts diseases using a variety of data. The fuzzy inference approach was proposed [29] for the destruction of the ECG signal. The MSE and transmission frequencies are boosted with the ANN. In 1974, Bezek devised and changed the furious clustering strategy of the FCM and was used by academics in several classification applications [30]. The contrasting color on FCM is also effective for the categorization of the ECG signal. In [31], ten distinct arrhythmias were classified by FCM from the ECG data. The results were compared with 92 patients. The FCM clustering decreased the number of segments that increased algorithm speed by combining comparable training samples segment. The clustering technique type 2 of the FCM is also utilized to classify ECG arrhythmia in [32]. The development/certification phase using FCM was made more efficient. They produced a fresh training dataset using the FCM type 2 by identifying the appropriate arrhythmia. A clustering-based methodology is used to obtain the 99 percent accuracy rate. In [33], FCM is utilized to categorize the ECG signals in the heartbeat situations. With 93.57 percent accuracy, the suggested approach was able to distinguish irregular and normal heartbeat. In [34] an ECG and a cardiac color ultrasonography were created to the FCM model spectral-based link-centric heart failure algorithm.

14.7 Fourier transform wavelet transforms

In the early 1980s, Morlet employed the wavelet transformation. The transformer of the wavelet can generate single- or multidimensional data that provide the Fourier transformation an additional answer. The wavelet transforms have a number of requests, for example, in the fields of data categorization and authentication, telecommunication, multichannel audio application development, face recognition and medical ML. The sliding window technique is used for a continuous time signal of duration and discontinuous period. Fourier modification is used for ECG signals since they are not stationary information. The transformation wavelet is determined by wrapping low-frequency and bandwidth filtering in the signals and then flowing straight downward. Thus, extracted features may assess minor differences from around piece of data. This wavelet characteristic is helpful in the ECG signal finding of tips or discontinuity.

The cached problems and problems of the ECG signals have a poor definition of the uninterrupted magnitude and phase compared with the transformed wavelet [35]. The wavelet transformation was used to detect the QRS complex wave [36]. The P and T impulses were also detected by the electrocardiogram disturbance. The reliability of the QRS categorization was more than 99.8 percent, including ECG signal drifting and distortions. The QRS detectors were designed [37] to transform the ECG signals of the dyadic waveform. In comparison to existing analytical techniques, the suggested approach offered improved results. In [38], the transforming wavelet is employed to lower the ECG signal dimensions and is then supplied into the neural network. The values achieved with the suggested wavelet are 99.28, 99.83, 99.97 and 99.21 percent correspondingly for *Ac*, *Sp*, *Se* and +*P* parameters of cardiac beat categorization. RR periods have been reconstructed from ECG data using this discreet wavelet approach [39]. The proposed structure minimized noninformative variables and lowered the classification data length. Several essential problems have been solved, such as overtime for scalability and stability.

To categorize a higher frequency from the ECG signal, the quick transform Fourier (FFT) and the discrete cosine transform are used [40]. In [41], a taxonomy of rhythmic utilizing its physicochemical features was suggested. The RR interval knowledge is described as the ECG signal dynamics. The method has been evaluated with MIT-BIH rhythmic databases and the reliability of the grading has been enhanced. The identification methodology for QRS complexes was created with the transformation of the adjustable Q wavelet [42]. Improved breakdown of the ECG signal is properly set as constants and substrands. About 99.88 percent of the suggested approach, 99.89 percent of the sensitivities and 99.83 percent of the positive ECG signals are present in the MIT-BIH arrhythmic database.

14.8 Combination of machine learning and statistical algorithms

A mixture of analytical techniques and other ML algorithms is employed for the ML-based algorithm. A proposed methodology to the ECG signal was referred to as a mixture of statistics algorithms and ML algorithms.

In [43], an intricate neural network has been created for ECG beat identification and categorization. The FCM and ANN were utilized to differentiate between several ECG-beat types with very effective results. In [44], wavelet transform is employed for the derivation of functions, and the ECG beats were classified using a fuzzy neural-based subscription algorithm. In addition to an ANN-based beat categorization of the ECG data, the integrative, independent assessment of the components (ICA) was suggested in [45]. The ECG signal is weighed downward here average, using ICA technique, of substantially mutually independent fundamental components. The back-propagative neural network is used for the classification of the data. The suggested approach provides more than 98 percent classification precision. The concept is applied to identify fuzzy neural networks (FNNs) for the use of involuntary muscle contraction (PVCs) using ECG data (FNNs). The ANN trains the ECG signals using weighty, fuzzy associations from the MIT-BIH PVC dataset. The ECG beat ensemble classifier was proposed in [46] for particle swarm optimization with radial functional neural network basis. A reduced network value was estimated with six distinct types of categorization beats. SVM, wavelet and ANN are employed for the fusion strategy. The ECG signal first came with the strong discrete transforming wavelet. The ML approach was next presented to discover arrhythmia, which attained an accuracy of 98.06 percent. The principal supervised learning of component analysis (PCA), in conjunction with the DNN, determines arrhythmia in the ECG data. The PCA was utilized to decrease the imbalance of the signal database system. With the hybrid technique, they attained a precision of 96.7 percent.

14.9 Conclusion and future work

This chapter examined different machine-based learning techniques and their implications for medical image analysis. First, we highlighted succinctly the relevance for the biological image processing of ML-based approaches. We concentrated mostly on ECG signal processing throughout the chapter. For reprocessing the ECG signal, database, many learning techniques for LMS-based optimization methods have been described. For the identification and categorization of ECG features, various ML-based approaches are briefly mentioned. Potential components and publications for an ECG waveform, ANN, FL, spectral and optimization techniques are used to investigate MI. Atheoretical notions of ML for biological image analysis applications have been demonstrated in real time. A decreased, elevated and reliable instrument may be developed by the ML-based methodology with a proper existing device for real-time biomedical clinical diagnostics.

References

[1] K.R. Foster, R. Koprowski, and J.D. Skufca, Machine learning, medical diagnosis, and biomedical engineering research – commentary, *Biomed. Eng. Online* 13(1) (2014).

[2] E. Ozpolat, B. Karakaya, T. Kaya, and A. Gulten, FPGA-based digital filter design for biomedical signal, *Perspect. Technol. Methods MEMS Des. MEMSTECH 2016 – Proc. 12th Int. Conf.* (2016) pp. 70–73.

[3] C.K. Roopa, and B.S. Harish, A survey on various machine learning approaches for ECG analysis, *Int. J. Comput. Appl.* 163(9) (2017) 25–33.

[4] G. John *Webster, Medical Instrumentation Application and Design*, 4th ed., Wiley, New York, 2010.

[5] A.L. Goldberger, L.A.N. Amaral, L. Glass, *et al.*, PhysioBank, PhysioToolkit, and PhysioNet: components of a new research resource for complex physiologic signals, *Circulation* 101 (2000) E215–E220.

[6] J. Zhang, B. Li, K. Xiang, and X. Shi, Method of diagnosing heart disease based on deep learning ECG signal, arXiv preprint arXiv:1907.01514 (2019).

[7] R. Qureshi, M. Uzair, and K. Khurshid, Multistage adaptive filter for ECG signal processing, *Proc. 2017 Int. Conf. Commun. Comput. Digit. Syst. C-CODE 2017* (2017) pp. 363–368.

[8] P.S. Halmiton, A comparison of adaptive and nonadaptive filters for reduction of power line interference in the ECG, *IEEE Trans. Biomed. Eng.* 43(1) (1996) 105–109.

[9] N.V. Thakor, and Y.-S. Zhu, Applications of adaptive filtering to ECG analysis: noise cancellation and arrhythmia detection, *IEEE Trans. Biomed. Eng.* 38(8) (1991) 785–794.

[10] C. Venkatesan, P. Karthigaikumar, and R. Varatharajan, FPGA implementation of modified error normalized LMS adaptive filter for ECG noise removal, *Cluster Comput.* (2018) 19.

[11] M.Z.U. Rahman, R.A. Shaik, and D.V.R.K. Reddy, Efficient and simplified adaptive noise cancelers for ECG sensor based remote health monitoring, *IEEE Sens. J.* 12(3) (2012) 566–573.

[12] G. Lu, J.S. Brittain, P. Holland, *et al.*, Removing ECG noise from surface EMG signals using adaptive filtering, *Neurosci. Lett.* 462(1) (2009) 14–19.

[13] F. Xiong, D. Chen, Z. Chen, and S. Dai, Cancellation of motion artifacts in ambulatory ECG signals using TD-LMS adaptive filtering techniques, *J. Visual Commun. Image Represent.* 58 (2019) 606–618.

[14] M. Alfaras, M.C. Soriano, and S. Ortín, A fast machine learning model for ECG-based heartbeat classification and arrhythmia detection, *Front. Phys.* 7 (2019).

[15] W. Jiang, and S.G. Kong, Block-based neural networks for personalized ECG signal classification, *IEEE Trans. Neural Netw.* 18(6) (2007) 1750–1761.

[16] T. Ince, S. Kiranyaz, and M. Gabbou, A generic and robust system for automated patient-specific classification of ECG signals, *IEEE Trans. Biomed. Eng.* 56(5) (2009) 1415–1426.

[17] E.D. Übeyli, Combining recurrent neural networks with eigenvector methods for classification of ECG beats, *Digital Signal Process.* 19(2) (2009) 320–329.

[18] T. Teijeiro, P. Félix, J. Presedo, and D. Castro, Heartbeat classification using abstract features from the abductive interpretation of the ECG, *IEEE J. Biomed. Health Inf.* 22(2) (2018) 409–420.

[19] M.M. Al Rahhal, Y. Bazi, H. AlHichri, N. Alajlan, F. Melgani, and R.R. Yager, Deep learning approach for active classification of electrocardiogram signals, *Inf. Sci.* 345 (2016) 340–354.

[20] U.R. Acharya, S.L. Oh, Y. Hagiwara, *et al.*, A deep convolutional neural network model to classify heartbeats, *Comput. Biol. Med.* 89 (2017) 389–396.

[21] L. Guo, G. Sim, and B. Matuszewski, Inter-patient ECG classification with convolutional and Recurrent Neural Networks, *Biocybern. Biomed. Eng.* 39(3) (2019) 868–879.

[22] S. Kiranyaz, T. Ince, and M. Gabbouj, Real-time patient-specific ECG classification by 1-D convolutional neural networks, *IEEE Trans. Biomed. Eng.* 63(3) (2016) 664–675.

[23] Ö. Yıldırım, P. Pławiak, R.S. Tan, and U.R. Acharya, Arrhythmia detection using deep convolutional neural network with long duration ECG signals, *Comput. Biol. Med.* 102 (2018) 411–420.

[24] U.R. Acharya, H. Fujita, S.L. Oh, Y. Hagiwara, J.H. Tan, and M. Adam, Application of deep convolutional neural network for automated detection of myocardial infarction using ECG signals, *Inf. Sci.* 415–416 (2017) 190–198.

[25] G. Wang, C. Zhang, Y. Liu, *et al.*, A global and updatable ECG beat classification system based on recurrent neural networks and active learning, *Inf. Sci.* 501 (2019) 523–542.

[26] S. Mitra, M. Mitra, and B.B. Chaudhuri, An approach to a rough set-based disease inference engine for ECG classification, In: Greco S. et al. (eds) *Rough Sets and Current Trends in Computing*. RSCTC 2006. Lecture Notes in Computer Science, vol 4259. Springer, Berlin, Heidelberg (2006).

[27] W.K. Lei, B.N. Li, M.C. Dong, and M.I. Vai, AFC-ECG: an adaptive fuzzy ECG classifier, *Soft Computing in Industrial Applications* (pp. 189–199), Springer, Berlin (2007).

[28] D. Pal, K.M. Mandana, S. Pal, D. Sarkar, and C. Chakraborty, Fuzzy expert system approach for coronary artery disease screening using clinical parameters, *Knowl.-Based Syst.* 36 (2012) 162–174.

[29] S. Goel, P. Tomar, and G. Kaur, A fuzzy based approach for denoising of ECG signal using wavelet transform, *Int. J. Bio-Sci. Bio-Technol.* 8(2) (2016) 143–156.

[30] A.K. Shah, and D.M. Adhyaru, Parameter identification of PWARX models using fuzzy distance weighted least squares method, *Appl. Soft Comput.* 25 (2014) 174–183.

[31] Y. Özbay, R. Ceylan, and B. Karlik, A fuzzy clustering neural network architecture for classification of ECG arrhythmias, *Comput. Biol. Med.* 36(4) (2006) 376–388.

[32] R. Ceylan, Y. Özbay, and B. Karlik, A novel approach for classification of ECG arrhythmias: type-2 fuzzy clustering neural network, *Expert Syst. Appl.* 36(3) (2009) 6721–6726. PART 2.

[33] Y.C. Yeh, W.J. Wang, and C.W. Chiou, A novel fuzzy c-means method for classifying heartbeat cases from ECG signals, *Meas. J. Int. Meas. Confed.* 43 (10) (2010) 1542–1555.

[34] J. Dongdong, N. Arunkumar, Z. Wenyu, L. Beibei, Z. Xinlei, and Z. Guangjian, Semantic clustering fuzzy c means spectral model based comparative analysis of cardiac color ultrasound and electrocardiogram in patients with left ventricular heart failure and cardiomyopathy, *Future Gener. Comput. Syst.* 92 (2019) 324–328.

[35] P.S. Addison, Wavelet transforms and the ECG: a review, *Physiol. Meas.* 26 (5) (2005) R155–R199.

[36] C. Li, C. Zheng, and C. Tai, Detection of ECG characteristic points using wavelet transforms, *IEEE Trans. Biomed. Eng.* 42 (1995) 21–28.

[37] S. Kadambe, R. Murray, and G.F. Boudreaux-Bartels, Wavelet transform-based QRS complex detector, *IEEE Trans. Biomed. Eng.* 46 (1999) 838–848.

[38] R.J. Martis, U.R. Acharya, and L.C. Min, ECG beat classification using PCA, LDA, ICA and discrete wavelet transform, *Biomed. Signal Process. Control.* 8(5) (2013) 437–448.

[39] M.M. Tantawi, K. Revett, A.B. Salem, and M.F. Tolba, A wavelet feature extraction method for electrocardiogram (ECG)-based biometric recognition, *Signal Image Video Process.* 9(6) (2015) 1271–1280.

[40] University Malaysia Perlis. School of Mechatronic Engineering, IEEE Malaysia Section, IEEE Engineering in Medicine and Biology Society.

Malaysia Chapter, and Institute of Electrical and Electronics Engineers, Proceedings, 2015 2nd International Conference on Biomedical Engineering (ICoBE 2015): 3031 (2015), Penang, Malaysia.

[41] S.M. Anwar, M. Gul, M. Majid, and M. Alnowami, Arrhythmia classification of ECG signals using hybrid features, *Comput. Math. Methods Med.* 2018 (2018).

[42] A. Sharma, S. Patidar, A. Upadhyay, and U. Rajendra Acharya, Accurate tunable-Q wavelet transforms-based method for QRS complex detection, *Comput. Electr. Eng.* 75 (2019) 101–111.

[43] S. Osowski, and T.H. Linh, ECG beat recognition using fuzzy hybrid neural network, *IEEE Trans. Biomed. Eng.* 48 (2001) 1265–1271.

[44] M. Engin, ECG beat classification using neuro-fuzzy network, *Pattern Recognit. Lett.* 25(15) (2004) 1715–1722.

[45] S.N. Yu, and K.T. Chou, Integration of independent component analysis and neural networks for ECG beat classification, *Expert Syst. Appl.* 34(4) (2008) 2841–2846.

[46] M. Korürek, and B. Dogan, ECG beat classification using particle swarm optimization and radial basis function neural network, *Expert Syst. Appl.* 37(12) (2010) 7563–7569.

Chapter 15

A survey and taxonomy on mutual interference mitigation techniques in wireless body area networks

Neethu Suman[1] and P.C. Neelakantan[2]

Abstract

Our world has evolved from the era when sensors were just used to measure certain basic physiological human body signals such as temperature and pressure during the late 1980s to the current era where we have wireless and miniaturized implanted sensors that can even monitor the operation of internal organs and transmit the health critical information to experts within seconds. Wireless body area network (WBAN) is the wireless sensor network in which the nodes can be emplaced in, on, or around the human body to measure the human biotic signals and ambient information. In dense areas such as hospitals, old age homes, marathons, etc., the number of WBAN users will be more and varies dynamically. This leads to the degradation of WBAN performance parameters such as throughput, latency, energy efficiency, and reliability due to the interference between the WBANs. Thus, dealing with interference issues is one of the most important challenges related to WBAN compared to other wireless networks, owing to the inter-WBAN short distances and dynamic nature. This chapter discusses the classification of the interference associated with the WBAN networks and a comparative study on existing mutual interference mitigation approaches in each use case.

Keywords: Wireless body area networks; Mutual interference mitigation techniques; MAC approach for mutual interference mitigation in WBAN

15.1 Introduction

Nowadays, the world is exploring the opportunity of being connected in every field of research. One such area is wireless body area networks (WBANs) where the

[1]Department of Electronics and Communication Engineering, Adi Shankara Institute of Engineering and Technology, APJ Abdul Kalam Technological University, Ernakulam, India
[2]Department of Electronics and Communication Engineering, Muthoot Institute of Technology and Science, APJ Abdul Kalam Technological University, Ernakulam, India

nodes can be emplaced in, on, or around the human body. The earlier stage of WBAN [1] was wireless personal area networks (WPANs) implemented first at Massachusetts Institute of Technology during the 1990s. This WPAN was to realize the data transmission using electric field modulation through the body and also to measure body positioning. Later, IEEE had approved an IEEE Standard 802.15.6 [2] stating directions for implementing low power, short distance, high data rate, and meeting the specific absorption rate (SAR) guidelines. The three physical-layer propagation methods [2] defined by IEEE 802.15.6 WBAN standard are narrowband communication, ultra-wideband [3] communications, and human-body communications, and four communication scenarios are off-body [4], on-body [5], in-body [6], and body-to-body [7–10] communications.

The general three-tier architecture of WBANs [11] includes (1) intra-BAN communications that represent the communications among the nodes and the coordinator of the WBAN, (2) inter-BAN communications which denote the communications among the coordinator node and access point (AP) to data collecting and storing system, and (3) beyond-BAN tier that links the AP to the Internet or the other end-user such as ambulance, doctors, and medical assistance. It uses Bluetooth [12], Wibree [13], ZigBee [12] (IEEE 802.15.4), and WBAN standard [14,15] (IEEE 802.15.6) for short-range communication and WiMAX, Wi-Fi, LTE, and LTE-advance for long-range communications. The limitations of existing WBAN architecture are vendor dependency, mobility, cloud integration, time-variant data volume, resource utilization, security, and privacy [12,16].

There are three categories of nodes based on their placement [17]. The first one is implant nodes (e.g. implantable glucometer), the nodes that are implanted below the human skin or even deeper inside. The second type is body surface nodes, the nodes emplaced on the human skin surface or at least 2 cm away from the body. The third one is the external nodes that are nodes placed in the range of few centimetres to 5 m away from the body. These acquire important human periodic or emergency signals such as EEG, blood pressure, ECG, blood glucose level, and heart rate. The collected information is analysed for any abnormality by medical personnel and computer program. This opens up a new opportunity for early detection of diseases, speedy post-surgery recovery, continuous monitoring of patients, and healthcare solutions for ageing. Apart from these medical applications, there are non-medical applications such as interactive gaming, fitness monitoring applications.

The WBANs can be classified into two major application areas: medical and non-medical. Continuous health monitoring [18] of elderly and diseased people are the main medical applications of WBAN. The typical examples count the timely detection and keep track of diseases, medical assistance for the patients, and post-surgery rehabilitation [19]. Typically, body sensors utilized in health monitoring can be either (1) human body vital signal measurement sensors like body temperature, blood pressure, ECG, EEG, oxygen saturation, capsule endoscope [20]; or (2) motion sensors use to measure human body movement-based signals as acceleration or angular rate of rotation. Apart from body sensors, ambient sensors are also used to measure environmental information like temperature, pressure, light, or humidity which is an add-on to the medical diagnosis and treatment. Based on device usage, medical applications can be further classified into the wearable, implant, and remote monitoring device categories [20]. Medical assistance in disaster management, interactive gaming, driving assistance and fitness monitoring [21], safety monitoring in the construction site [22], fire-fighters' and soldiers' vital signal monitoring [23], biometric authentication [24] are the few non-medical applications of WBAN. For example, a smartwatch is capable of keeping track of how much calorie is burnt and the distance walked per day. The technical requirement that should be considered for a WBAN application scenario includes movement, location, energy and processing capacity, data rate, and node temperature. Jones and Katzis [25] discuss the possibility of integrating the latest 5G wireless technology with WBAN networks, including the architecture, energy efficiency, interference mitigation, data rate, communication frequency ranges, and security issues.

An introduction to the interference conditions on the coexisting WBANs is discussed in Section 15.2. We present a survey on existing mutual interference mitigation methods in Section 15.3, and our conclusions based on the survey are presented in Section 15.4.

15.2 Interference issues in WBAN [11]

In crowded scenarios like hospitals, marathons, buses, many WBANs are randomly and dynamically distributed in the restricted area. The network efficiency of individual WBANs will be reduced owing to the transmission signals interfering with each other and the limited transmission channel. Interference is the one of important design concerns associated with WBAN. The interference on the coexisting WBANs can be either intra- or inter-network interference. The concurrent transmission (CCT) of nodes within a single WBAN causes intra- and inter-network interference occurs due to the transmission of nodes within the multiple WBANs. Inter-network interference can be further categorized into mutual interference and cross interference. Mutual interference is due to the interference between the nodes of multiple WBANs within a short-range and cross interference is the interference caused due to the presence of different other wireless networks operated in the same frequency as the WBAN operating frequency. Figure 15.1 shows the intra-interference, mutual interference [11], and cross interference scenario in WBAN.

The study conducted by the authors of [21,26] on interference shows that the interference generated by dynamic WBANs highly decreases the throughput and SINR values and increases the average packet delay of the emergency signal compared with the WBAN without the interference and power consumption. The node placement and mobility, path loss and shadowing, medium access control (MAC) layer access mechanism, and channel frequency are the various sources of interference in WBAN. The analysis in [27] has shown that the numbers of WBANs, path loss exponent, and transmission power of sensors influence the interference level. In the next section, we present a comparative study of the various mutual interference mitigation schemes; their relative performance metrics and features.

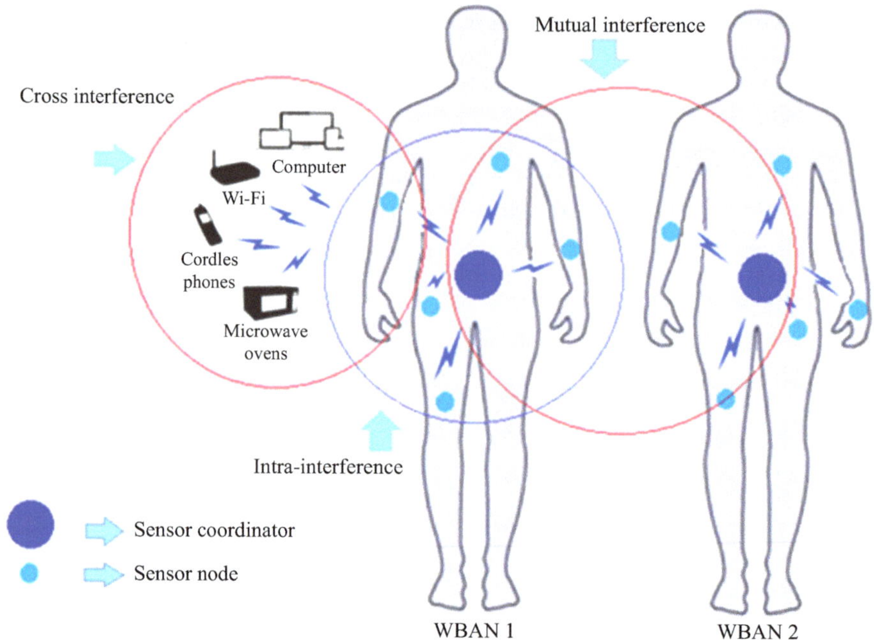

Figure 15.1 Intra-network interference (blue circle) [11] and inter-network interference – cross interference (red circle left) and mutual interference (red circle right) in WBAN

15.3 Mutual interference mitigation schemes

The traditional scheduling schemes such as TDMA and CSMA/CA and hybrid MAC protocols can be used for avoiding the intra-network interference of a single WBAN. The topology of a single-WBAN network is much more stable compared to multiple-WBAN network. But the mutual interference mitigation is more challenging as WBAN is a decentralized network and so normal centralized interference mitigation used in cellular networks cannot be used in WBAN.

The CCT/cooperative/opportunistic scheduling and non-CCT (NCCT) scheduling are two basic classifications of scheduling for mutual interference mitigation. In CCT [28], the multiple nodes transmit concurrently in the same time slot (TS)-based dynamic variation in the channel condition of sensors like sensors count, traffic signal strength, and the priority of the applications. In NCCT, the resources are distributed among the adjacent WBAN; for example, in [29,30], using on vertex colouring techniques, different times are allocated to adjacent WBANs based on their sensor data priority and data traffic requirement.

15.3.1 MAC approach

2L-MAC [31]: Chen *et al.* proposed a MAC protocol with two-layer solutions for interference mitigation in WBAN. Within the first layer, the coordinator coordinates the intra-WBAN communication using a distributed polling-based protocol. In the second layer, it employs CSMA techniques to avoid inter-BAN interference. The proposed protocol also allows WBANs to change their operating channel and prioritizes sensors for satisfying quality of service (QoS) requirements. In the simulations, Chen *et al.* [31] compare 2L-MAC with beacon shifting, channel hopping, and B2IRS.

Adaptive CSMA/CA MAC protocol: In [32], Huang and Quek propose an adaptive CSMA/CA MAC protocol to avoid inter-WBAN interference for WBAN. Compared to [31], the proposed protocol is adaptive and improves throughput and delay performance. Intra-WBAN interference is avoided by using interference adaptive polling period/MAC frame length. The coordinator reduces MAC frame length when it notices the interference from other WBAN to reduce the transmission delay. Similarly, it increases the frame length if there is less interference. The inter-WBAN interference mitigation method is similar to [31], i.e. CSMA/CA.

isMAC [33]: The isMAC is an adaptive multi-channel interference mitigation scheme for WBAN. In this scheme, both TDMA- and multichannel-based protocol are used to allocate the channel requirement of the neighbouring WBANs. The WBAN coordinator node (WCN) role rotation mechanism is also used to reduce the overall energy consumption. The central node listens to the channel information and decides and informs all the available different WBAN node members about their current WCN based on the residual energy level, number of terms of WCN, and sensor node priority.

Hybrid multi-channel medium access control (HM-MAC) protocol for WBANs [34]: The high priority user data transmission with high reliability and low latency are performed during the random access phase of superframe. The periodic data are transmitted in the scheduled phase also with high reliability. The inter-WBAN interference is controlled by the channel selection algorithm. Using this algorithm, the coordinator selects the idle channel by sensing the channel energy periodically and the idle channels are allocated to WBANs based on the idle channel information and WBAN sensor priority orders with one-hop neighbour WBANs.

Three-dimensional Markov chain model based CSMA/CA protocol [3D-MCM] [35]: 3D-MCM analyse the dynamic and multi-WBAN coexistence interference performance. A health critical index taking into account the WBANs priority, data traffic differentiates, and severity had been designed to ensure the transmission privilege of emergency data with lower delay and high reliability.

QoS-based MAC scheduling and fuzzy interference engine [QoS MAC] [36]: The inter-WBAN interference was avoided by using a modified priority pre-emptive scheduling algorithm. The coordinator broadcasts in the contention-free period of the superframe assigned the TS to the sensor node according to their priority order. The coordinator in the range of each WBAN communicates in the same frequency compares the priority level of its sensor data, pre-empts the low priority data, and thus avoids interference. The pre-empted data are transmitted later.

15.3.1.1 Summary and discussion on MAC approach

The various parameters used for the analysis of the MAC approach are summarized in Table 15.1. A comparative study based on the different network performance metrics

Table 15.1 Parameters considered for the analysis of mutual interference mitigation methods (by default, the parameter is considered in the simulation analysis)

	Mutual interference mitigation methods	Parameters considered for the analysis
1	MAC approach	
	2L-MAC [31]	Data delivery rate, data delivery latency, energy saving
	Adaptive CSMA/CA [32]	Average throughput, average delay, average number of sensing actions
	isMAC [33]	Average end-to-end delay (EED), energy consumption of WBAN coordinator node, total throughput value of the network
	HM-MAC [34]	Packet delivery ratio, average EED, average throughput, energy consumption
		Average throughput, average EED (used for mathematical analysis)
	3D-MCM [35]	Normalized throughput and average access delay
	QoS MAC [36]	SNR, BER, Eb/No
2	Transmission power control	
	PAPU [37]	Network utility, power consumption (used for experimental analysis)
	LRL [38,39]	SINR
	QPC [40]	Transmission power, SINR (used for experimental analysis)
	APLDR [27]	Packet loss ratio (PLR)
	Bayesian game [41]	Average power level, average throughput
3	Adaptive spectrum allocation	
	AIM [42]	Average reuse factor, average delay
		Average reuse factor (used for mathematical analysis)
	ACESS [43]	Packet reception rate (PRR)
	Inter-ACS [43]	Average data rate, interference count
	RIC [30]	Time complexity, spatial reuse, convergence speed, channel utilization
	CEVC [29]	Efficiency
4	Cooperative scheduling for interference mitigation	
	DCS [28]	Packet reception rate (PRR), fairness
	FTMH [45]	Throughput, average EED, energy consumption, packet drop rate

such as latency, collision rate, spatial reuse, power consumption, throughput, channel access, QoS support, and reliability is given in Table 15.2. In the simulations, the authors of [31] compare 2L-MAC with beacon shifting, channel hopping, and B2IRS. The results show that the 2L-MAC protocol has shown better delivery performance and energy efficiency. The proposed protocol has lowered the energy consumption of sensors by 44.1% and 78%, respectively, compared to beacon shifting and B2IRS. Compared to [31], the adaptive CSMA/CA MAC protocol [32] is adaptive and improves throughput and delay performance. The simulation results show that the required sensing power has been reduced without much performance loss.

Table 15.2 Comparison of mutual interference mitigation schemes

		Collision rate	Power consumption	Latency	Throughput	Spatial reuse	Channel access	QoS support	Reliability
1	MAC approach								
	2L-MAC [31]	Medium	Low	Low	High	No	CSMA/CA	Yes	Medium
	Adaptive CSMA/CA [32]	Low	Low	Medium	High	No	CSMA/CA	Yes	High
	isMAC [33]	Low	Low	Low	High	No	TDMA	Yes	Medium
	HM-MAC [34]	Low	Low	Low	High	No	CSMA/CA, TDMA	Yes	High
	3D-MCM [35]	Low		Low	High	No	CSMA/CA	Yes	Medium
	QoS MAC [36]	Low	Low	Medium	Medium	No	TDMA	Yes	Medium
2	Transmission power control								
	PAPU [37]	Medium	Low	Low	Medium	No	TDMA	Yes	Medium
	LRL [38,39]	Medium	Low	Medium	High	No	–	Yes	Medium
	QPC [40]	Low	Low	Medium	Medium	No	–	Yes	High
	APLDR [27]	Low	Medium	Low	High	No	CDMA	Yes	Medium
	Bayesian game [41]	Low	Low	Low	High	No	TDMA	Yes	High
3	Adaptive spectrum allocation								
	AIM [42]	Low	Medium	Low	High	Yes	TDMA	Yes	High
	ACCESS [43]	Medium	Low	Low	High	No	CSMA/CA	Yes	Medium
	Inter-ACS [44]	Low	Medium	High	Medium	No	TDMA	Yes	Medium
	RIC [30]	Low	Medium	Low	High	Yes	TDMA	Yes	Medium
	CEVC [29]	Low	Low	Low	High	Yes	TDMA	Yes	High
4	Cooperative scheduling for interference mitigation								
	DCS [28]	Low	Medium	Low	Medium	Yes	TDMA	Yes	Medium
	FTMH [45]	Low	Low	Low	High	Yes	TDMA	Yes	High

The iMAC protocol [33] has shown an almost constant value of 4 ms, 3.78 J and 1 packet per slot for the average end-to-end delay (EED), energy consumption of WCN, and total throughput value of the network, respectively, for the WBAN count varying from 5 to 40. According to the simulation results, HM-MAC [34] achieves low-energy consumption, and EED, high throughput, and PDR for higher priority users compared to MC-MAC protocol. The simulation using OMNeT++ simulator showed that the QoS-based MAC scheduling approach [36] has reduced the latency of the high priority data along with reducing the mutual interference. The normalized throughput and average access delay under different interference conditions have been evaluated using the 3D-MCM [35]. The simulation results demonstrate the 70% reduction in normalized throughput and twice increased in average access delay for general medical data and emergency data in the presence of interference due to dynamic adjust WBANs compared with single WBAN.

15.3.2 Transmission power control

In most of the applications, WBAN may vary its transmission power based on its assumption of coexisting WBANs. Battery energy, one of the key parameters, may be degraded faster by the interference. The mutual interference can be reduced by minimizing the average transmit power. The different approaches to minimize the transmission power using game theory, reinforcement learning (RL), etc. are discussed in the following.

Pro-active power update (PAPU): In PAPU [37] method, game theory is applied to control the transmission power and minimize the network utility and the energy consumption of each sensor node in each WBAN, based on the transmission power and SINR of the other nearby WBANs. The transmission power of each link is varied and broadcasted to nearby WBAN whenever there is a change in the transmission power and SINR of the nearby WBAN. PAPU algorithm converges the transmission power of the node to the Nash equilibrium (NE) condition.

Lightweight RL power controller (LRL): A dynamic power controller using RL proposed in [38,39] to control transmission power in a distributed manner. The proposed controller reduces mutual interference by controlling the transmission power level based on the SINR at each sensor node. The multi-agents in this *Q*-algorithm converge to NE without its prior knowledge.

QoS-based adaptive power control (QPC) scheme [40]: Wang *et al.* introduced QPC based on the Nash bargaining game model where the transmission power of the interfering nodes are adjusted actively according to the different QoS requirements and SINR of the high priority data.

Adaptive power level and data rate–based interference mitigation (APLDR) [27]: Ghare and Kothari proposed a run-time adaptive data rate along with a run time adaptive power level interference mitigation method. The default data rate value of a particular sensor considered is 250 kbps and its value varies to 200, 150, and 100 kbps based on the packet loss ratio and sensor node priority. The power level is varied based on the SAR values for WBAN, the initial energy, and power handling capabilities of the sensors.

Bayesian game–based power control scheme [41]: In this scheme, the WBAN is modelled as the players and its active links as player types. The harmonic algorithm is used to control transmission power level to reduce the mutual interference. The payoff prices the trade-off between power consumption and throughput.

15.3.2.1 Summary and discussion on transmission power control

The various parameters used for the analysis of the transmission power control approach are summarized in Table 15.1. A comparative study based on the different network performance metrics such as latency, collision rate, spatial reuse, power consumption, throughput, channel access, QoS support, and reliability is given in Table 15.2. Based on the experimental study, PAPU algorithm [37] has shown a reduction in the transmission power by 50%–80% with only a 10%–30% rise in the network utility compared to asynchronous distributed pricing algorithm for wireless sensor networks. An experimental study conducted on LRL [38] by varying the WBAN count suggests setting the initial learning rate and the eligibility trace parameter to 1 and the discount factor to 0. The result also confirmed that even without any prior knowledge of NE, agents in the proposed algorithm based system can converge to the NE and deliver almost the same throughput and lesser transmission power as compared to the non-cooperative game power control method. Comparing the LRL algorithm [39] with other RL algorithms such as Sarsa and OLSPI, LRL achieves lesser energy consumption with slightly lesser throughput.

The experimental simulation using the QoS-aware power control scheme [40] shows that when the transmission power of abnormal data increases then the transmission power of other sensor nodes decreases to avoid interference and thus SINR values also improve linearly. By this method, the reliability and real-time transmission factor of abnormal data transmission also increases. The transmission power and SINR decrease to compensate for the rise in energy consumption. Using the run-time adaptive power level and date rate mechanism [27] simultaneously, the packet loss rate has reduced up to 26% compared to that without using any interference mitigation method. The Bayesian game approach [41] for power control reaches the Bayesian equilibrium and payoff balance between power consumption and throughput.

15.3.3 Adaptive spectrum allocation

Adaptive internetwork interference mitigation (AIM): Based on the traffic priority, SINR, packet length, and the number of WBAN nodes, Movassaghi *et al.* [42] had proposed an adaptive interference mitigation method for coinciding WBANs. The interference level value was calculated by the coexisting WBAN coordinators by considering the received power, packet length, and priority of its sensor nodes. Inter-interference list was generated by adding the sensor with received power lesser than the threshold value. Based on the list, channels are allocated to the highest priority sensor node and all other nodes in the inter-interference list remain silent for the packet length of the transmitting node. All other nodes that are not in the list can transmit simultaneously.

ACESS [43]: Kim *et al.* proposed an adaptive channel estimation using the two-state Markov model. The coordinator maintains a history table containing the information about the channel ID, transit status from the busy state to the idle state, and the channel stability criterion. The coordinator selects the best channel based on the channel transit probability from the idle state to the busy state.

Inter ACS [44]: Interference-aware channel switching algorithm is an interference deduction algorithm based on the SINR. When more WBANs using the same frequency, range come closer and have been there for a longer period, then the channel available for the transmission reduces. This causes the SINR reduction of the system. According to the observed SINR value, the coordinator node of the WBAN switches the channel to the next 2–4 hop channels.

Adaptive time allocation based on vertex colouring: In vertex colouring problem, WBAN represents the vertex, and interference between the WBANs represents the edges; according to the colouring rule, no two adjacent WBANs are allocated with the same TS to communicate. Distributed vertex colouring (DVC) [29], random incomplete colouring (RIC) [29,30], extended vertex colouring (EVC) [29], and cooperative resource allocation method based on extended vertex colouring (CEVC) [29] are the different proposed vertex colouring algorithm used for TS allocation in WBAN network. DVC assigns the available resource equally to all WBANs. In DVC, all WBANs are first synchronized and broadcast a chosen TS until it wins the TS. RIC colouring algorithm is similar to DVC, but it has two concepts. The first is the random colouring concept where WBAN with higher uniformly distributed random value wins the TS. In RIC, the number of colours is less than the chromatic number of the graph and so the second concept incomplete colouring as all WBANs may not get TS during all cycles. EVC improves the TS allocation efficiency irrespective of the number of colours used and the method used to colour. CEVC consists of three stages: Hello-Hubs, Declare-Neighbours, and TS allocation and synchronization phases. In the Hello-Hubs phase, each hub instigates itself to its neighbours with Hello-Hubs frame comprising the sender's ID, timer, traffic, and priority. In the next phase, each hub transmits a Declare-Neighbours frame which consists of the sender's information, neighbours' address, and a timer. In the last phase, the Local Masters (LM) start TS allocation using the BEGINNER TS allocation algorithm and broadcasts the Allocation Message (AMSG), and LM which receives the AMSG uses a non-BEGINNER TS allocation algorithm.

15.3.3.1 Summary and discussion on adaptive spectrum allocation

The various parameters used for the analysis of the adaptive spectrum allocation are summarized in Table 15.1. A comparative study based on the different network performance metrics such as latency, collision rate, spatial reuse, power consumption, throughput, channel access, QoS support, and reliability is given in Table 15.2. The mathematical analysis and simulation results show that the proposed AIM scheme [42] improves the average reuse rate by keeping the critical minimum delay requirements. In [43], the ACCESS scheme was compared with the existing IEEE 802.15.6 single channel scheme and random channel selection, and the simulation shows that the packet reception rate of the ACCESS scheme is higher than the other schemes. The inter ACS [44] algorithm was simulated using an NS-3 simulator and compared to a uniformly channel switching approach; this algorithm shows better interference count versus average data rate performance. DVC has low efficiency, requires synchronization among the WBANs, and so consumes more time and energy for message exchange. RIC has more communication complexity and fast convergence time compared to DVC. The simulation analysis using OPNET [29] and an eight-WBAN scenario shows that the TS allocation efficiency of CEVC has increased by 19.7%, 79%, and 43.2% compared to 4-colouring, 6-colouring, and RIC, respectively. In the case of priority-based CEVC, its efficiency was enhanced by 17.8%, 76.6%, and 38.4% compared to 4-colouring, 6-colouring, and RIC, respectively. CEVC also has a better TS allocation efficiency compared to DVC with lesser transmission complexity.

15.3.4 Cooperative scheduling for interference mitigation

Distributed cooperative scheduling (DCS): Wang *et al.* [28] proposed a horse racing (HR) algorithm to schedule a single WBAN, and based on it, they also proposed DCS to handle multi-WBAN concurrent scheduling. In DCS, first, each BAN creates a table containing the BAN ID of its and all its neighbours' using superframe, and BAN with the lowest ID becomes the master and performs the HR scheduling for the next superframe. All BANs remove the master's ID from the ID table upon receiving the update message indicating the master's BAN ID. After a few superframe transmissions, several groups of masters are formed and appear repeatedly.

Fairness-based throughput maximization heuristic (FTMH) algorithm [45]: In the FTMH algorithm, the WBAN coordinator finds and sorts the QoS and the interference signal strength (ISS) from the other WBANs into different sets based on the threshold value. Then the TSs with large ISS values are allocated to sensor set with large QoS and similarly do the allocation till they allocate week ISS to set with lesser QoS. Finally, the scheduling strategy is obtained by optimizing the throughput of each sensor set.

15.3.4.1 Summary and discussion on cooperative scheduling for interference mitigation

The various parameters used for the analysis of the cooperative scheduling approach are summarized in Table 15.1. A comparative study based on the different network performance metrics such as latency, collision rate, spatial reuse, power consumption, throughput, channel access, QoS support, and reliability is given in Table 15.2. When compared to the Hungarian algorithm and greedy algorithm, the HR algorithm and DCS [28] achieved a near optimal PRR for single- and multi-BAN scheduling, respectively. FTMH [45] algorithm was evaluated by comparing it with the iteration algorithm and the HR algorithm [28]. Similar to [28], two scenarios were considered

Table 15.3 Network simulator used for each mutual interference mitigation scheme

Sl. no	Simulator	Mutual-interference mitigation schemes
1	OMNeT++	QoS MAC [36], 2L-MAC [31], adaptive CSMA/CA [32], HM-MAC [34]
2	C++ simulator	ACCESS [43]
3	OPNET modeller	isMAC [33], CEVC [29]
4	NS3	Inter ACS [44]
5	WSNet	DCS [28]
6	NetSim	APLDR [27]
7	NS2	FTMH [45]

that contain two WBANs and eight WBANs and in each scenario, each WBAN was equipped with 12 sensors. The performance was analysed using energy efficiency, throughput, and QoS of each sensor. In both cases, FTMH obtains greater optimal throughput and QoS compared to the other algorithms.

15.4 Conclusion and future scope

The mutual interference of WBAN is an important challenging problem associated with it as it degrades the network performance and is caused due to mobility, the same frequency data transmission within a short range. Of late, researchers have shown keen interest in the various mutual interference mitigation methods. In this chapter, we have discussed the various approaches used in mutual interference mitigation. The various parameters used for the analysis of the different approaches are also summarized. Further, the comparison study based on the different network performance parameters such as latency, collision rate, spatial reuse, power consumption, throughput, channel access, QoS support, and reliability of the different mutual interference avoidance schemes is presented. The different network simulators used for the simulation and validation of the various approaches is also catalogued in Table 15.3.

References

[1] Movassaghi, S., Abolhasan, M., Lipman, J., Smith, D., and Jamalipour, A. (2014). Wireless body area networks: A survey. *IEEE Communications Surveys & Tutorials*, 16(3), 1658–1686.

[2] Smith, D. B., Miniutti, D., Lamahewa, T. A., and Hanlen, L. W. (2013). Propagation models for body-area networks: A survey and new outlook. *IEEE Antennas and Propagation Magazine*, 55(5), 97–117.

[3] Ho, C. K., See, T. S., and Yuce, M. R. (2012). An ultra-wideband wireless body area network: Evaluation in static and dynamic channel conditions. *Sensors and Actuators A: Physical*, 180, 137–147.

[4] Sarestoniemi, M., Hamalainen, M., and Iinatti, J. (2017). An overview of the electromagnetic simulation-based channel modelling techniques for wireless body area network applications. *IEEE Access*, 5, 10622–10632.

[5] Meharouech, A., Elias, J., Paris, S., and Mehaoua, A. (2015, June). A game theoretical approach for interference mitigation in body-to-body networks. In *2015 IEEE International Conference on Communication Workshop (ICCW)* (pp. 259–264). IEEE.

[6] Kumpuniemi, T., Hamalainen, M., Yazdandoost, K. Y., and Iinatti, J. (2017). Human body shadowing effect on dynamic UWB on-body radio channels. *IEEE Antennas and Wireless Propagation Letters*, 16, 1871–1874.

[7] Elias, J., Paris, S., and Krunz, M. (2014). Cross-technology interference mitigation in body area networks: An optimization approach. *IEEE Transactions on Vehicular Technology*, 64(9), 4144–4157.

[8] Paris, S., Elias, J., and Mehaoua, A. (2013, June). Cross technology interference mitigation in body-to-body area networks. In *2013 IEEE 14th International Symposium on "A World of Wireless, Mobile and Multimedia Networks" (WoWMoM)* (pp. 1–9). IEEE.

[9] Meharouech, A., Elias, J., and Mehaoua, A. (2016). A two-stage game theoretical approach for interference mitigation in body-to-body networks. *Computer Networks*, 95, 15–34.

[10] Meharouech, A., Elias, J., Paris, S., and Mehaoua, A. (2014, October). Socially-aware interference mitigation game in body-to-body networks. In *2014 7th International Conference on Network Games, Control and Optimization (NetGCoop)* (pp. 162–163). IEEE.

[11] Shaik, M. F., Komanapalli, V. L. N., and Subashini, M. M. (2018). A comparative study of interference and mitigation techniques in wireless body area networks. *Wireless Personal Communications*, 98(2), 2333–2365.

[12] Hasan, K., Biswas, K., Ahmed, K., Nafi, N. S., and Islam, M. S. (2019). A comprehensive review of wireless body area network. *Journal of Network and Computer Applications*, 143, 178–198.

[13] Hayajneh, T., Almashaqbeh, G., Ullah, S., and Vasilakos, A. V. (2014). A survey of wireless technologies coexistence in WBAN: Analysis and open research issues. *Wireless Networks*, 20(8), 2165–2199.

[14] Kwak, K. S., Ullah, S., and Ullah, N. (2010, November). An overview of IEEE 802.15.6 standard. In *2010 3rd International Symposium on Applied Sciences in Biomedical and Communication Technologies (ISABEL 2010)* (pp. 1–6). IEEE.

[15] Astrin A. (2012).IEEE Standard for Local and metropolitan area networks – Part 15.6: Wireless Body Area Networks, in *IEEE Std 802.15.6-2012*, pp. 1–271, 29 Feb. 2012.

[16] Al Shayokh, M., Abeshu, A., Satrya, G. B., and Nugroho, M. A. (2016, September). Efficient and secure data delivery in software defined WBAN for virtual hospital. In *2016 International Conference on Control, Electronics, Renewable Energy and Communications (ICCEREC)* (pp. 12–16). IEEE.

[17] Yazdandoost, K., and Sayrafian, K. (2010). Channel Model for Body Area Network (BAN). IEEE 802.15.6 technical contribution, document ID: IEEE P802.15-08-0780-12-0006.

[18] Otto, C. A., Jovanov, E., and Milenkovic, A. (2006, September). A WBAN-based system for health monitoring at home. In *2006 3rd IEEE/EMBS International Summer School on Medical Devices and Biosensors* (pp. 20–23). IEEE.

[19] Negra, R., Jemili, I., and Belghith, A. (2016). Wireless body area networks: Applications and technologies. *Procedia Computer Science*, 83, 1274–1281.

[20] Bouazizi, A., Zaibi, G., Samet, M., and Kachouri, A. (2017, February). Wireless body area network for e-health applications: Overview. In *2017 International Conference on Smart, Monitored and Controlled Cities (SM2C)* (pp. 64–68). IEEE.

[21] Gangwar, D. S. (2013, January). Biomedical sensor network for cardiovascular fitness and activity monitoring. In *2013 IEEE Point-of-Care Healthcare Technologies (PHT)* (pp. 279–282). IEEE.

[22] Wu, F., Wu, T., and Yuce, M. R. (2019). An internet-of-things (IoT) network system for connected safety and health monitoring applications. *Sensors*, 19 (1), 21.

[23] Saboor, A., Ahmad, R., Ahmed, W., Kiani, A. K., Le Moullec, Y., and Alam, M. M. (2018). On research challenges in hybrid medium-access control protocols for IEEE 802.15.6 WBANs. *IEEE Sensors Journal*, 19(19), 8543–8555.

[24] Sarkar, S., and Misra, S. (2016). From micro to nano: The evolution of wireless sensor-based health care. *IEEE Pulse*, 7(1), 21–25.

[25] Jones, R. W., and Katzis, K. (2018, April). 5G and wireless body area networks. In *2018 IEEE Wireless Communications and Networking Conference Workshops (WCNCW)* (pp. 373–378). IEEE.

[26] Yuan, X., Li, C., Zhang, K., *et al.* (2018, May). Dynamic interference analysis of coexisting mobile WBANs for health monitoring. In *2018 IEEE International Conference on Communications (ICC)* (pp. 1–6). IEEE.

[27] Ghare, P. H., and Kothari, A. G. (2017). Interference analysis and mitigation techniques in wireless body area networks. *Wireless Personal Communications*, 96(3), 3333–3344.

[28] Wang, L., Goursaud, C., Nikaein, N., Cottatellucci, L., and Gorce, J. M. (2012). Cooperative scheduling for coexisting body area networks. *IEEE Transactions on Wireless Communications*, 12(1), 123–133.

[29] Miri, M., Mohamedpour, K., Darmani, Y., Sarkar, M., and Tummala, R. L. (2019). An efficient resource allocation algorithm based on vertex colouring to mitigate interference among coexisting WBANs. *Computer Networks*, 151, 132–146.

[30] Cheng, S. H., and Huang, C. Y. (2012). Colouring-based inter-WBAN scheduling for mobile wireless body area networks. *IEEE Transactions on Parallel and Distributed Systems*, 24(2), 250–259.

[31] Chen, G. T., Chen, W. T., and Shen, S. H. (2014, June). 2L-MAC: A MAC protocol with two-layer interference mitigation in wireless body area networks for medical applications. In *2014 IEEE International Conference on Communications (ICC)* (pp. 3523–3528). IEEE.

[32] Huang, W., and Quek, T. Q. (2015, June). Adaptive CSMA/CA MAC protocol to reduce inter-WBAN interference for wireless body area networks. In *2015 IEEE 12th International Conference on Wearable and Implantable Body Sensor Networks (BSN)* (pp. 1–6). IEEE.

[33] Kirbas, I., Karahan, A., Sevin, A., and Bayilmis, C. (2013). isMAC: An adaptive and energy-efficient MAC protocol based on multi-channel communication for wireless body area networks. *KSII Transactions on Internet & Information Systems*, 7(8).

[34] Le, T., and Moh, S. (2018). Hybrid multi-channel MAC protocol for WBANs with inter-WBAN interference mitigation. *Sensors*, 18(5), 1373.

[35] Yuan, X., Li, C., Ye, Q., *et al.* (2018). Performance analysis of IEEE 802.15.6-based coexisting mobile WBANs with prioritized traffic and dynamic interference. *IEEE Transactions on Wireless Communications*, 17(8), 5637–5652.

[36] Jamthe, A., Mishra, A., and Agrawal, D. P. (2014, June). Scheduling schemes for interference suppression in healthcare sensor networks. In *2014 IEEE International Conference on Communications (ICC)* (pp. 391–396). IEEE.

[37] Fang, G., Dutkiewicz, E., Yu, K., Vesilo, R., and Yu, Y. (2010, December). Distributed inter-network interference coordination for wireless body area networks. In *2010 IEEE Global Telecommunications Conference GLOBECOM 2010* (pp. 1–5). IEEE.

[38] Kazemi, R., Vesilo, R., Dutkiewicz, E., and Liu, R. P. (2012, September). Design considerations of reinforcement learning power controllers in wireless body area networks. In *2012 IEEE 23rd International Symposium on Personal, Indoor and Mobile Radio Communications—(PIMRC)* (pp. 2030–2036). IEEE.

[39] Kazemi, R., Vesilo, R., Dutkiewicz, E., and Liu, R. P. (2012, October). Reinforcement learning in power control games for internetwork interference mitigation in wireless body area networks. In *2012 International Symposium on Communications and Information Technologies (ISCIT)* (pp. 256–262). IEEE.

[40] Wang, J., Sun, Y., and Ji, Y. (2018). QoS-based adaptive power control scheme for co-located WBANs: A cooperative bargaining game theoretic perspective. *Wireless Networks*, 24(8), 3129–3139.

[41] Zou, L., Liu, B., Chen, C., and Chen, C. W. (2014, December). Bayesian game based power control scheme for inter-WBAN interference mitigation. In *2014 IEEE Global Communications Conference* (pp. 240–245). IEEE.

[42] Movassaghi, S., Abolhasan, M., Smith, D., and Jamalipour, A. (2014, December). AIM: Adaptive internetwork interference mitigation amongst

co-existing wireless body area networks. In *2014 IEEE Global Communications Conference* (pp. 2460–2465). IEEE.

[43] Kim, B., Cho, J., Kim, D. Y., and Lee, B. (2016, January). ACESS: Adaptive channel estimation and selection scheme for coexistence mitigation in WBANs. In *Proceedings of the 10th International Conference on Ubiquitous Information Management and Communication* (pp. 1–4).

[44] Mahapatro, J., Misra, S., Manjunatha, M., and Islam, N. (2012, December). Interference-aware channel switching for use in WBAN with human-sensor interface. In *2012 4th International Conference on Intelligent Human Computer Interaction (IHCI)* (pp. 1–5). IEEE.

[45] Li, M., Liu, J., Ma, Z., Yuan, C., and Yuan, B. (2015, June). Throughput optimization with fairness consideration for coexisting WBANs. In *2015 IEEE International Conference on Communications (ICC)* (pp. 6418–6423). IEEE.

Chapter 16

Predicting COVID cases using machine learning, android, and firebase cloud storage

Ritesh Kumar Sinha[1], Sukant Kishoro Bisoy[1], Saurabh Kumar[1], Sai Prasad Sarangi[1] and Utku Kose[2]

Abstract

In machine learning (ML), many prediction strategies are being popularly made to handle prediction and forecasting issues. Our study demonstrates the potential of ML models to forecast the quantity of forthcoming patients plagued by COVID-19 that is presently thought of as a possible threat to human kind. Four commonly used prediction models such as linear regression, random forest, support vector machine (SVM), and decision-tree classifier are employed in this study to predict the COVID-19 cases under different scenarios. Three styles of predictions were created by every model such as quantity of fresh infected cases, quantity of deaths, and also the range of recoveries within the next 10 days. The results created by the study prove it as efficient mechanism to use these strategies for the present situation of the COVID-19. In this work, we have collected the dataset from the Indian Council of Medical Research website and have applied train test split method to train the model and test the model. We have taken 80% data to train our model and 20% to test our model. In this work, we have applied four ML models for predicting the active cases, recovered cases, confirmed cases, and deceased cases. The four models that we have applied were linear regression, SVM, random forest classifier, and decision tree. After applying these models, we found that linear regression model gives the highest accuracy. In this work, we have also made an android app where we stored all the data of our prediction in firebase cloud storage. When the user opens the app it shows two buttons where one button is for ML prediction and the other for knowing the numerical value of the COVID cases. Thus when a user clicks for the numerical value, it asks for the day and month, and after mentioning the day and month, all the numeric details of active cases, recovered/deceased cases, and confirmed cases are displayed. If a user clicks for ML prediction, then it

[1]Department of Computer Engineering, C.V. Raman Global University, Bhubaneswar, India
[2]Department of Computer Engineering, Faculty of Engineering, Suleyman Demirel University, Isparta, Turkey

gives a pop-up for all the types of ML models and thus it displays the graph of that model that the user has clicked.

Keywords: ML; COVID; SVM; DT

16.1 Introduction

Disease found over some defined period of time is termed pandemic and epidemic [1]. Coronaviruses are RNA viruses groups found in birds, which causes respiratory tract infections ranging from mild to lethal conditions in humans and birds, while in dairy animals and pigs they cause loose bowels, hepatitis, and encephalopathy in mice. COVID-19 pandemic has been caused by SARS-COV2, and most serious public emergency as it spreads rapidly [2]. The spread trends show transmission through human interaction through tiny droplets formed through coughing, sneezing, talking where contact with an affected exterior is becoming one of primary reasons for the transmission. They are enclosed infections with a positive-sense single-stranded RNA genome and a helical evened nucleocapsid. The world is facing a great crisis since post–World War Two leading to 792,457 deaths and more than 87,589,017 confirmed cases as of November 21, 2020 and its effect would be felt for many upcoming years. According to the sources [2], the epidemic started from Wuhan, China in December, 2019 as a pneumonia outbreak that was further found to be a novel strain of coronavirus and was called 2019-nCoV by the WHO, at that point changed to SARS-COV2 by the International Committee on Taxonomy of Viruses [3]. On March 1, WHO declared the pandemic that has spread over the world [2,4–7]. This pandemic has brought about movement limitations and lockdowns in numerous nations. There have been 9,095,910 confirmed cases in over 29 states and 5 union territories with a total of 133,263 deaths in India as of November 21, 2020 [2]. India's index case was reported on January 30, 2020 in Thrissur, Kerala (10°31′39″N 76°12′52″E) and the country is facing the pandemic since 9 months, 3 weeks, and 1 day as on November 21, 2020. The country underwent a series of lockdowns since March 22, 2020 as directed by the Government of India. India's fatality rate stands at 2.41% with a steady decline and recovery rate of 81.18% as on October 23, 2020 [2]. The lockdown in India has started in the month of March, 2020 to stop the active cases looking at the high speed rate of growth of Italy [8]. As per the report given by Indian Government, Maharashtra state of India is severely affected by coronavirus [9].

Different models have been utilized for foreseeing the life cycle of COVID-19 for determining the trends with data for outbreak severity, observing the agitation, correlating susceptible-infected removed (SIR) and susceptible exposed infectious removed, predicting the spread and death rate and its impact. Author in [10] developed a theoretical approach to investigate the spreading of Corona using the SIR model. Daily expected COVID cases are forecasted in Saudi Arab for 4 weeks using the model that is named ARIMA which stands for autoregressive integrated moving average model [11]. Machine learning (ML) can be variably used in many of the fields that also include detecting malwares [12,13], detecting the malwares present in mobiles [14,15], medicine [16–18], and to retrieve information [19,20].

Lately, statistical and time series models are also used to create models for predicting the duration of the global crisis caused by coronavirus. Authors have utilized the information of affirmed cases in Nigeria in bend measurable estimation models as well as utilized the linear regression model to anticipate the rate of demises in India due to coronavirus. Due to the rapid growth of the number of active cases, it has become difficult for doctors to diagnose within a short time. There is a need for techniques that can predict the number of active cases, recovery cases, and deceased cases. Due to advent of many machine tools, it is possible to analyze the large volume of data and predict the cases. Our aim is to predict the number of active cases in the next 30 days using linear regression, random forest, support vector machine (SVM), decision tree for being prepared in advance to take some preventive measures.

The pandemic, termed COVID-19, has now emerged as a global pandemic that has spread in almost all over the world. It has become a major challenge to find the person suffering from this disease because the symptoms are shown in very rare cases. Thus, now it has become necessary to ascertain a suitable method to estimate the number of persons getting infected from this to take appropriate precautions regularly. In the place of other traditional time-consuming methods, we better opt for AI and ML, which also results in lower cost. Although there are many studies over the topic named COVID-19, this study basically focuses on the use of ML in predicting the cases of COVID-19.

ML is now used efficiently in many fields such as detecting malware, ATM fraud detection, medicine and information retrieval, and weather forecasting. In the year 2012, an artificial neural network–based modern system was introduced, which is named deep learning. Here we have used the train-test split method to divide our dataset into training data and testing data and thus we applied our ML models to it. Further, in Section 16.2, we will explain the libraries that we have used for designing our android app and detailed discussion on firebase cloud storage.

16.2 Literature survey

For the last 15 years, digital technologies and their advancements are playing crucial roles in the majority of the healthcare sector issues as well as illness bar, this worldwide global health issue additionally seeking advancement in technology to support the control of COVID-19 [4]. In some papers, authors also highlighted some attainable applications of digital technologies such as AI, IoT, big data analytics, which also stand for deep learning, and blockchain technology to find certain ways for watching, detecting, and a bar of the epidemic; additionally, to spot the wound of the epidemic in healthcare sector, during an investigation work supportive of presented by Benvenuto *et al.*, creators arranged partner autoregressive coordinated moving normal model to anticipate the unfurl of COVID-19. In this particular paper, the creator anticipated the differed boundaries for the succeeding 2 days anticipating the investigation in regards to the pervasiveness and frequency of the COVID-19. This exploration work moreover shows the correlogram and ARIMA gauge chart for the scourge frequency and commonness [8]. Deb *et al.* arranged a measurement procedure to explore frequency pattern and furthermore the measurable copy assortment of COVID-19 events. They performed measurements and numerical examination to investigate the patterns of the pandemic to highlight this epidemiologic phase of an area altogether that various arrangements will be known to manage COVID-19 pandemic in a few nations [11]. According to this situation, it is crucial to handle the first unfurl examples of the contamination to set up and the board successfully measures the well-being. Toward this path, Kucharski arranged a logical model of vital transmission of SARS-COV2 by exploiting totally unique datasets to check the COVID-19 regular occasion in Wuhan [10]. With this, they investigated the achievable unfurl of sickness on regular occasions outside the city. As of late, their square measure numerous investigations directed on the epidemiologic outbreak of COVID-19 through alpha information examination upheld various accessible datasets. The examinations in the primary focus on the pervasiveness of affirmed, demise, and recuperated cases in the city and furthermore the rest of earth to get a handle on the speculated dangers and ensuant concocting of control exercises. Later, in their examination the work has raised the trouble of the criticality of the hatching time frame for COVID-19 [9].

They considered 181 affirmed cases and recognized that the timeframe may fluctuate from 5 to 14 days and upheld this higher perception, and the executive's exercises will be arranged. In ongoing examination work, Singer broke down information on 25 tainted provinces to follow momentary expectations concerning the COVID-19 pandemic. The examination featured that the area explicit pace of sickness unfurl follows either consistent or dangerous force law development with totally extraordinary scaling types. With this arrangement, the creators dissected the effect of lockdown in various parts of the planet. In light of the top of writing, it is obvious that good work is offered on exploratory information examination to get a handle on the overarching pattern of the pandemic anyway; still there are huge loads of extensions to create and investigate prudent AI essentially based expectation models altogether that proactive ways might be known to cook the quick needs.

The AI has changed the disposition of distinguishing proof by giving pleasant outcomes to illnesses like polygenic issues and cerebrum issues. Chakraborti *et al.* recognized mind issues through AI, where signals, such as EEG/EOG, are utilized for the discovery of ordinary and epileptic conditions through fake neural organizations [12]. Sarwar *et al.* diagnosing polygenic turmoil utilizing AI and outfit learning methods results demonstrated that group strategy guaranteed a precision of 98.60%. Firm and real diagnosing of COVID-19 will save a ton of lives and will produce a huge data where AI (ML) model will be prepared. AI could offer accommodating contribution during this respect, explicitly in making analyze upheld clinical content, radiography pictures, and so on in sync with Bullock *et al.* The ML will supplant people by giving the right diagnosis. The correct conclusion will save the time of radiologist and may be more effective than other traditional tests. X-beams, processed tomography (CT) outputs will be used for training the model. Numerous works are currently performed in the similar manner. Wang and Wong created COVID-Net, which is a type of profound CNN organization and can analyze the disease of COVID from chest radiography pictures. When COVID-19 is distinguished, the inquiry is whether the manner in which seriously that individual will be influenced [5].

Not all the COVID-19 patients who are positive can need complete consideration. Being able to forecast that will be influenced a ton with proper attention will encourage in mandate help and by arranging the clinical asset distribution and usage. Yan *et al.* build a model to predict and check the mortality of an individual, through information from patients at Tongji Hospital in Wuhan, China. Jiang *et al.* proposed an AI model that will anticipate a person influenced by COVID-19 and has the probability to create an intense metastasis trouble condition (ARDS) [16]. The proposed model brought about 80th of exactness. ML will be needed to analyze COVID-19 that requires a lot of attempts; however, it is not widely operational. Since a very small amount of work is being performed on recognizable proof and anticipating through text, we used AI and some other learning models to characterize the medical reports into four classes of infections.

16.3 Implementation and methodology

Currently, the detection of COVID-19 cases in the world is one of the biggest challenges that lead to the exponential spread of the deadly disease. Recent global trends and statistics show that the number of people diagnosed with the recent deadly disease is increasing exponentially, with not less than 11.2 million confirmed cases; the disease is spreading to almost all the countries across the globe. We have collected the number of active, recovered, deceased daily dataset from the WHO site. In this, data is collected from the period March 16, 2020 to November 20, 2020. USA and India are the most affected countries in the world. India has taken initiative from much earlier and imposed the lockdown in the country from March 23, 2020. The prediction of a number of active, recovered, and deceased cases is shown for Odisha and India in Figures 16.1 and 16.2, respectively. It is observed that the numbers of active, recovered, and deceased cases are increasing linearly from the month of November. However, the disease is increasing rapidly in Maharashtra in the month of November.

The main obstacle faced by the doctors and government is to detect the infected persons where no symptoms are found. Thus, it becomes very important to find a method that will estimate the infected persons' number to adopt the preventive measures.

Hence, the correlation and distribution of a number of active cases are analyzed later. After collecting the data, the cleaning process of data is done and correlation analysis is performed using Python. The correlation analysis describes the relationship between two variables. Currently, we rely on decision-making trends and seasonality on the active cases in different states of India. The trend and seasonality of the active cases for the different states of India dataset are shown in

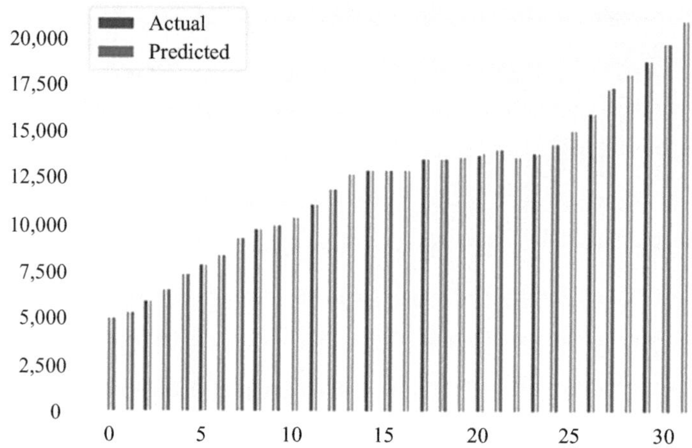

Figure 16.1 Output of linear regression for dataset of Odisha

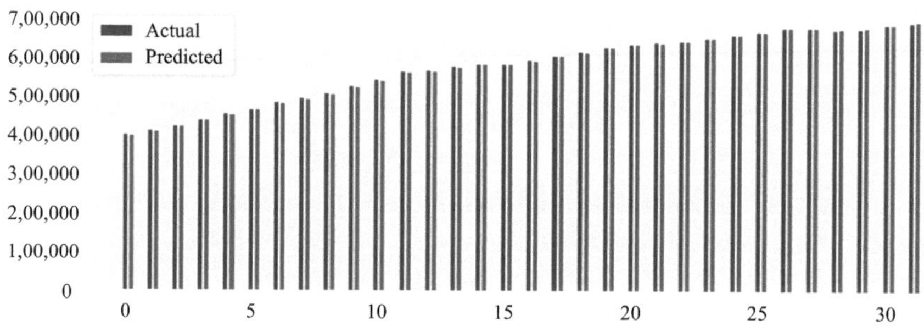

Figure 16.2 Output of linear regression for dataset of India

Figures 16.1 and 16.3. From this figure, we can say that there is a growing trend of active cases and also less impact of seasonality in the active cases [21]. The author analyzed the association of census features and weather data on a number of active cases and found that mortality cases depend on weather data.

After implementing the ML techniques, we have designed an android app where the user can get the details of the active, recovered, confirmed, and deceased cases graphically or through numbers. The first page of our app asks the user to enter the name of the country, state, and date on which they want to know the cases count. After filling in the details, there are two buttons on the screen for numerical presentation of cases and ML prediction. If the user enters for a numerical count, then a second screen appears, which shows the total details of active, confirmed, recovered, and deceased cases. If the user presses the ML prediction button then the next screen appears, which asks the user to select the type of model for which they want to see the prediction of those four

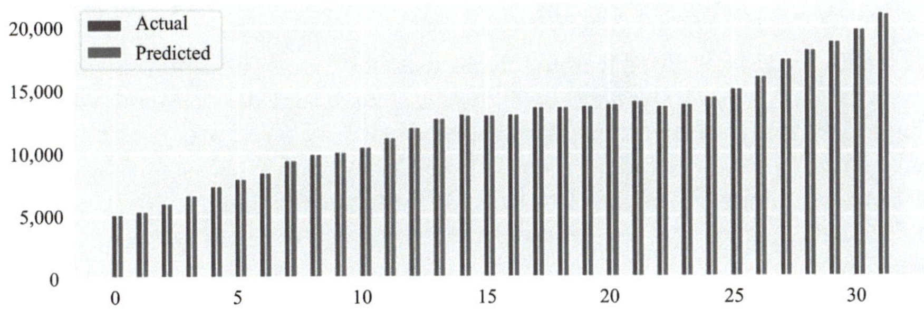

Figure 16.3 Output of linear regression for dataset of Maharashtra

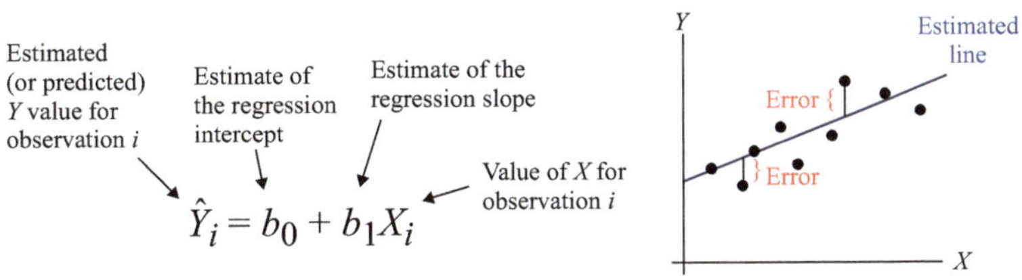

Figure 16.4 The equation of linear regression

models. After selecting one of the models from the previous user needs to press the "Submit" button then the next screen comes, which graphically shows the COVID trends.

16.4 Machine learning models

16.4.1 Linear regression

It is one of the most uncomplicated algorithms, which is used all around the globe. This method consists of two types of variables, i.e. response and explanatory. The linear regression model is used to predict the response variable by attaching the linear relation between them as

$$Yi = b0 + b1Xi \tag{16.1}$$

where the graph in Figure 16.4 establishes a linear relationship between the response variable and the explanatory variable. In common words, we can write the linear regression formula as

$$Y = MX + C \tag{16.2}$$

where Y is the response variable, X is the explanatory variable, C is the intercept (estimate of regression), and M is the estimate of the regression slope.

16.4.2 Support vector machine

This model lies in supervised learning that is used for the classification and analysis of regression. Suppose we have two types a square and a circle and we have training data that is labeled, then the process carried by SVM occurs as shown in Figure 16.5.

Here the training data is labeled; hence the result or the output of the algorithm is a decision boundary that divides the plane into two parts where each class lays at either side.

In the graph of Figure 16.6, we observe that there are two classes: a square and a rectangle split by many lines. The work that SVM performs is that it finds the decision boundary that provides the smallest distance to the training. Therefore, the increase in the ideal separating decision boundary increases the margin of the training data. SVM works well with explicit margin disunion. It is usually most

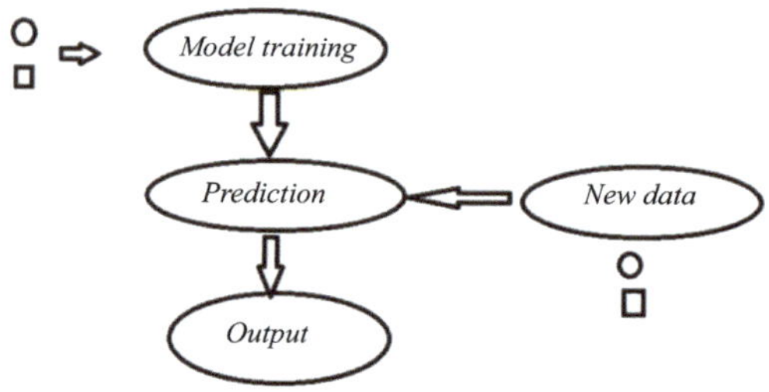

Figure 16.5 A label diagram of the working of support vector machine

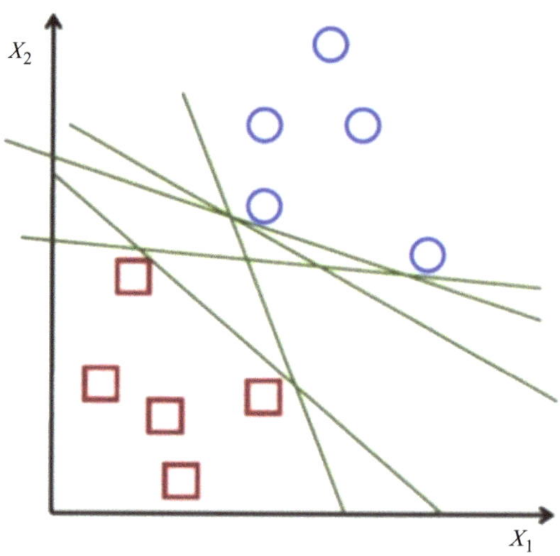

Figure 16.6 Graph indicating two classes split by many lines

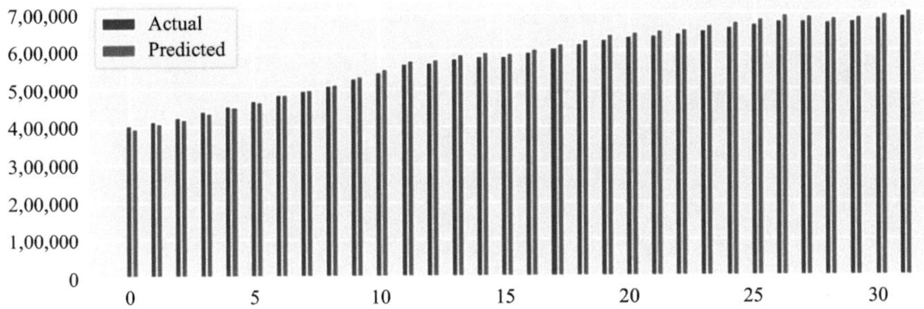

Figure 16.7 SVM output for dataset of India

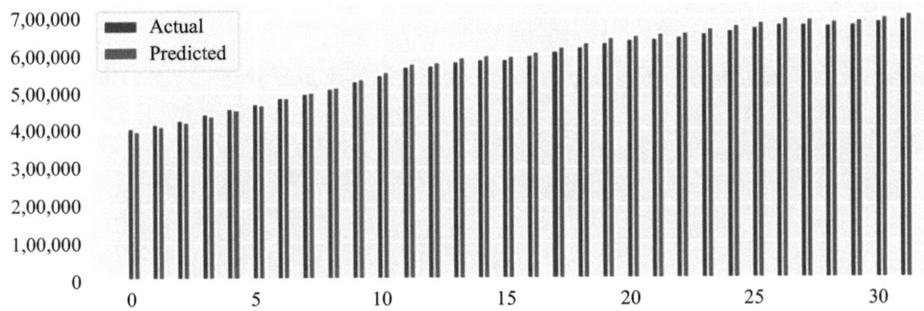

Figure 16.8 SVM output for dataset of Odisha

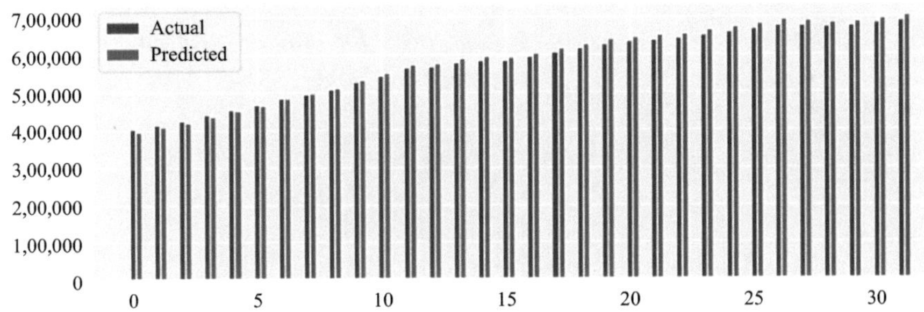

Figure 16.9 SVM output for dataset of Maharashtra

productive where the counting of dimensions is higher than the number of samples (Figures 16.7–16.9).

16.4.3 Random forest

It is one of the most famous supervised ML models. To understand the concept of random forest, one should have the basic idea about decision trees because it is the

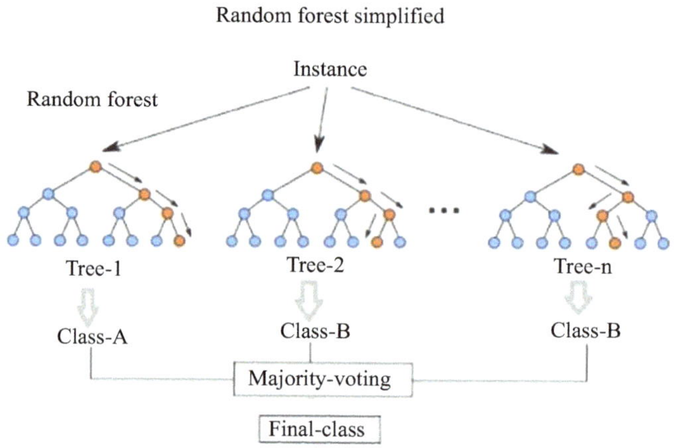

Figure 16.10 Diagram showing the division of class and tree in random forest

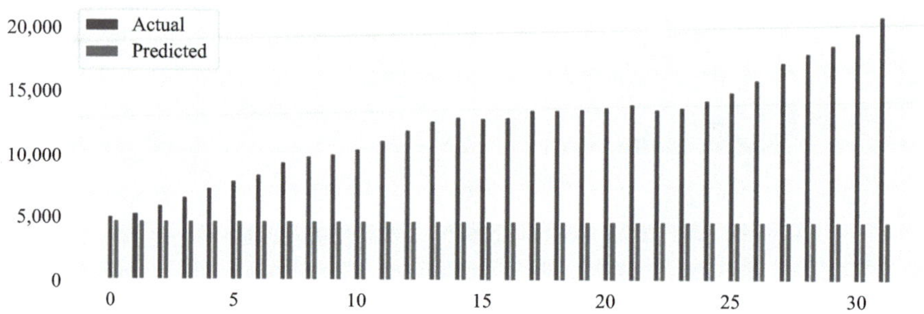

Figure 16.11 Output of random forest for dataset of India

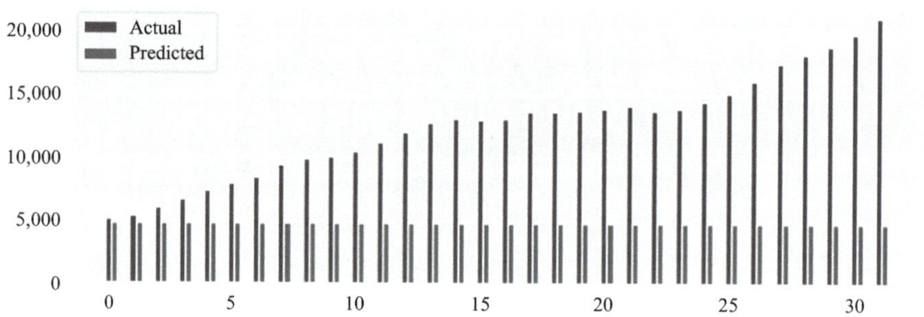

Figure 16.12 Output of random forest for dataset of Odisha

basic part of this model. Random forest is a kind of ensemble classifier that uses a decision tree algorithm in a randomized manner (Figure 16.10).

It basically works by forming a crowd of decision trees at training time and producing the class, which is either the mode of classes or the mean of the single tree (Figures 16.11–16.13).

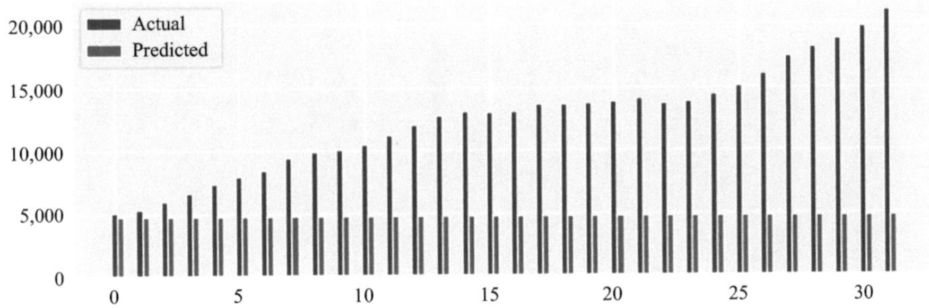

Figure 16.13 Output of random forest for dataset of Maharashtra

16.4.4 Decision tree

This model utilizes a tree-like structure of decisions and their potential outcome. It includes chance occasion results, asset expenses, and utility. It is a supervised AI strategy for actuating a decision tree from information prepared (Figures 16.14–16.16).

16.5 Introduction to android app

We have designed an android app that helps the end users to check the status of COVID on their phones. The user has just to visit our app and when the app opens up, it asks the user to select the particular state whose COVID cases they want to see. Once the user selects the state it asks the user to enter the date on which they want to see the COVID cases. After entering the date, there are two buttons available: one that shows the COVID cases in numerals and the other one that shows the cases graphically through ML prediction.

If the user presses the numerical button, then another activity opens up, which shows complete details of confirmed cases, active cases, recovered cases, and deceased cases. If the user presses the ML prediction button, then another activity opens up, which asks the user to select the ML models like linear regression, random forest, SVM, and decision tree. Once the user selects the model, then presses ok, and it shows the graph of that particular model.

For designing the APP, we have written the codes in java, and layout is made in XML. We have used implicit intent to move from one activity to another. We have stored all the images of graphs and numerical figures of COVID cases in firebase cloud storage (Figure 16.17).

16.6 Result analysis

Many state-of-art models are used to predict the number of coronavirus cases using ML and deep learning models [22]. To analyze the number of infected diseases, statistics plays an important role. In [23] the author analyzed the effect of lockdown

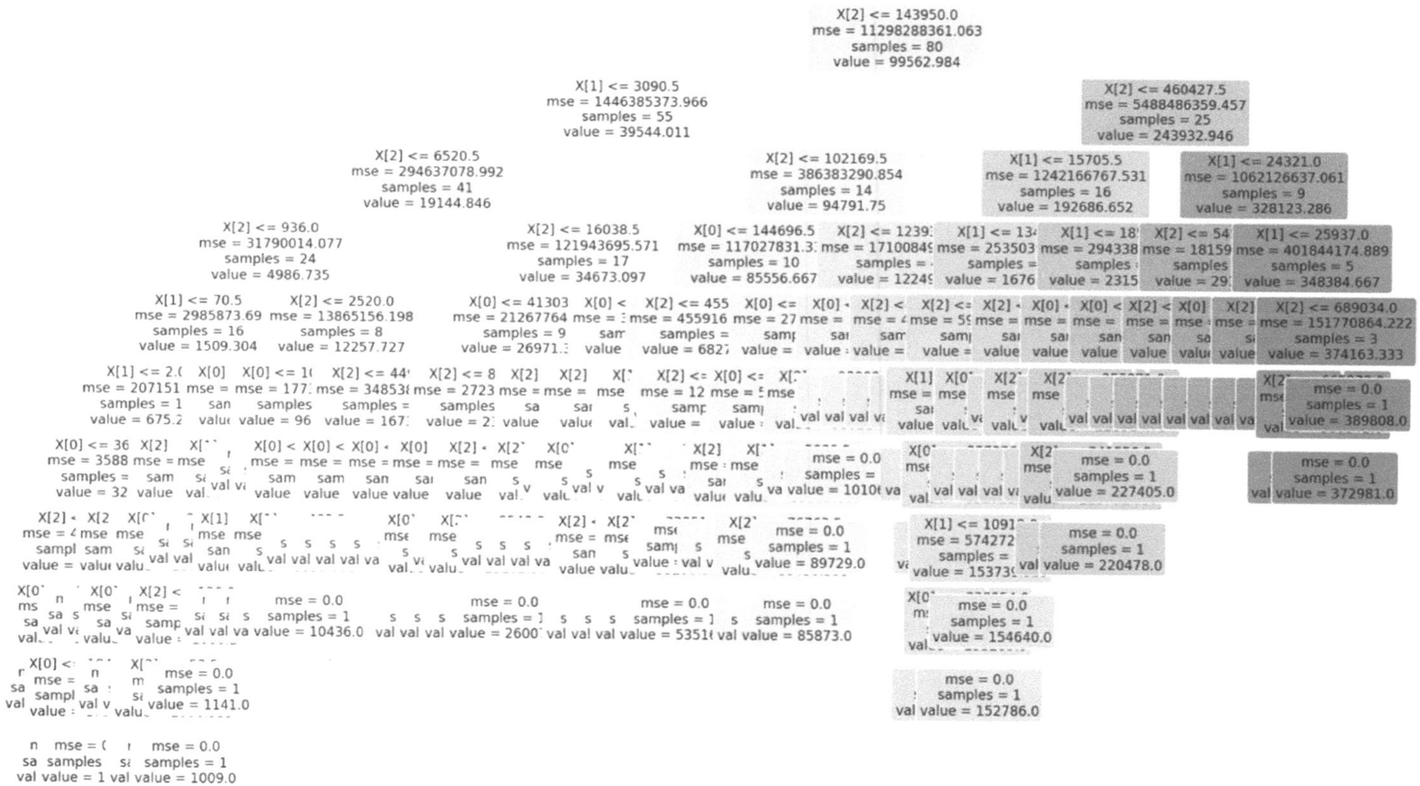

Figure 16.14 Decision tree graph of India

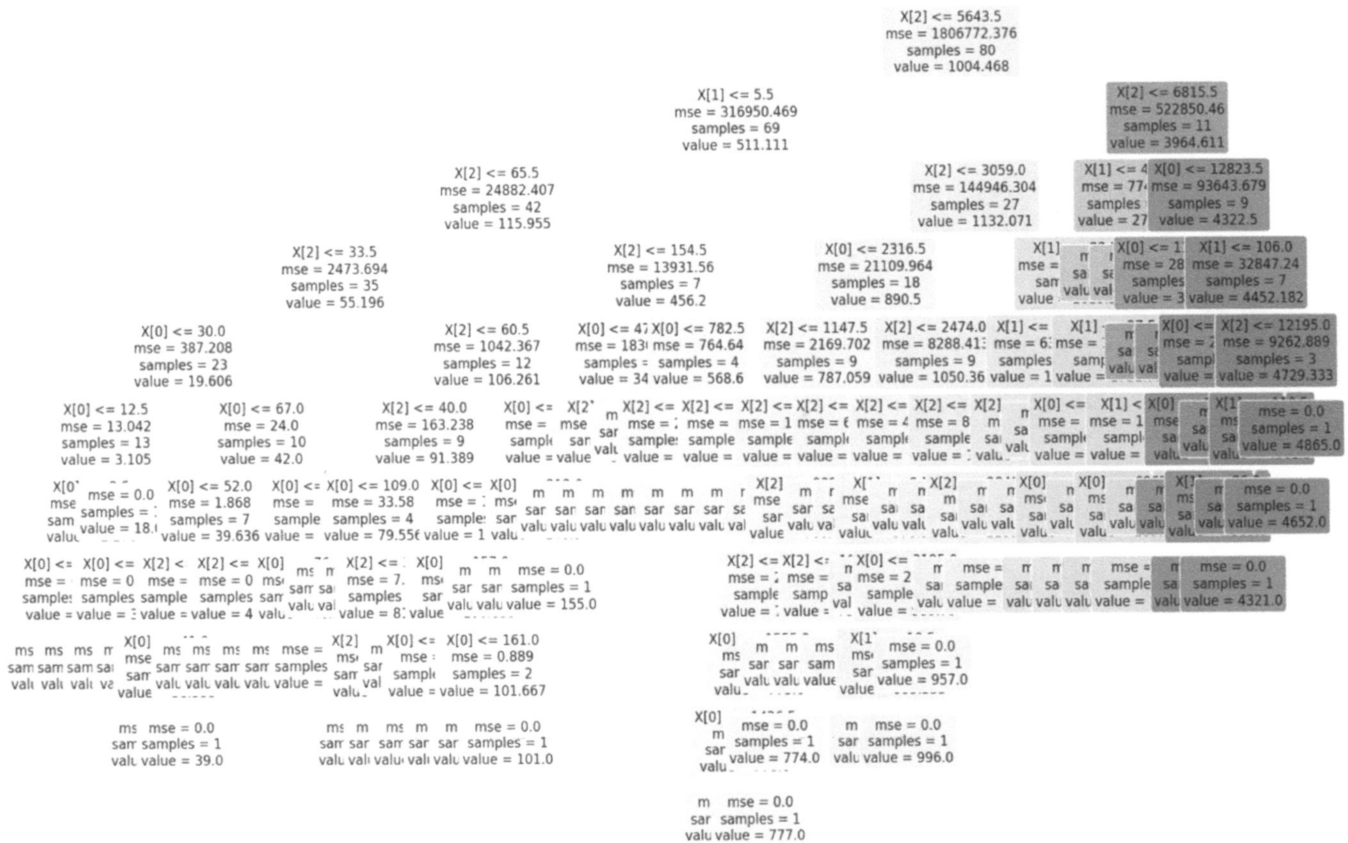

Figure 16.15 Decision tree graph of Odisha

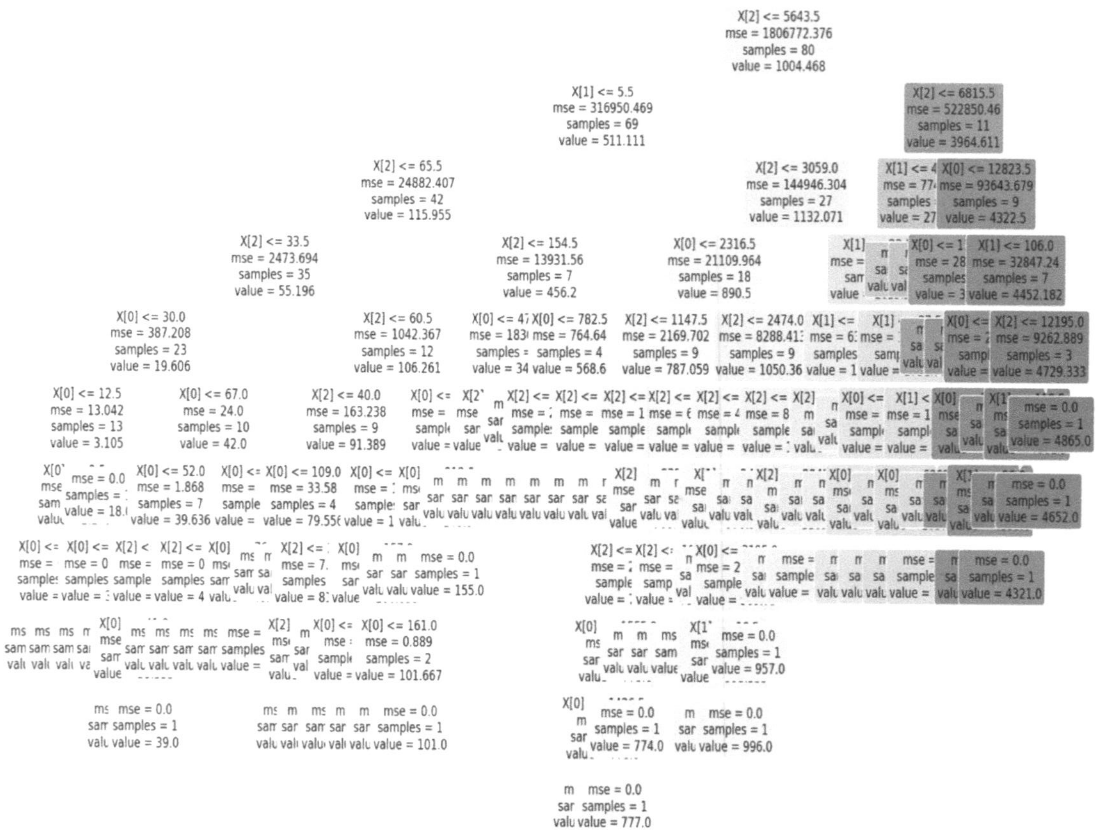

Figure 16.16 Decision tree graph of Maharashtra

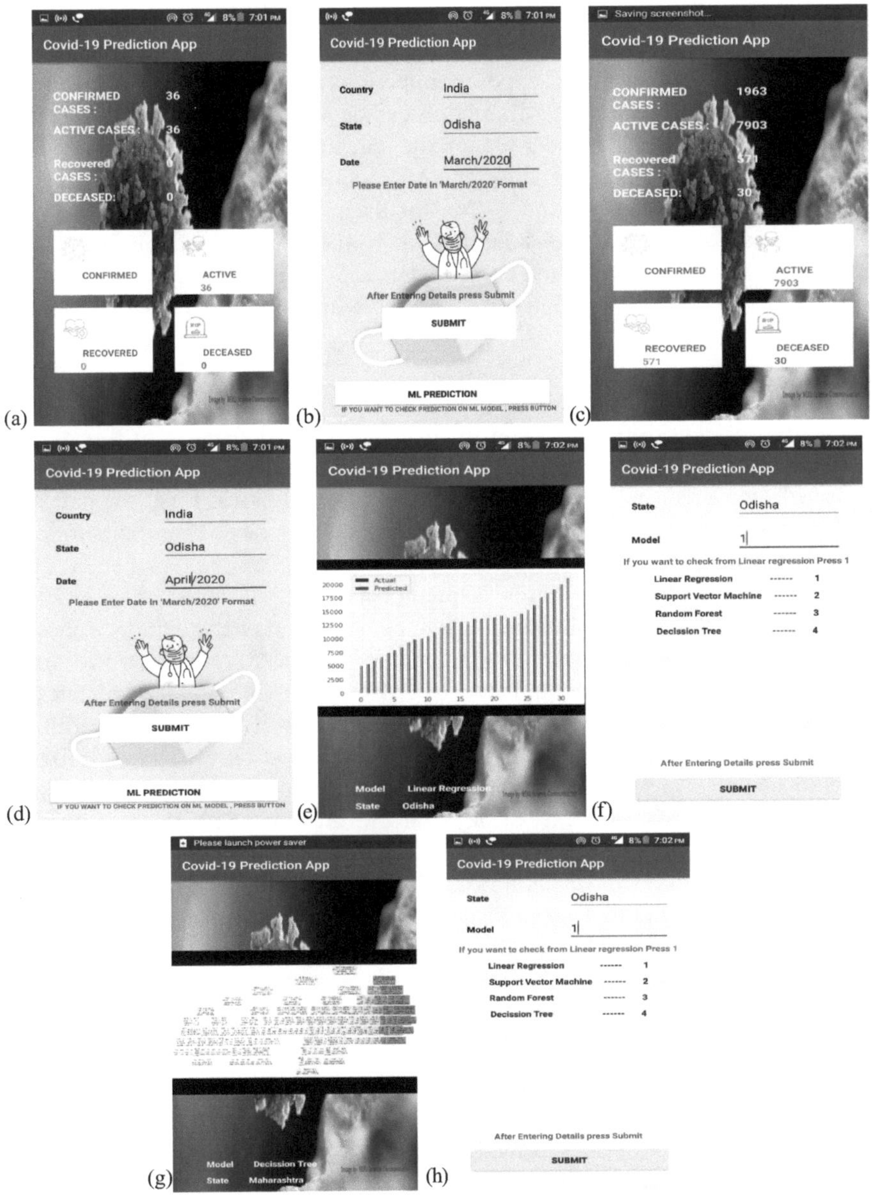

Figure 16.17 *(a) Numerical presentation of the amount of cases of the state that user has entered and (b) the user interface of the app where user needs to click on "Submit" for numerical presentation and ML prediction for graphical presentation. (c) Graphical output for active case prediction using linear regression in Odisha. (d) The user interface that asks the user to choose between four machine learning models. (e) Graphical representation for decision tree model and (f) the model that user has entered. (g) The figure shows Decision Tree model and (h) the figure shows which model to be used for prediction*

and implemented susceptible–exposed–infectious–recovered model to predict number of active cases in India. ML models can be helpful to analyze the behaviors of the newly found cases in order to stop the spread of the disease.

We have considered four different ML models such as linear regression, decision tree, random forest, and SVMs for the prediction of COVID cases. As mentioned earlier, we have considered data from the period March 16, 2020 to November 20, 2020 and classified into two datasets. From these, 80% data has been used for training and 20% for testing. We have analyzed the case of Odisha in Case-1 and India in Case-2.

Case-1:

This section provides the performances of linear regression, random forest, decision tree, and SVM models to predict the number of active cases, the number of confirmed recovered and deceased cases and recovered cases. First, the dataset is divided into training set and testing set. All the models have been trained on the first 138 instances of the dataset that is from March 16, 2020 to October 31, 2020. Then, the number of active cases is predicted for 20 instances that are from November 1, 2020 to November 20, 2020 to evaluate and analyze the performance of the different models. The values of parameters for linear regressions after fitting on the training set are shown in Table 16.1. Here, the value of R2 indicates the linear regression models as the strong fitted model. Similarly, random forest and SVMs are trained on the same training set and evaluated on the same testing set. The comparison of actual and predicted values of random forest, multiple linear regression, and SVMs for next 20 days on the different datasets are shown in Figures 16.18–16.20. The prediction performances of all these models are evaluated based on mean error, mean absolute error, mean absolute percentage error, mean squared error, and root-mean-squared error. The values of these performance metrics are provided in Table 16.2. From Table 16.2, we can conclude that the SVM has outperformed all the models in all the performance metrics for the prediction of active cases in different states.

16.6.1 Odisha analysis

Case-2:

The actual and predicted values of random forest, decision tree, and linear regression and SVMs on different dataset are shown in Figure 16.19. The prediction performances of all these models are evaluated based on mean error, absolute mean error,

Table 16.1 Analysis of linear regression

Mean absolute error (in %)	0.9094964300984387
Mean-squared error	3,774.501697282683
Mean absolute error	54.40728328005709
Mean error	−54.40728328005709
Root-mean-squared error	61.436973373390416

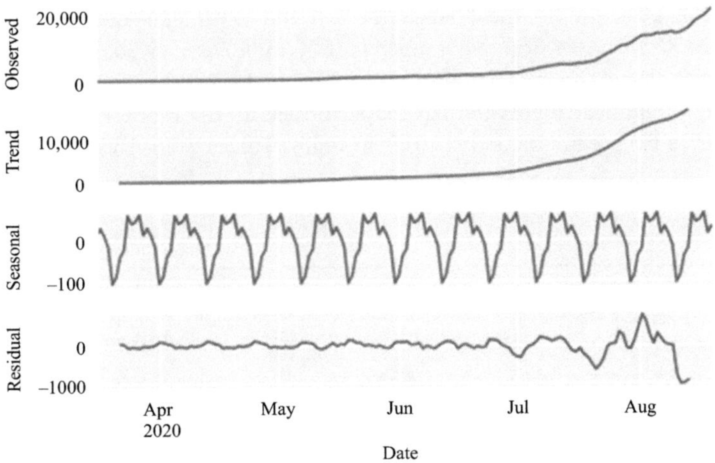

Figure 16.18 Seasonal trend for dataset of Odisha

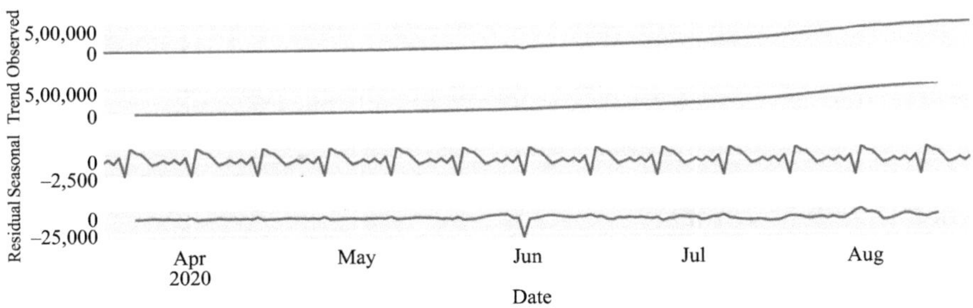

Figure 16.19 Seasonal trend for dataset of India

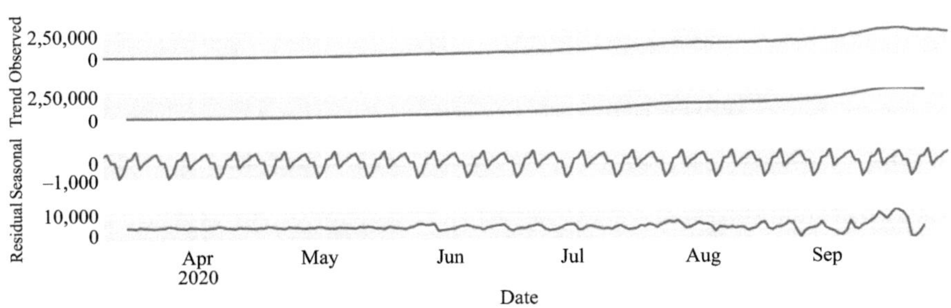

Figure 16.20 Seasonal trend for dataset of Maharashtra

mean absolute error (in %), mean squared error, and root-mean-squared error for the prediction of active cases from November 1, 2020 to November 20, 2020. The values of these performance metrics are provided in Table 16.3. From Table 16.4, we can conclude that the linear regression has outperformed all the models in all the performance metrics for prediction active cases in India (Tables 16.5–16.9).

Table 16.2 Analysis of support vector regression

Mean absolute error (in %)	0.14417560953898045
Mean-squared error	100.77708155781197
Mean absolute error	8.793622275305292
Mean error	−8.793622275305292
Root-mean-squared error	10.038778887783712

Table 16.3 Analysis of random forest

Mean absolute error (in %)	54.38628892838645
Mean-squared error	18,631,195.07867186
Mean absolute error	3,519.773
Mean error	3,519.773
Root-mean-squared error	4,316.386808277482

16.6.2 Delhi analysis

Table 16.4 Linear regression analysis

Mean absolute error (in %)	0.19405347012519197
Mean-squared error	1,495,872.0518280012
Mean absolute error	1,092.4727433862572
Mean error	551.5540571806923
Root-mean-squared error	1,223.0584825869944

Table 16.5 Support vector regression analysis

Mean absolute error (in %)	1.4533423138760877
Mean-squared error	91.3541581736475
Mean absolute error	8.712695355665368
Mean error	−6,917.536236677668
Root-mean-squared error	95.56956409724005

Table 16.6 Random forest analysis

Mean absolute error (in %)	32.27907985356206
Mean-squared-error	196,557.08125
Mean absolute error	46,519,491,113.14313
Mean error	196,557.08125
Root-mean-squared error	215,683.77572998652

16.6.3 Maharashtra analysis

Table 16.7 Linear regression analysis

Mean absolute error (in %)	15.144353129178628
Mean-squared error	1,685,554,805.040623
Mean absolute error	34,289.752536078304
Mean error	549.5540571806923
Root-mean-squared error	1,123.0584825869944

Table 16.8 Support vector regression analysis

Mean absolute error (in %)	1.0533423138760877
Mean-squared-error	87.3541581736475
Mean absolute error	7.712695355665368
Mean error	−6,217.536236677668
Root-mean-squared error	87.56956409724005

Table 16.9 Random forest analysis

Mean absolute error (in %)	35.27907985356206
Mean squared error	186,557.08125
Mean absolute error	485,976,842.14313
Mean error	201,589.08125
Root-mean-squared error	245,683.77572998652

16.7 Conclusion and future work

In this work, we have analyzed the number of active cases of different states of India and used four different models to predict the COVID cased for next 25 days. Out of the data collected from WHO, 80% was used for testing and 20% for testing. It is observed that SVM gives better result for Odisha and linear regression provides better result for India as the number cases are very high. Our result shows that the *R*2 value of linear regression model is 1 for states, which indicates prediction is robust. Our prediction model could help the medical professional to take appropriate plan so that future cases in COVID-19 can be minimized.

References

[1] Carolyn O, Sattenspiel L, Miller E, and Dimka J. Defining epidemics in computer simulation models: How do definitions influence conclusions? *Epidemics* 2017; 19: 24–32.

[2] World Health Organization. Coronavirus disease (COVID-19) pandemic. Available at https://who.int/emergencies/diseases/novel-coronavirus-2019. Accessed on 17 June 2020.

[3] Wang W, Tang J, and Wei F. Updated understanding of the outbreak of 2019 novel coronavirus (2019-nCoV) in Wuhan, China. *J Med Virol* 2020; 92(4): 441e7.

[4] Wu JT, Leung K, and Leung GM. Nowcasting and forecasting the potential domestic and international spread of the 2019-nCoV outbreak originating in Wuhan, china: A modelling study. *Lancet* 2020; 395(10225): 689–97.

[5] Novel coronavirus (COVID-19) cases, provided by JHU CSSE. Available at https://github.com/CSSEGISandData/COVID-19. Accessed on 26 March 2021.

[6] Tang B, Wang X, Li Q, *et al*. Estimation of the transmission risk of the 2019-nCoV and its implication for public health interventions. *J Clin Med* 2020; 9 (2): 462.

[7] Kraemer MU, Yang CH, Gutierrez B, *et al*. The effect of human mobility and control measures on the COVID-19 epidemic in china. *Science* 2020; 368(6490): 493–7.

[8] Barkur G, and Vibha GBK. Sentiment analysis of nationwide lockdown due to COVID 19 outbreak: Evidence from India. *Asian J Psychiatry* 2020; 51: 102089.

[9] India COVID-19 TRACKER. 2020 [online]. Available at https://covid19india.org/. Accessed on: 11th September 2020.

[10] Cooper I, Mondal A, and Antonopoulos CG. A SIR model assumption for the spread of COVID-19 in different communities. *Chaos Solitons Fractals* 2020; 139: 110057.

[11] Alzahrani SI, Aljamaan IA, and Al-Fakih EA. Forecasting the spread of the COVID-19 pandemic in Saudi Arabia using ARIMA prediction model under current public health interventions. *J Infect Public Health* 2020; 13: 914–19.

[12] Alazab A, Hobbs M, Abawajy J, and Alazab M. Using feature selection for intrusion detection system. In *2012 International Symposium on Communications and Information Technologies (ISCIT)*, 2012, pp. 296–301.

[13] Alazab A, Alazab M, Abawajy J, and Hobbs M. Web application protection against SQL injection attack. In *Proceedings of the 7th International Conference on Information Technology and Applications*, 2011, pp. 1–7.

[14] Alazab M, Alazab A, and Batten L. Smartphone malware based on synchronisation vulnerabilities. In *ICITA 2011: Proceedings of the 7th International Conference on Information Technology and Applications*, Sydney, Australia, 2012, pp. 1–6.

[15] Alazab M, Monsamy V, Batten L, Lantz P, and Tian R. Analysis of malicious and benign android applications. In *International Conference on Distributed Computing Systems Workshops (ICDCSW)*, 2012 32nd, 2012, pp. 608–16.

[16] Xu Y, Wang Y, Yuan J, Cheng Q, Wang X, and Carson PL. Medical breast ultrasound image segmentation by machine learning. *Ultrasonics* 2019; 91: 1–9.

[17] Mesleh A. Lung cancer detection using multi-layer neural networks with independent component analysis: A comparative study of training algorithms. *Jordan J Biol Sci* 2017; 10.

[18] Mesleh A, Skopin D, Baglikov S, and Quteishat A. Heart rate extraction from vowel speech signals. *J Comput Sci Technol* 2012; 27: 1243–51.

[19] Mesleh A. Chi square feature extraction based SVMs Arabic language text categorization system. *J Comput Sci* 2007; 3: 430–5.

[20] Mesleh A. Feature sub-set selection metrics for Arabic text classification. *Pattern Recognit Lett* 2011; 32: 1922–9.

[21] Malki Z, Atlam ES, Hassanien AE, Dagnew G, Elhosseini MA, and Gad A. Association between weather data and COVID-19 pandemic predicting mortality rate: Machine learning approaches. *Chaos Solitons Fractals* 2020; 138: 110137.

[22] Swapnarekha H, Behera HS, Nayak J, and Naik B. Role of intelligent computing in COVID-19 prognosis: A state-of-the-art review. *Chaos Solitons Fractals* 2020; 138: 109947.

[23] Pai P, Bhaskar A, and Rawoot V. Investigating the dynamics of COVID-19 pandemic in India under lockdown. *Chaos Solitons Fractals* 2020; 138: 109988.

Chapter 17

Technological advancement with artificial intelligence in healthcare

Manas Kumar Yogi[1], Jyotsna Garikipati[2] and Jyotir Moy Chatterjee[3]

Abstract

Machine learning (ML) techniques in healthcare are very much useful in the early diagnosis of various diseases, discovery of new drugs for the new viruses or diseases that are spreading, predicting the diseases and maintaining the huge volumes of data that is being generated in an easily accessible manner. The accuracy of different algorithms for the diagnosis of various diseases has been compared. Drug development using support vector machine and random forest is compared. The differences between the electronic medical record and electronic health record (EHR) are discussed, and case studies are discussed to understand the use of EHR. Finally, robust disease prediction frameworks are also presented in this chapter. This chapter will act as a readymade guide to persons who want to pursue using ML principles in the healthcare domain.

Keywords: AI; ML; Healthcare; Deep learning; Medical

17.1 Introduction

NetFlix, Alexa, Siri and other websites that recommend products/services to their customers based on their previous choices are the real-world examples of machine learning (ML). Advances in ML techniques have skyrocketed in the recent past leading to a great impact on various domains such as the Finance, Media, Travel, Retail, Healthcare sector. As per Gartner, the global artificial intelligence (AI)-based economic activity will be about \$3.9 trillion in 2022 from \$1.2 trillion in 2018 [1]. Advances in AI and ML techniques help to unfold complex data patterns, thereby providing quality treatment. When integrated with AI tools, there can be a

[1]CSE Department, Pragati Engineering College (Autonomous), Surampalem, India
[2]CSE Department, Andhra University, Visakhapatnam, India
[3]Department of IT, Lord Buddha Education Foundation, Kathmandu, Nepal

considerable paradigm change in medical decision-making. Even though the usage of many of the systems is under discussion for decades, only a few have come up with successful implementation. AI and ML are quite confusing for many people. AI can be understood as a machine or a technology that can act smart by taking appropriate decisions [2]. ML is a subset of AI, and deep learning (DL) is a subset of ML. Figure 17.1 clarifies this notion.

In simple words, ML can be defined as making the computer (machine) to learn on its own. For that we need to train the machine through a model. The model is nothing but a mathematical formula that can be applied to the data that is provided to the machine as input. This differs from the traditional programming where we need to tell the computer what to do with the data provided through a program [3] (Figure 17.2).

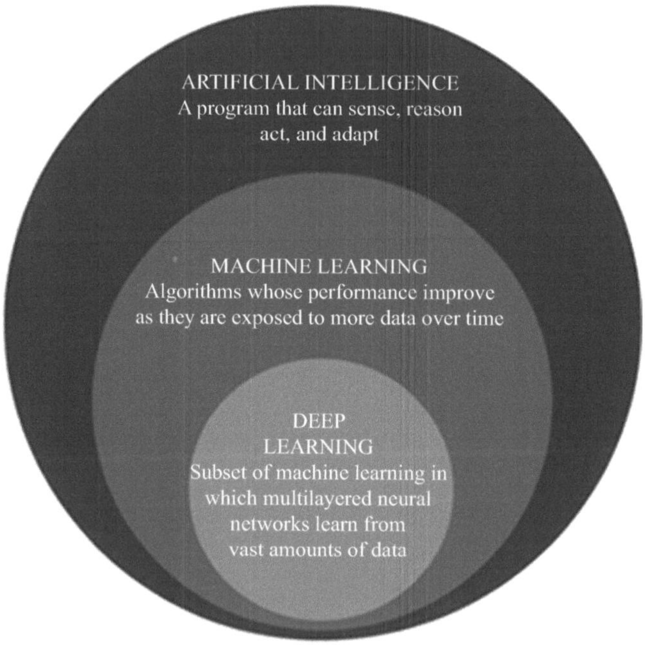

Figure 17.1 Hierarchy of AI, ML and DL

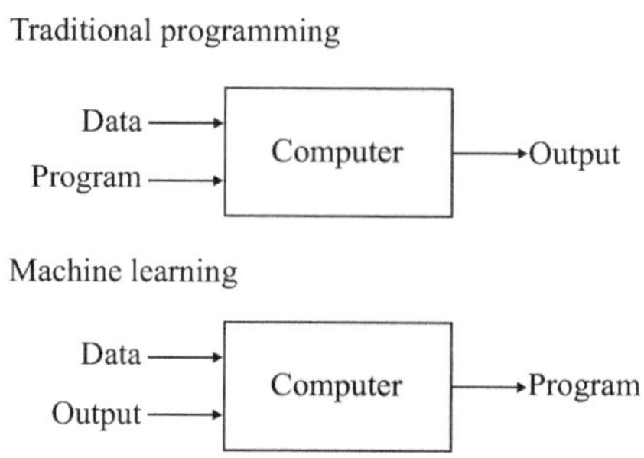

Figure 17.2 Traditional programming vs machine learning

17.1.1 Steps to build a machine learning model

The following are the sequence of steps to build an ML model [4]:

1. Problem definition: Problem statement should be clear and concise.
2. Data collection: Collect the data from the primary sources or from the repositories.
3. Data preprocessing: Refine data to eliminate any missing values, redundant values, etc.
4. Feature selection: Only required features will be chosen.
5. Algorithm selection: Depending on the given input and the required output, choose the best ML algorithm.
6. Model training: Train the model by dividing data into training data and test data.
7. Model evaluation: The model will be evaluated by changing the training and the test data from the same dataset(s) that is used in the step 5.

17.1.2 Machine learning terminology

Before proceeding further, let us understand a few terms that are used in ML frequently (Figure 17.3).

17.1.2.1 Overfitting

The fitting includes all the noise points as well into the model. This has a negative impact on the performance of the model, thereby reducing the accuracy [5].

17.1.2.2 Underfitting

The model is too simple that it fails to fit all the data points correctly from the training set, thereby leaving most of the points in the testing data as outliers or noise.

17.1.2.3 Data split

The given input data is split into training, test and validation data. The training data is used by the model for learning [6]. Validation data is used to evaluate the model to fine-tune the hyperparameters of the model. The final model is obtained from the test data. To understand better, training data can be taken as the lecture (information)

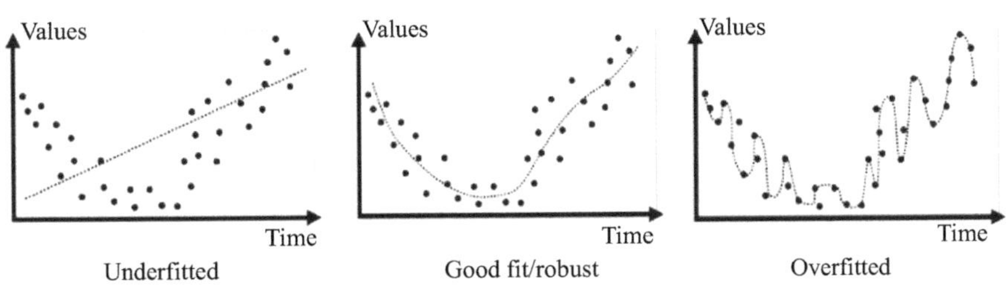

Figure 17.3 Overfitting, good fit, underfitting

delivered during a classroom session, validation data is the test conducted in the class by the instructor or the trainer and the test data is the final board exam.

17.1.3 ML algorithms

ML algorithms are mainly categorized as follows [7] (Figure 17.4):

1. Supervised learning [8]: The input will be mapped to one among the predefined classes. Next, the approximation of the mapping function should be performed in such a way that we can be able to predict the output for the given new data. The correct answers are known in advance and the model will guide us in making the right predictions. On achieving good performance, learning will be stopped. Most important supervised ML algorithms are linear regression, random forest (RF), support vector machine (SVM), etc.
2. Unsupervised learning: Here, there will not be any correct answers, and also no supervision. The obvious aim is to construct the underlying structure based on the given input data. Some popular unsupervised ML algorithms are *K*-means, apriori algorithm, etc.
3. Semi-supervised learning: This stands in the middle of supervised and the unsupervised learning. From the large input data, some of the input data is labeled and some is not. Most of the real-world ML problems belong to this category.

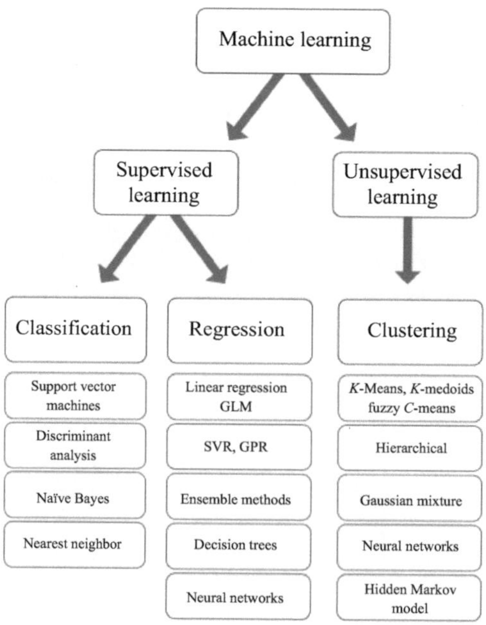

Figure 17.4 Various machine learning algorithms

Supervised learning techniques are used to predict the unlabeled data and the unsupervised learning techniques are used to discover the structure of the input.

4. Reinforcement learning: In this type of learning, the machines will learn from the environment and will be rewarded for each action either a positive reward or a negative reward. The popular ones are *Q*-learning, temporal difference, deep adversarial networks.

17.2 Literature review

The authors in [9,10] discussed various tools for single-nucleotide polymorphism analysis and target discovery respectively and concluded that the SVM and RF showed better performance over other algorithms in both the scenarios. In the survey paper [11], RFs, ensemble models and naïve Bayes have performed well in predicting heart disease. The framework in [12] used a combined dataset with hybrid classifiers by combining traditional ones with the bagging and achieved highest accuracy of 99.05% using random forest bagging method and relief feature selection methods for predicting cardiovascular diseases, whereas the framework in [13], where traditional methods like *K*-nearest neighbor (*K*-NN), AdaBoost, RF, naïve Bayes and logistic regression are used, a positive prediction accuracy of only 94% is achieved. Using the RF, XGBoost and ResNet [14], creatinine value is predicted with an area under receiver operating characteristic curve (AUC) of 0.76 in classifying the samples for chronic kidney disease. In [15], XGBoost, SVM and logistic regression are compared and concluded that XGBoost gave the best accuracy in predicting the chronic kidney disease. In [16], the researchers studied the electronic health record (EHR)'s of New York City, which has 24 cancers in total with 28 features. In [17], 366 398 EHR's of 1 694 colorectal cancer patients CRC and 3 458 breast cancer BC patients are studied post chemotherapy and observed that the patients with Type 2 diabetes showed more symptoms like the anxiety, depression and neuropathic symptoms. Sreekanth and Suryakanthi [18] have taken a dataset with 1 500 observations, built the CART and RF-predictive models to predict the variables that are responsible for chronic diabetes. Singh *et al.* [19] combined *K*-means clustering with improved ensemble methods to diagnose liver disease and achieved accuracy as high as 99.35%. The automated heart disease diagnosis system proposed in [20] integrates convolutional neural networks, genetic algorithms, SVM and NB and achieves 85.3% accuracy. In [21], a new improved *K*-means clustering algorithm is used by setting the seed value depending on the minimal clustering error.

17.2.1 Applications of machine learning in healthcare

There are numerous applications of ML in the healthcare sector. These include

1. Disease identification and diagnosis
2. Drug discovery and manufacturing
3. Electronic health records
4. Disease prediction

5. Radiology and radiopathy
6. Robotic surgery and so on

In the current chapter, we will be discussing in detail about the first four applications listed.

17.3 Disease identification and diagnosis

Major changes have come in the computer-aided diagnosis applications because a small error can lead to a wrong treatment, which in adverse cases may result in loss of patient's life. In identifying the diseases, ML algorithms can be used for pattern recognition and hence improve the perception accuracy, thus leading to better diagnosis. Huge data will be generated for each and every patient that needs to be classified for the medical data analysis [22] and the disease detection. First, the medical data will be analyzed and then used for diagnosing the diseases. This analyzed data will be the input to the ML algorithm and the results will be obtained by using the previously solved cases. These results will be taken by the physicians to diagnose a novel patient at a much higher speed and enhanced accuracy.

Many diseases can be diagnosed using ML. Figure 17.6 shows some of the diseases that can be diagnosed using different ML algorithms. In the medical domain it is mostly required to do either classification or regression. Now let us see the accuracy of various ML algorithms for each of the diseases depicted in Figure 17.5.

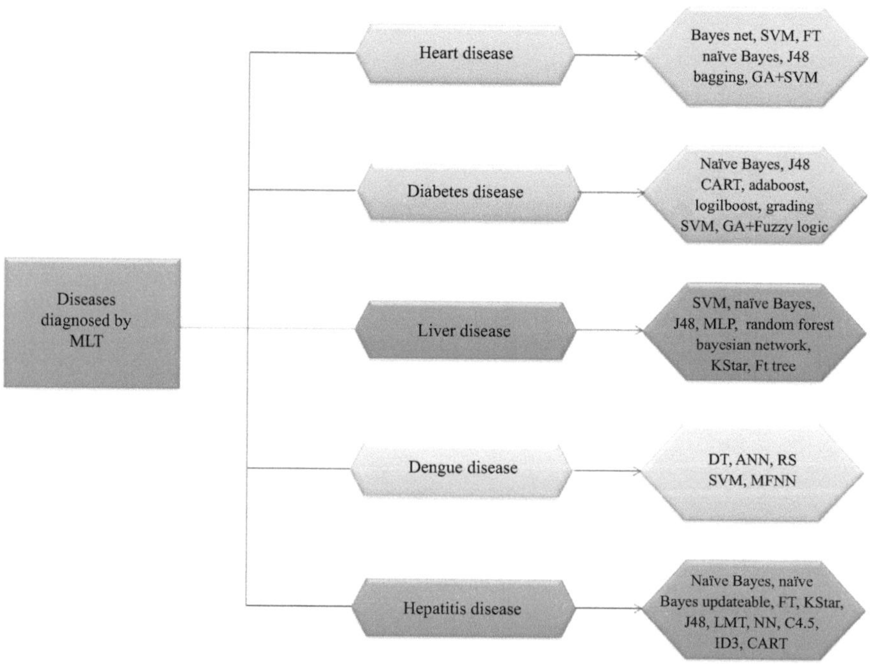

Figure 17.5 Diseases diagnosed using machine learning algorithms

17.3.1 Heart disease

Various researchers have proposed different systems for detecting heart diseases [23]. As per Figure 17.6, SVM provides highest accuracy. The advantage of SVM over other techniques is that it constructs the classifiers correctly with less overfitting and robustness to noise. Its main drawback is, it is a binary classifier, with high computational cost and its running time is also high.

17.3.2 Diabetes

It occurs when insufficient supply or improper utilization of insulin is taking place in the body. The various types of diabetes are Type 1 (less or no insulin supply), Type 2 (inefficient use of insulin) and gestational diabetes (high blood glucose during pregnancy). In the diabetes disease diagnosis, the research shows that the naïve Bayes algorithm gives a better accuracy over the other algorithms as shown in Figure 17.7. Naïve Bayes on different datasets achieved 79.56% and 95% with the WEKA tool and MATLAB® with SQL Server, respectively. The naïve Bayes algorithm eliminates the unnecessary features, thereby enhancing the performance with less computational time. But we need to give enormous input to get a better output.

17.3.3 Liver disease

Liver disease is also called hepatic disease. As shown in Figure 17.8, the functional tree (FT) algorithm gave better results. On the UCI dataset using the WEKA tool, it gave 97.10% accuracy. The FT algorithm has a very easy interpretation and also its prediction is faster. But the calculations involved will be complex if the values are uncertain.

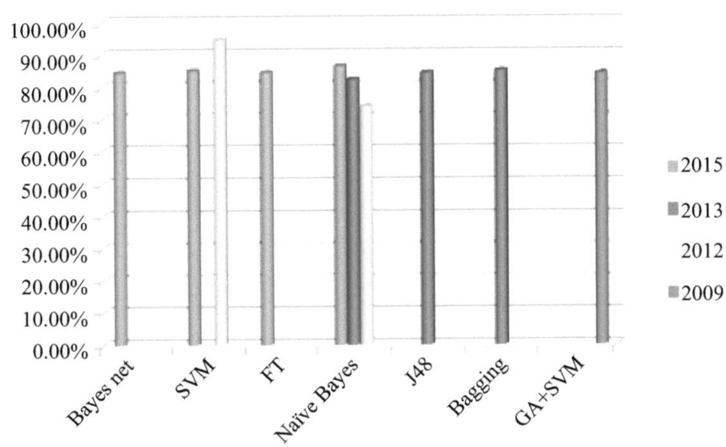

Figure 17.6 Accuracy of ML algorithms for heart disease

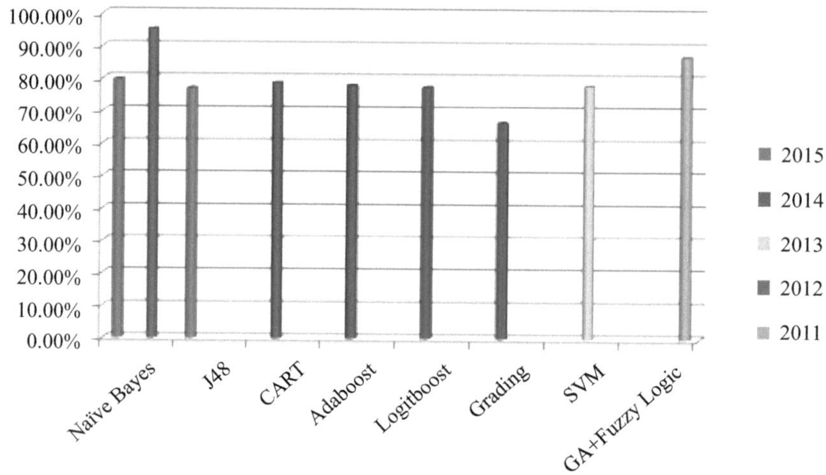

Figure 17.7 Accuracy of ML algorithms for diabetes disease

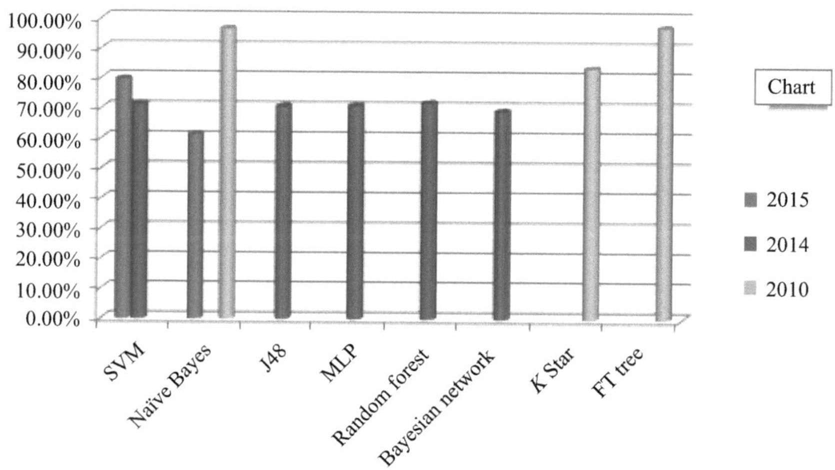

Figure 17.8 Accuracy of ML algorithms for liver disease

17.3.4 Dengue disease

This problem is caused due to mosquitos that result into viral infection subsequently leading to serious illness and death. Rough set (RS) theory shows promising results of 100% accuracy as shown in Figure 17.9. Uncertain problems can be solved using RS theory. Although it is very easy to understand and applies for both qualitative and quantitative, it is not widely used.

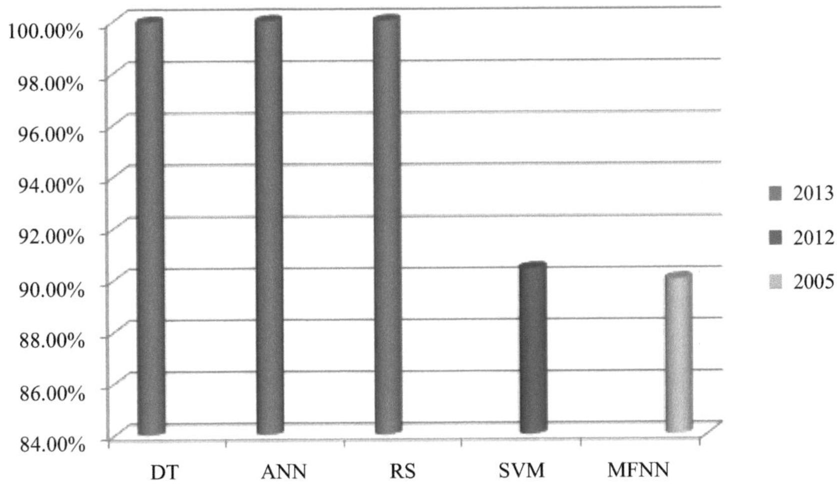

Figure 17.9 Accuracy of ML algorithms for dengue disease

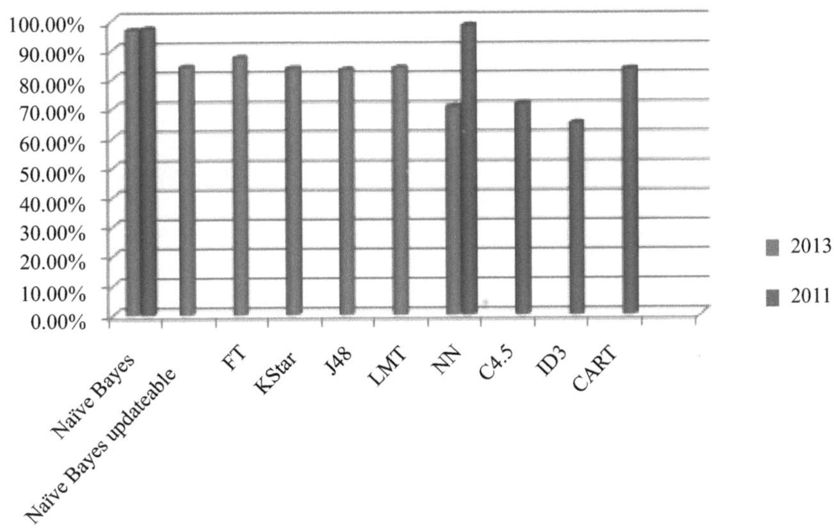

Figure 17.10 Accuracy of ML algorithms for hepatitis disease

17.3.5 Hepatitis disease

Various ML algorithms have been used to diagnose hepatitis disease, which is due to the inflammation of the liver. Feed-forward neural networks with back-propagation technique using the RapidMiner tool gave results with 98% accuracy. The results are depicted in Figure 17.10. Neural networks are known for adaptive learning and self-organization. Overall the naïve Bayes algorithm and the SVM are mostly used and have better results.

17.4 Drug discovery and manufacturing

For a drug to come into the market, it will take more than 10 years after extensive research with an average cost of 2.6 billion dollars. Consequently, for most of the rare diseases, effective treatment is not getting done. Traditional approaches to drug discovery focus mainly on overall treatment of the body. With the drastic increase in the cost of the drug discovery, alternative approaches using ML techniques are being used. Now, let us first see the various steps involved in drug discovery and then how we can speed up the process using ML. The steps involved in the drug discovery are [10] as follows:

Step 1: Target identification: First we identify the possible targets for the diseases. These DNA mutations are included along with misfolded proteins and other potential disease biomarkers. Roughly 2 years are needed for this. But it is extremely difficult for us to find out all the possible combinations manually.

Step 2: Lead discovery: The main chemical compound that can be used for the treatment of the disease will be identified. Here, we need to narrow down to the actual potential compounds in 1–2 years.

Step 3: Medicinal chemistry: Need to test the potential compounds for their reactions with the targets identified in step 1. Based on outputs, the compounds will be further optimized for the intended targets, which needs 1–2 years.

Step 4: In vitro studies: The optimized set of the compounds will be tested in an in vitro model of the disease in which the cells and the microbes behave in a restricted environment, which is different from the actual behavior of the microbes. It takes around 2 years for this area of study.

Step 5: In vivo studies: Now the compounds will be tested on animal models like mice, etc. Again, the failure rate will be high with a completion period of 1–2 years.

Step 6: Clinical trials: Now that the compound is showing promising results in the previous stages, it will be tested in human settings to validate the usefulness and safety of the compound on humans. This takes nearly 6 years.

Step 7: Only those drugs that complete the previous tests will be submitted to FDA for approval. Once this is done, the drug will be commercially available in the market. This step roughly takes 1 year.

As the overall process is taking more than 10 years, we need to speed up the process except for the clinical trials. Lead compounds can be discovered and then optimized using digital techniques for studying the molecular structures, their bindings, relation between the structure and the activity, etc. ML techniques can be used in various stages of drug discovery, like in predicting how different drugs are binded with the proteins, discovering the optimal response of a drug, making sure that the body responds well to a medication or treatment and optimizing the effect of the chemical/drug on the molecules. Various ML methods can be used for the drug–target interaction that can be based on either similarity/distance, DL, feature, matrix factorization, network based or hybrid methods [24]. An alternative for in vitro is to use the in silico where computer simulation will be done [25]. Some of the companies that were using AI and ML techniques for the drug manufacturing are Pfizer, Janssen Pharmaceutica, Sanofi, Novartis, Bayer, etc.

Of all the algorithms that are listed in Figure 17.11 [26], the algorithms RF and SVM are discussed in this chapter because of their wide usage [10]. The RF is explicitly used for huge multifeatured datasets. The key factors of RF that are helpful for discovering the drugs are as follows: RF accelerates the training of the model, with minimal parameters, dealing with the missing and nonparametric data. Another version of it is the multivariant RF, which limits the error by various error estimating techniques. RF is used to generate the regression tree nodes and the leaf nodes. Leaf nodes will make the predictions regarding the dose-specific profile and also store the functional data.

SVMs are used not to relate different classes of compounds using the feature selector by getting a hyperplane. The count of hyperplanes is not finite. In the case of linear data, depending on the selected features, the classes of compounds are projected into a chemical feature space. For *N*-dimensional space, optimal hyperplane is obtained by maximizing the margin between the classes of compounds. SVM can separate the active compounds from the available compounds and give them rankings in the database, etc. These regression models help us to find the

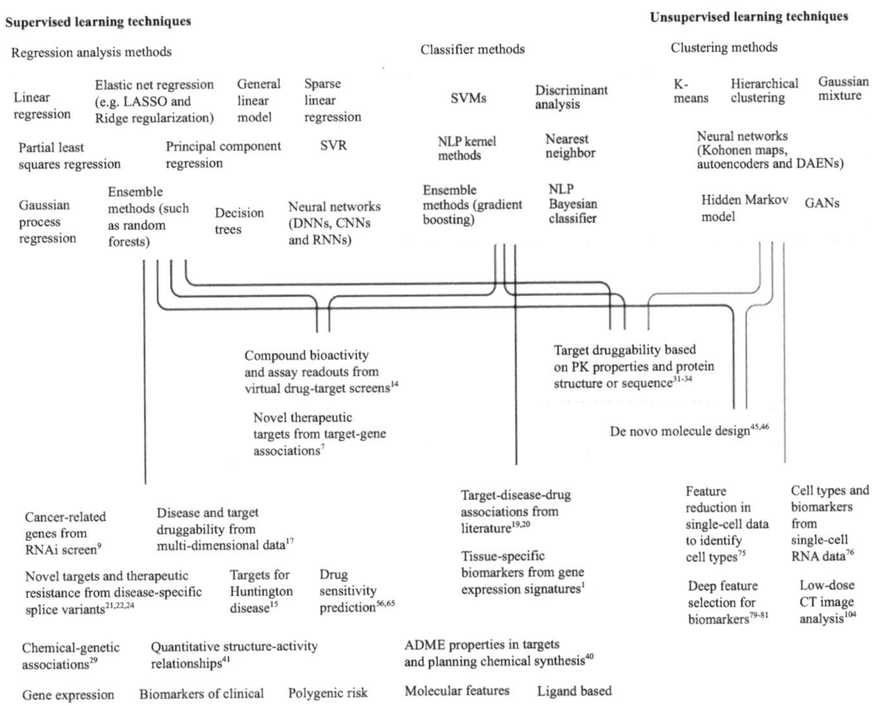

Figure 17.11 Machine learning algorithms for drug discovery and manufacturing

relation between the drug and the ligand. SVM can also differentiate the active and inactive molecules. In Figures 17.12 and 17.13 [10], how the drugs can be developed using RF, and SVM is shown, respectively.

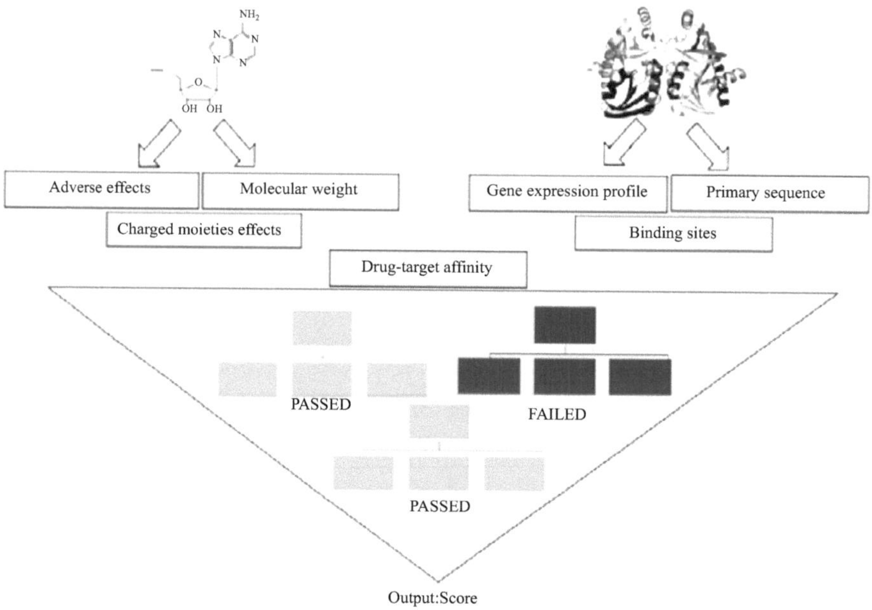

Figure 17.12 Drug development using random forest

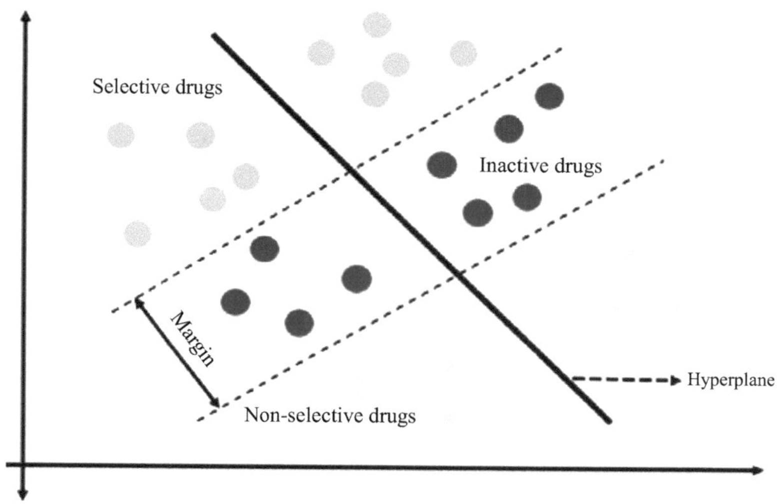

Figure 17.13 Drug development using support vector machine

17.5 Electronic health records

An EHR is a digital version of the patient's health/treatment data. They store the real-world data of the patient during and after the meeting with the medical professional. The data from all the smart devices like the sensors on the patient's body, smart homes, robots will be collected and shared among the authorized users for a better diagnosis, monitoring, early detection and treatment of the patient. Smart health system that takes data from the EHR includes acquiring data from different sources, interconnecting between different devices using different technologies by ensuring the security and privacy issues and processing the data and data dissemination.

First, we have to remove the ambiguity between the terms. EHR and electronic medical record (EMR) are often confused. EMR will store the medical and treatment history of a patient from a single physician in digital form. It is not shared among the various doctors. On the contrary, EHR will store the patient's data from various doctors. It will give a holistic view of the patient's health [27].

The EMRs help us to discover the phenotype–genotype associations, detect the adverse drug event, quicken precision medicine research, etc. EMR will contain the real-world data of the patient's clinical and private data, which can either be in structured or unstructured form. Analyzing the unstructured data is relatively difficult and time-consuming when compared to the structured data [28]. These EMRs are integrated for a long-term view of a particular patient. With a standardized EHR system, if a patient wants to switch to a different doctor, the patient's data can be homogeneously transferred to different hospitals. This reduces record duplication, identifies missing data, thereby reducing the time spent on the clinical care and hence improving the quality of care.

Statistical ML methods such as logistic regression, SVM, RF are used for mining reliable predictive patterns using EHR data. Natural language processing approach [29] can also be used for retrieving useful data from EHR. Now let us take some of the case studies to understand the use of EHR in a better way.

CASE 1 [16]: Cancerous tumors when detected and treated at an early stage can improve the chances of the survival of the patients. Delayed detection or treatment may result in shorter survival periods. Even though ML algorithms are used in the diagnosis and prediction of cancer, wrong or biased data leads to a wrong prediction and hence to a wrong treatment. SVM can be used for both the linear and nonlinear relationships between the predictors and the outcomes. Generally, EHRs might contain missing data due to various reasons like the availability of different testing equipment, how the disease progresses and others. Because of the missing data problems, the accuracy in the classification and prediction of diseases using ML algorithms will be reduced drastically. The data is stored in the form of vectors and the missing values are filled with the mean values. Kernels are used in SVM to manipulate the data. By plotting the testing scores for the linear kernel SVM and RBF (radial basis function) kernel SVM in K-fold cross-validation, it is observed that the RBF kernel SVM is more efficient than the linear SVM.

CASE 2 [18]: As more and more data is being stored in the enterprise databases and in the cloud storage for the EHR, we now have to deal with big data. Big data can be described with 4V characteristics. They are the volume, variety, velocity and veracity. Predictive analysis is needed by the doctors to identify the admission of the patient at an early stage. The main challenge is to find the strong indicators for the accurate prediction. Predictive modelling takes help of a mathematical model for the prediction of the future. Independent variables are identified and a mathematical model is designed. Among the CART, RF and the scalable RF models, the scalable RF model gave a better accuracy of 87.5%. Figure 17.14 shows different levels of the classification tree for diabetes.

CASE 3 [30]: As EHRs contain data from different hospitals, it might not have the data in a computable fashion. To elaborate further, a medication might be used for various conditions, and the condition for which this medication is being used for a particular patient may not be listed in the EHR. Even if the medication and the conditions were listed in the same note, they might not be linked properly. The simplest statistical method to store the medications and the conditions is the tabulation method. Regression is better than tabulation and can differentiate the medications for hypertension. Regression also gives information regarding some medications that are preferred over the other medications depending upon the patient's condition. Least absolute shrinkage and selection operator (LASSO) logistic regression is used to reduce overfitting with simple functions. Using LASSO, the logistic regression will be performed by keeping the summation of the absolute values of the regression coefficients less than the given threshold value.

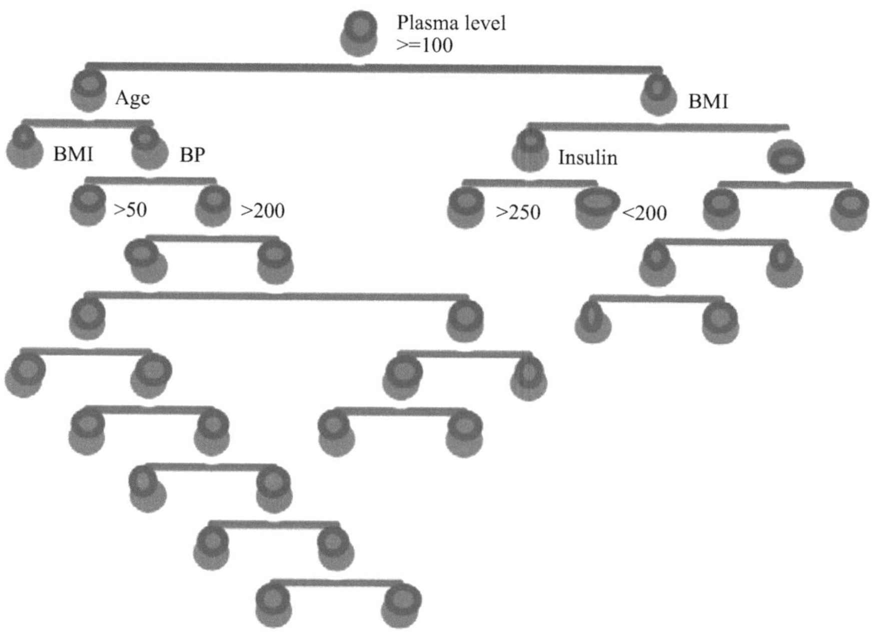

Figure 17.14 Classification tree for diabetes

There are few problems with EHRs in the healthcare systems [31]. These are significantly related to the implementation and the workflow disturbances. Only affordable hospitals can implement an EHR system. For small-scale practices, implementing EHR systems is not financially viable. Also, the workflow will be disturbed because the clinicians have to spend their valuable time filling up the documents. Also, we need to have up-to-date technology to store the data.

17.6 Disease prediction using machine learning

Classical diagnosis requires that the patients have to undergo various medical tests and based on the reports obtained, the medical supervisor will start treating the patient. This is a very laborious, costly and time-consuming process. To speed up, the process ML techniques can be used. The general workflow of any disease prediction system with ML starts with the user input as the symptoms the patient is exhibiting, which then compared with the dataset having various diseases and their symptoms and then using ML techniques, the disease will be predicted. Now we will be discussing a few disease prediction frameworks.

SVM and the bootstrap aggregation (bagging) using reduced error pruning tree can be used for the disease prediction [32]. Minimum redundancy and maximum relevance feature selection algorithm is used for extracting only the relevant features and also with less repetition. Three datasets, namely, the diabetes dataset, breast cancer dataset and hypothyroid dataset were used. The training data is classified by means of operations related to SVM and bagging. The test data will first be classified using SVM. If a positive output is obtained, it will be validated. Otherwise, the remaining test data will be classified using bagging. This tool is not specific to any disease type.

Apriori association algorithm is used to select the ten best rules from the dataset to implement different classification algorithms [33]. Then the performance of the five classifiers, namely, *K*-NN, naïve Bayes, Zero R, OneR and J48 is evaluated using the WEKA tool. Their study emphasized on the usage of feature selection with the classification algorithms. In WEKA, IBk (instance-based learner) with apriori association algorithm predicted chronic kidney disease with 99% accuracy.

ML techniques like the *K*-nearest neighborhood and RF are used to predict whether a person has heart disease or not [34]. Depending on the attributes like the severity of the chest pain, cholesterol level, age of the person, the analysis was done. The *K*-NN and RF have been predicted with accuracy of 86.885% and 81.967%, respectively.

17.7 Fairness

It is useless to use biased ML in any field. Many applications of ML will have the potential for life-changing consequences and obviously its importance is supreme in healthcare [35], judicial system, etc. Thus, fairness in ML plays a crucial role. The need for fairness in ML is stimulated by the inclination to stick to the legislative rules. ML models are to be built in such a way that they ensure trust and transparency. Fairness is critically needed in all the domains in which automated systems are used. Even though everyone agrees upon the need for fairness in ML, there is no single idea that can be applicable in all the scenarios. Fairness in ML on the classification parity due to the protected features such as age, gender and race can be calculated.

17.7.1 Fairness in the dataset

Even with a larger training dataset, which has either outdated or understated or has unintentional support or has historical skewed attributes, then the ML methods outcomes might be unfair. Yuan *et al.* applied an oversampling of protected features to have a fair dataset.

17.7.2 Fairness in model or algorithm

The biasing in the ML algorithms can be due to the biasing in the dataset or in the preprocessing stage or in the design of the algorithm like resource allocation.

17.7.3 Fairness in the metrics/results

This comes in the post-processing stage where metrics are used for calculating the efficiency of the used algorithms. The threshold is determined to have an unbiased outcome. The AUC scores of the logistic regression, RF and XGBoost methods are compared and observed that the output of an accurate model does not infer a fair outcome.

17.8 Data analytics role in healthcare

In healthcare [36], suppliers and officials are confronted with the undertaking of settling on the most ideal choices for patients and the business in general. From picking the best medicines, to deciding the best approaches to use assets, pioneers are settling on choices consistently that can affect well-being results and expenses. With the entirety of this data to consider, it is no big surprise that enormous information investigation apparatuses have assumed an undeniably critical part in healthcare dynamic. Specialists, suppliers and policymakers are going to large information examination models to assist with further developing consideration conveyance, allotment of assets and preventive well-being measures. As the business proceeds to improve and refine these instruments, information-driven choices will before long become standard, prompting more proactive, fruitful healthcare activities.

17.8.1 Predictive modeling

Predictive modeling is the most common way of analyzing current and historical information to anticipate future results. Models use information mining, AI and insights to recognize designs and anticipate results. Predictive models worked-off of the well-being information being gathered give arrangements on the full-scale and miniature level. The utilization of predictive analytics can make medical services experts aware of possible dangers. By analyzing social information, we can anticipate therapy results, possible dangers for ongoing sickness and even foresee hazard of self-hurt. The well-being information gathered can be utilized for hazard scoring, readmission forecast and anticipation, foreseeing contamination and disintegration and quite a lot more at the singular patient level. Predictive modeling can likewise be utilized on a lot bigger scope. Populace well-being the board is incomprehensible without the utilization of these models. Episodes can be anticipated, results can be anticipated, and in realizing what is to come, preventive measures can be taken. Predictive modeling can even be utilized in authoritative applications to build proficiency and lower costs for all.

17.8.2 Reduction in healthcare costs

Medical services are costly. And, those costs just keep on expanding in all cases. We are, be that as it may, seeing a shift from expense for administration installment models to esteem-based consideration. Using predictive and prescriptive analytics, medical care associations and specialists can get nitty-gritty models for bringing down costs and patient danger. Notwithstanding the patient-driven advantages referenced earlier, well-being information analytics can diminish arrangement flake-outs, oversee inventory network costs, and forestall gear breakdowns and lessening extortion.

17.8.3 Empowering advanced chronic disease prevention

As well as observing and getting ready for COVID-19 floods, healthcare specialists have progressively gone to enormous information analytics apparatuses to further develop chronic disease recognition and therapy. In fostering these models, examiners look to assess explicit clinical and nonclinical elements that might add to an individual's danger of fostering a chronic disease. At the College of Information Sciences and Technology at Penn State, analysts have fostered a computerized reasoning calculation to anticipate defenselessness to substance use issue among youthful destitute people. The model could assist with illuminating authorities about customized recovery programs for exceptionally helpless youngsters. To help policymakers in concocting successful projects and approaches in a principled way, it is gainful to foster AI and AI arrangements that can consequently uncover an extensive arrangement of elements related with substance use issue among destitute youth.

17.9 Deep learning applications in healthcare

DL is helping medical experts and scientists to find the secret chances in information and to serve the healthcare business better. DL in healthcare gives doctors the examination of any sickness precisely and assists them with treating them better, accordingly, bringing about better medical choices.

17.9.1 Drug discovery

DL in healthcare helps in discovery of drugs and their turn of events. The innovation examines the patient's medical history and gives the best therapy to them.

Also, this innovation is acquiring bits of knowledge from patient side effects and tests.

17.9.1.1 Medical imaging

Medical imaging procedures, for example, MRI scans, CT scans, ECG, are utilized to analyze unpleasant sicknesses such as coronary illness, disease, mind growth. Subsequently, DL assists doctors with investigating the illness better and give patients the best treatment.

17.9.1.2 Insurance fraud

DL is utilized to dissect the medical insurance fraud claims. With predictive analytics, it can predict fraud guarantees that are probably going to occur later on. Additionally, DL helps insurance industry to convey limits and offers to their objective patients.

17.9.1.3 Alzheimer's sickness

Alzheimer is one of the huge difficulties that medical industry faces. DL strategy is utilized to detect Alzheimer's infection at a beginning phase.

17.9.1.4 Genome

DL strategy is utilized to comprehend a genome and assist patients with finding out with regards to infection that may affect them. DL has a promising future in genomics.

17.9.2 Challenges faced by deep learning applications in healthcare

In spite of the promising outcomes that got utilizing deep designs, there stay a few strange difficulties confronting the clinical utilization of DL to healthcare. Specifically, we feature the accompanying central points of contention.

17.9.2.1 Volume of information

As the data volume pertaining to the application of DL models in healthcare is increasing, the crucial challenge is how to manage the data, in terms of cost-effective factors. Preparing an exhaustive DL model is quite a task for the engineers working in this area. This leads to a restricted viewpoint for the researchers where further research work is essential in coming time.

17.9.2.2 Degree of temporality

The DL mechanisms cannot infer with non-static data. They need massive amount of time for learning the trends in the medical datasets, so this angle of temporal data modelling needs to be further investigated. Efficient planning is the key task in achieving this goal.

17.9.2.3 Complexity of domain specialization

Each domain has its own design challenges and more so in healthcare as privacy of the patients must also be taken into consideration in this domain. Privacy preserving DL algorithms are being actively worked on by researchers worldwide and the concept of synthetic data is being implemented. But in big data medical systems, the efficiency of such mechanisms is not so encouraging till date.

17.9.2.4 Human difficulties for adopting AI techniques for healthcare

In order to gain maximum benefits from the AI techniques, focus must be on patient disease detection and the degree of clinical applicability must also be high. These two factors are to be considered prominently by the research community.

17.9.2.5 Algorithmic bias

The ML algorithms may suffer from discriminatory bias on the basis of race, color, community, socio-economic status, etc. The designers have to focus on this aspect with great care and study the harmful effects.

17.10 Conclusion and future scope

As per the Frost and Sullivan report, by the year 2025, AI systems will be part of everything from population health management to digital avatars that can answer particular patient queries. With so many applications of AI and ML in the healthcare industry, many startups are now entering healthcare with ML and AI. Some of these include SigTuple, Qure.ai, Tricog, OncoStem, Nirami Health Analytics, Predible Health, CARING (Centre for Advanced Research Imaging, NeuroScience and Genomics). Due to the lack of trained doctors and the population explosion, the healthcare industry is getting overburdened. In India, the doctor patient ratio is 1:1 700, a very higher value than the recommendation by WHO which is 1:1 000. Various applications of ML in healthcare were discussed. The various algorithms that can be used in the drug discovery, disease identification and diagnosis, and prediction of diseases were explained. We have also understood how the big data generated in the EHR will be processed. Various tools that can be used in the prediction of the diseases were explained. Finally, the aspect of fairness in ML and the dimensions for fairness were discussed. The COVID-19 pandemic has stimulated the usage of AI and ML techniques in various domains, mainly in the healthcare sector. The pandemic resulted in the generation of enormous amounts of data about patients, which then be used for various analyses. This helps in speeding up the drug development process and also for a better and early diagnosis. Usage of ML and AI techniques will improve the productivity and fidelity of the existing systems, thereby helping in attending more patients in less time with greater healthcare outcomes and limited cost.

References

[1] K. Costello and M. Rimol. "Gartner Forecasts Worldwide IT Spending to Grow 6.2% in 2021." January 25, 2021. https://gartner.com/en/newsroom/

press-releases/2020-01-25-gartner-forecasts-worldwide-it-spending-to-grow-6-point-2-percent-in-2021. Accessed 1 September 2021.

[2] S. Singh. "Cousins of Artificial Intelligence." Towards Data Science. https://towardsdatascience.com/cousins-of-artificial-intelligence-dda4edc27b55 (accessed on May 27, 2018).

[3] P. Shah. "Insights into Machine Learning." OpenSource For U. https://opensourceforu.com/2018/01/insights-machine-learning/ (accessed on Jan 16, 2018).

[4] R. Smith. "The 7 Key Steps to build Your Machine Learning Model." https://becominghuman.ai/the-7-key-steps-to-build-your-machine-learning-model-2739d85b0cef (accessed on Aug 12, 2020).

[5] A. Bhande. "What Is Underfitting and Overfitting in Machine Learning and How to Deal It." GREYATOM. https://medium.com/greyatom/what-is-underfitting-and-overfitting-in-machine-learning-and-how-to-deal-with-it-6803a989c76 (accessed on Mar 12, 2018).

[6] Widsse. "Splitting Data Folders Into Training, Validation and Testing Folders Using Shuffling With Python and Scikit-Learn." Widsse. https://medium.com/@Ana_Caballero_H/splitting-data-folders-into-training-validation-and-testing-folders-using-shuffling-with-python-63cabcd997dd (accessed on May 8, 2020).

[7] D. Fumo. "Types of Machine Learning Algorithms You Should Know." Towards Data Science. https://towardsdatascience.com/types-of-machine-learning-algorithms-you-should-know-953a08248861 (accessed on June 15, 2017).

[8] J. Bhattacharjee. "Popular Machine Learning Algorithms." NINELEAPS. https://medium.com/technology-nineleaps/popular-machine-learning-algorithms-a574e3835ebb (accessed on Nov 10, 2017).

[9] A. Nayarisseri, R. Khandelwal, G. Thakur and A. S. Planche. "Artificial Intelligence, Big Data, Machine Learning Approaches in Precision Medicine and Drug Discovery." https://researchgate.net/publication/348234715_Artificial_Intelligence_Big_data_and_Machine_Learning_approaches_in_Precision_Medicine_Drug_Discovery (accessed on Jan, 2021).

[10] T. Lauv Patel, X. Shukla, D. W. Huang and S. W. Ussery. "Machine Learning Methods in Drug Discovery." *Molecules*, 25, no. 22 (2020): 5277.

[11] V. V. Ramalingam, A. Dandapath and M. Karthik Raja. "Heart Disease Prediction Using Machine Learning Techniques: A Survey." *International Journal of Engineering and Technology*, 7 (2018): 684–687.

[12] P. Ghosh, S. Azam, M. Jonkman, *et al.* "Efficient Prediction of Cardio Vascular Disease Using Machine Learning Algorithms with Relief and LASSO Feature Selection Techniques." *IEEE Access*, 9 (2021): 19304–19326.

[13] E. Maini, B. Venkateswarulu, B. Maini and D. Marwaha. "Machine Learning-Based Heart Disease Prediction System for Indian Population: An Exploratory Study Done in South India." *Medical Journal Armed Forces India*, 77 (2021): 302–311.

[14] W. Wang, G. Chakraborty and B. Chakraborty. "Predicting the Risk of Chronic Kidney Disease (CKD) Using Machine Learning Algorithms." *Applied Sciences*, 11, no. 1 (2020): 202.

[15] H. You. "Predictive Analysis of Chronic Kidney Disease Based on Machine Learning." *Engineering and Applied Science Letters*, 11, no. 1 (2021): 62.

[16] X. Zang, F. Gu and J. Xiao. "Applying Support Vector machines to electronic health records for cancer classification." In *Proceedings of MSM'19* (2019): 1–9.

[17] X. Luo, S. Storey, P. Gandhi, *et al.* "Analysing the Symptoms in Colorectal and Breast Cancer Patients With or Without Type 2 Diabetes Using EHR Data." *Health Informatics Journal*, 27, no. 1 (2021): 1–20.

[18] S. Rallapalli and T. Suryakanthi. "Predicting the risk of diabetes in big data electronic health records by using scalable random forest classification algorithm." *2016 International Conference on Advances in Computing and Communication Engineering (ICACCE) (2016)*: 281–284.

[19] A. Singh, J. C. Mehta, D. Anand, P. Nath, B. Pandey and A. Kamparia. "An Intelligent Hybrid Approach for Hepatitis Disease Diagnosis: Combining Enhanced k-Means Clustering and Improved Ensemble Learning." *Expert Systems*, 38 (2021): https://doi.org/10.1111/exsy.12526.

[20] M. Elhoseny, M. A. Mohammed, S. A. Mostafa, *et al.* "A New Multi-Agent Feature Wrapper Machine Learning Approach for Heart Disease Diagnosis." *Computers, Materials & Continua*, 67, no. 1 (2021): 51–71.

[21] R. Thanga Selvi and I. MuthuLakshmi. "Modelling the Map Reduce Based Optimal Gradient Boosted Tree Classification Algorithm for Diabetes Mellitus Diagnosis System." *Journal of Ambient Intelligence and Humanized Computing*, 12 (2021): 1717–1730.

[22] R. Sujatha, S. Nathiya and J. M. Chatterjee (2020). Clinical Data Analysis Using IoT Data Analytics Platforms. *Internet of Things Use Cases for the Healthcare Industry*. Cham: Springer.

[23] M. Fathima and M. Pasha. "Survey of Machine Learning Algorithms for Disease Diagnostic." *Journal of Intelligent Learning Systems and Applications*, 9, no. 1 (2017): 1.

[24] M. Bagherian, E. Sabeti, K. Wang, *et al.* "Machine Learning Approaches and Databases for Prediction of Drug-Target Interaction – A Survey Paper." *Briefings in Bioinformatics*, 22, no. 1 (2021): 247–269.

[25] Sallieq. "Differences Between In Vitro, In Vivo and In Silico Studies." Jan, 09, 2019. https://mpkb.org/home/patients/assessing_literature/in_vitro_studies#:~:text=Bacterial%20sequencing%20techniques%20%E2%80%93%20As%20an,polymerase%20chain%20reaction%20(PCR). Accessed 5 September 2021.

[26] J. Vamathevan, D. Clark, P. Czodrowski, *et al.* "Applications of Machine Learning in Drug Discovery and Development." *PMC*, 18, no. 6 (2019): 463.

[27] "Understanding EMR Vs EHR". nextgen. https://nextgen.com/insights/emr-vs-ehr/emr-vs-ehr. Accessed 5 September 2021.

[28] M. Tayefi, P. Ngo, T. Chomutare, *et al.* "Challenges and Opportunities Beyond Structured Data in Analysis of Electronic Health Records." *WIREs Computational Statistics*, 13 (2021): e1549.

[29] J. Zeng, I. Banerjee, A. Solomon Henry, *et al.* "Natural Language Processing to Identify Cancer Treatments with Electronic Medical Records." *JCO Clinical Cancer Informatics*, 5 (2021): 379–393.

[30] D. Backenroth, H. S. Chase, Y. Wei, *et al.* "Monitoring Prescribing Patterns Using Regression and Electronic Health Records." *BMC Medical Informatics and Decision Making*, 17, no. 17 (2017): 175.

[31] V. Jain, R. Wason, J. M. Chatterjee and D. N. Le (Eds.). (2020). *Ontology-Based Information Retrieval for Healthcare Systems*. New York: John Wiley & Sons, Scrivener Publishing. ISBN: 978-1-119-64139-1.

[32] M. Rathi and V. Pareek. "Disease Prediction Tool: An Integrated Hybrid Data Mining Approach for Healthcare." *IRACST – International Journal of Computer Science and Information Technology & Security*, 6, no. 6 (2019).

[33] Z. Wang, J. W. Chung, X. Jiang, *et al.* "Machine-Learning based PRediction System for Chronic kidney Disease using Associative Classification Technique." *International Journal of Engineering and Technology*, 7, no. 4.36 (2018): 1161–1167.

[34] A. Garg, B. Sharma and R. Khan. "Heart Disease Prediction Using Machine Learning Techniques." *IOP Conference Series Material Science and Engineering*, 1022, no. 1 (2021): 1757.

[35] R. Agrawal, J. M. Chatterjee, A. Kumar, P. S. Rathore and D. N. Le (Eds.). (2020). *Machine Learning for Healthcare: Handling and Managing Data*. London/Boca Raton, FL: Chapman and Hall/CRC Press.

[36] V. Jain and J. M. Chatterjee (2020). *Machine Learning with Health Care Perspective*. Cham: Springer.

Chapter 18

Changing dynamics on the Internet of Medical Things: challenges and opportunities

Imtiaz Ali Brohi[1], Najma Imtiaz Ali[2] and Pardeep Kumar[3]

Abstract

Internet of Medical Things (IoMT) manages a large number of medical devices and these devices generate, collect, analyze, and transmit a huge amount of data over the network. The collection of medical devices, software applications, services, and healthcare system forms the IoMT healthcare system. The connectivity of sensors and devices has enabled healthcare services to modernize their clinical operations within the boundary of hospitals and from remote locations. The modernization of healthcare system has also posed new threats to security and privacy of sensitive healthcare data, and digitization, automation, new regulations, data analytics, and the development of value-based healthcare system represent some of numerous challenges and opportunities for the IoMT-based healthcare system. Thus, this chapter offers a brief introduction to the IoMT, and its impact on improving the quality of healthcare system. This chapter also provides insights into the emerging issues, i.e., security, privacy, trust, and risk due to the deployment of IoMT at large scale.

Keywords: Internet of Medical Things (IoMT); Healthcare; Security; Privacy; Trust; Risk; Challenges

18.1 Introduction

The Internet of Things (IoT) is referred to as the connectivity of various objects through Internet in order to gather, process, and analyze the data. Additionally, with the time, the number of devices connected per person is increasing, and

[1]Department of Information and Communication Technologies, The Begum Nusrat Bhutto Women University, Sukkur, Pakistan
[2]Institute of Mathematics and Computer Science, University of Sindh, Jamshoro, Pakistan
[3]Department of Software Engineering, Quaid-e-Awam University of Engineering, Science and Technology, Nawabshah, Pakistan

organizations will rely on devices connected with Internet to perform their daily activities [1]. According to Singh and Kapoor [2], the widespread usage of IoT is due to increase in embedded devices. The focus of IoT has attracted many, including researchers, practitioners, companies, and governments since few years. Industry 4.0, health 2.0, and medicine 4.0 incorporate the integration of IoT in manufacturing and consumer sector. It not only enables devices to be stronger, smarter, and effective but also covers a range of software and hardware, including wearable devices, sensors, cloud computing, information and communication technology, and actuators [3,4]. The IoT has already revolutionized many industries and has improved the lives of people in entertainment, learning, and the way they live and also IoT has made the people more proactive than reactive [1].

The mankind has always tried to find the ways to keep themselves healthy and update the status of facilities associated with healthcare system. Nowadays, hospitals are equipped with advanced technological equipment that not only help the healthcare practitioners but keep the patients' records for future as well. The integration of IoT has enabled the healthcare practitioners to monitor the health of patient with advanced methods is one of the key areas in healthcare. Moreover, people are willingly ingesting Internet-enabled devices into their bodies in order to diagnose the disease [1]. While fitness wearables have been adopted widely around the world, such devices are also used for treatments, diagnosis, and early warnings. According to Sadoughi *et al.* [4], diabetics was initial focus of IoT, later, 13 submedical fields were incorporated in order to take advantages of IoT devices, including cardiovascular, neurological, and mental diseases. Thus, the healthcare innovations have supported the healthcare industry in order to reduce the mortality rate and cost.

The healthcare addresses one of the top difficulties that each nation is confronting today. In spite of the fact that healthcare industry puts intensely in embracing most recent innovation, yet the guaranteed improvements in understanding safety and efficiency have not been acknowledged up to the norms [5–7]. While the majority of the hospitals depend on paper and written by hand records in less-developed nations to inform or make notes for future references, the data is being shared among applications and sections of the hospitals based on accessibility measures. The sharing of complex data between departments, doctors, and patients is not easily carried out. The integration of IoT and cloud in medical care might work on the sharing of data between the stakeholders that could further develop the disease monitoring, findings, and therapy in more viable and effective manner [8]. The IoT can possibly carry advantages to medical care because of the utilization of NFC/RFID labels, keen gadgets, and sensors. It empowers the online record-keeping of patients that assist doctors with the actual physical area of patient and clinical records [2,9].

According to Karunarathne *et al.* [10], in hospitals, the IoT empowers the healthcare practitioners to acquire fast access to data that can help with the finding of conditions or the progress of appropriate treatment plans. It can make patient records, test results, and suggested treatment available from the diagnostic room. It can likewise permit healthcare practitioners to talk with one another remotely about the treatment plans or usable techniques available to the stakeholders [11]. Simultaneously, the IoT upholds a shift toward more understanding focused consideration, empowering end-users to keep health-related data by themselves; to impart with healthcare suppliers, doctors, and different stakeholders; and even to get healthcare at home. However, the record-keeping and accessing does not satisfy the needs of doctors to analyze the chronic diseases. In addition, the potential data breach is another matter of concern due to vulnerability of sensitive medical data over the Internet [7].

According to report by [12], one of the key five functional elements should be part of IoT architecture such as security, privacy, ease of access, cost, performance, and agility in order to be considered as good architecture for the organization. The security and privacy have always been a challenge for any organizations and it has been addressed in healthcare industry as well due to confidentiality and sensitivity of data [13].

This chapter presents an overview of issues related with privacy and security of IoT in clinical care, consumer healthcare, and medical records. This chapter also identifies the policy and organizational level issues that will have a profound effect on the deployment of IoT.

18.2 The applications of Internet of Things

Healthcare industry have changed significantly due to information and communication technology [5]. Whereas any change in technology requires a sound ecosystem of hardware and software suppliers, buyers, consultants, implementers, and talented individuals, the challenging phase in adoption of IoT is that most of the organizations do not know the application of it [12]. According to the report by [14] by integrating IoT in ecosystem does not discontinue the existing system, but it will enhance the output of existing investments in OT, IT, and processes. IoT will reshape the economy by transforming many businesses into new digital business models by improving their efficiency in business and consumer engagement; and by 2020 there will be 20 billion devices connected with Internet performing dedicated functions such as connected cars, vending machines, jet engines, and improved human well-being system.

While we have been witnessing firms making huge investments in engaging the latest technologies to enhance efficiencies and decreasing downtime and cost, the pandemic has caused the shutdown of many enterprises and disturbance in supply chain around the world. However, the new concept of remote work environment has been practiced due to social distancing [13]. However, there is surge in adoption of IoT in social care, health, and well-being. The induction of IoT will help to improve healthcare system from episodic treatment of disease to well-being solutions and preventive care. Using IoT in healthcare has been practiced for few years in various countries, but the availability of advanced IoT devices has enabled healthcare services to provide better services and improve the way of healthcare overall ecosystem [15].

The IoT connects all physical objects that are being used such as wearables, drivable, readable/writable, even the humans are connected, addressed, and controlled remotely. This connectivity shares the data over cyberspace. Millions of intelligent devices will be connected every year, and these are components of wireless sensor network, wireless, and wearables, and it is embedded with traffic congestion, security, structural health, smart cities, waste management, logistics, emergency services, automated controls, retails, and healthcare [16].

18.3 Healthcare and Internet of Things

The application of IoT in healthcare and medicine is referred to as Internet of Medical Things (IoMT) [17]. The implementation of IoMT would bring sustainable improvements in healthcare due to the induction of new advanced devices such as biosensors architecture, microprocessors, intelligent health devices, and 5G technologies [18,19]. It is a vibrant activity that enables actions such as drugs management, tracking patients, staff surveillance, and remote medical assistance [15]. According to the report by Intel [20], by 2025, 6.2 trillion worth of IoT technology will consist of 40% of active devices under the IoT umbrella. This trend will increase day by day as most of the healthcare appliances and activities will move toward the usage of smart devices. Artificial intelligence is also being understood by the IoT-based system as it produces data intelligently that plays a role of input for the devices and translates that information into meaningful data for another. This type of system enables the healthcare practitioners to receive timely data pertaining to patients and provide remote monitoring system as well. Nowadays, a vast range of medical assistance is being provided through the usage of IoT-enabled devices such as fitness programs, medication at home, health monitoring systems and IoT-based devices such as actuators, services, sensors, and diagnostic devices in order to help the consumer and practitioner [15].

Yang *et al.* [21] fostered a nonintrusive breath checking framework for diabetic patients to consequently screen the indications of ketoacidosis. The work showed positive results in the test outcomes. The planned framework utilized C-band detecting to empower the element of 5G that is not normal in numerous nations these days. Furthermore, an S-band monitoring system based on frequency was developed for dementia patients. They used technique to monitor the patterns, i.e., random, pacing, and lapping of the patients [22]. Thus, the IoT is significant enabler of consumer health that not only provides better health services but also provides health monitoring services. The IoT initiatives would drive significant changes in the ecosystem of healthcare industry; with these changes, the duration of patient and doctor consultancy and visits are also declining. Such initiatives are helpful for stakeholders especially for consumers who remain informed and automated due to use of IoT devices such as wrist watches and other wearables [15,23].

18.4 Security in Internet of Medical Things

Availability of active devices and huge amount of data that is being produced by these devices indicate a problem that is associated with security, and keeping the confidentiality of medical records is one of the prevailing problems faced by various healthcare organizations using IoT-enabled devices in their business operations [24]. IoMT is emerging as a field and providing solutions that reduce cost and operational process at maximum level; along with the IoT solutions, it highlights prevailing security concerns such as confidentiality, integrity, and availability of data [25]. According to Marr [26], while its biggest application is the implementation of doctors' recommendations with the large-scale data acquisition for better diagnoses and treatment plans in order to reduce the waste and inefficiencies in healthcare system, IoT is being used within the healthcare to help inventory management, workflow optimization, and medical device integration. The expansion of IoT becomes one of the integral part of our every daily lives, which becomes one of the important components of national infrastructure, and its security is one of the top priorities, while, in recent years, most of the attacks were on healthcare industry. In addition, medical data is of more concern due to a potential threat of identity theft and fraud [27]. According to a survey conducted by Irdeto *et al.*, it was reported that only 13% of IoMT leaders of the USA are sure that their organizations are protected against cybersecurity attacks, while 88% of the companies are not prepared enough. Furthermore,

> This is concerning when considering that 80% of our survey participants report having suffered at least one cyberattack in the past five years, and it is all but certain that they face at least dozens of additional threats on a daily basis. The breadth of attacks targeting IoMT companies is also problematic. Our survey revealed that organizations have fallen victim to several attack techniques, including ransomware, malware, phishing, spoofing and DDoS, with customer databases, employee information and even R&D platforms being exploited [28].

The increase in connected devices in healthcare is putting more pressure to improve their cybersecurity methods, which is a challenge nowadays [29]. Many of the organizations are facing cyberattacks and concerned about the future of IoT devices. Irdeto [30] reported that 83% of the organization are concerned about IoT devices, including 82% organizations involved in producing IoT devices that are unsure about the security of devices. About 99% agree that security should be of top priority due to the sensitivity of the data. Additionally, there is a lack of IoT security standards; hence additional efforts are required to regulate security standards in the IoMT. The nature of healthcare services requires extra security measure due to sensitivity of medical data [31].

18.5 Privacy in Internet of Medical Things

The type of devices used in IoMT is typically attached with human body and collects and disseminates confidential and sensitive data. The data processed by IoMT-enabled devices helps in monitoring the health condition of humans and guides to take time-driven decisions [32]. According to Seničar *et al.* [33],

> A person has privacy when two factors are in place; first an ability to control information about oneself, and second, be able to exercise that control consistent with oneself values.

The sharing of sensitive data over Internet requires serious concerns in terms of privacy and security of IoMT-based healthcare infrastructure. The outcome of inadequate security and privacy mechanism could lead to compromising highly confidential data of patients and delay in detection of life-threating diseases due to hindrance in normal operations. The transaction of data over IoT network involves multiple devices at the same time that are administrated and owned by various stakeholders [10,34,35]. This makes it difficult for the ownership of data in the case of data leakage due to cyberattack and also it is a reasonably difficult situation in order to identify the source of data breach. This makes IoT sensors less reliable due to the involvement of multiple stakeholders in the system and the measures should be taken in terms of integrity of devices by securing it from external interventions [36]. According to a survey conducted by IBM report [37], with rapid digital transformation of companies during the pandemic and consumers, careless approach toward privacy and security might open a new window for the attackers to propagate data theft and ransomware cyberattacks. They reported that 51% of respondents would prefer to use insecure application or website that leads to more security and privacy concerns. During pandemic, 63% of respondents engaged in healthcare services were found using mobile, email, web, and text messages, as telemedicine was pushed further by healthcare required to redesign the security protocols in order to protect sensitive patients' data and IT systems. The privacy concerns are major drawbacks of IoMT-enabled devices. Within IoMT systems, various types of attacks are possible due to unauthorized tracking of devices, and misuse of personal information without individuals' consent is main threat nowadays for the humans in healthcare system due to the availability of data at large scale and involvement of multiple organizations [8,29]. Quantity of information is variable in different IoMT systems, and sensitivity of information could be different in terms of context to context and person to person. However, the researchers have identified the existence of privacy concerns in IoMT, designing effective and long-term solutions to address these concerns remain challenging [28,38].

The main threat in healthcare is the use of someone information without the owner's knowledge or consent. While the technology has improved the functions, capabilities, and features of medical record systems, it increases the number of stakeholders who might have unauthorized access to records such as insurance companies, pharmaceutical companies, marketing agencies, and employers. This type of ecosystem is the main source of concern for health information privacy. Whereas long-distance care and mobility of devices pose a serious threat in terms of security and privacy of the information that require vigilance [36], IoMT devices manages a large amount of healthcare data, including patient's financial data, patient tracking system, and clinical results. While healthcare organizations are abided by certain policies and procedures to ensure the privacy of consumer, within digital healthcare system, these features are not enough. Additionally, the main barrier to adoption of IoMT is outpacing of healthcare systems and regulations [39]. The application of IoMT linked with clinical databases and electronic medical records is growing concern regarding the security and privacy of individuals' health and financial information. Many countries like China, Canada, the United Kingdom, the USA, and Australia are taking IoT-based healthcare system seriously and investing huge amount in order to make improved healthcare services. This requires more flexible method for users to specify their personal information concerns rather than simply accepting or rejecting certain policies stated by the healthcare service provider as it only requires a single point of entry to attack all devices connected to centralized network, including wearable and implanted medical devices. Five million IoMT- and IoT-based unmanaged devices were in use by healthcare, retail, manufacturing, and life sciences between 2019 and 2020 that is a real world risk which requires a comprehensive approach in order to secure all these devices [40].

18.6 Perception of trust and risk in IoMT

The perception of human risk is reliant on trust. Whether it is trust in an organization, technology, and person to keep the shared information secure, organization- and technology-based trust is one of the concepts associated with attitudes and performance. The trust and privacy interplay in respect of technology and services. Jaigirdar *et al.* [41] state that the success of healthcare devices strongly depends on transmission of data through secure medium. Within healthcare environment, trust depends on device, communication channel, and acquired/delivered data. According to Lin and Dong [42], the trustworthiness of data is highly important in medical decisions as the reliability of data and source of the information related with the patient is an important factor for healthcare experts and technology experts; when the source of information is not trustworthy, it will lead to an unwanted situation. The ubiquity of IoMT devices and risk of personal data loss or misuse demand for a protection of personal data in the context of patients. Moreover, within the healthcare system, it is necessary that a patient should be well aware of by whom, how, and type of data shall be used for treatment [5,43]. In real-life scenarios, patients do not have a choice but to share their personal information that leads to put the personal information in danger of being exposed to third-party entities. IoMT devices are connected to cloud-based app that might be at the risk of being exposed to malware and other cyberattacks. Healthcare organizations are vulnerable and are responsible for protecting critical assets of patients, including health records and personal information that is connected to devices. In order to increase end-user trust and remove the risk factor, service providers should ensure that the application, cloud services, and platform should be based on shared responsibility mechanism for cybersecurity resilience and performance. Healthcare systems security is challenging and unique because of its reliance on different and shared technology platforms and outcome of it is related with possible errors and susceptibilities. Accordingly, there is major need of collaboration to form a common framework with regards to risk management and security governance between departments, partners, and functions across the stakeholders to mitigate the risk and improving human trust on IoT-based healthcare systems [44].

18.7 Conclusion and future scope

People always try to find ways to improve its resources on earth in order to make their lives better and better.

According to Evans [1],

> People desire to live healthy, fulfilling, and comfortable lives for themselves, their families, and those they care about. By combining the ability of the next evolution of the Internet (IoT) to sense, collect, transmit, analyze, and distribute data on a massive scale with the way people process information, humanity will have the knowledge and wisdom it needs not only to survive, but to thrive in the coming months, years, decades, and centuries

The advances in devices opened a way for lower healthcare cost and drive better outcomes in healthcare industry. The IoMT devices are capable of collecting, analyzing, and transmitting data for patients and doctors in order to track and prevent chronic illness and its capability to transform the healthcare system is unignorable. The large amount of data generated by medical devices and sensors over the web manages clinical workflow and guiding to overall improvement in healthcare system within the hospitals and in remote locations. The accurate diagnoses, lower costs, and fewer errors are benefits of IoMT devices and the real-time data sharing between patient and doctors makes it more suitable to surveil diseases, prevent, and track chronic illness as well. Protecting and assuring patients from cyber threats represents an ever evolving challenge and the future work might consider the disparity in the quality of the data and what data types, sources, and network security initiatives can ensure security and privacy of patients' data handled by unmanaged smart devices and sensors.

References

[1] Evans, D. (2011). The Internet of Things How the Next Evolution of the Internet Is Changing Everything. *Cisco Internet Business Solutions Group (IBSG)*. Retrieved from http://cisco.com/web/about/ac79/docs/innov/IoT_IBSG_0411FINAL.pdf. Accessed 5 September 2021.

[2] Singh, K. J., and Kapoor, D. S. (2017). Create Your Own Internet of Things: A Survey of IoT Platforms. *IEEE Consumer Electronics Magazine*, 6, 57–68.

[3] Bhatia, M., and Sood, S. K. (2017). A Comprehensive Health Assessment Framework to Facilitate IoT-Assisted Smart Workouts: A Predictive Healthcare Perspective. *Computers in Industry*, 92–93, 50–66.

[4] Sadoughi, F., Behmanesh, A., and Sayfouri, N. (2020). Internet of Things in Medicine: A Systematic Mapping Study. *Journal of Biomedical Informatics*, 103, 103383.

[5] Garale, R. B. (2019). Internet of Things in Healthcare. *International Journal for Research in Applied Science and Engineering Technology*, 7(6), 1549–1554.

[6] Panchatcharam, P., and Vivekanandan, S. (2019). Internet of Things (IoT) in Healthcare – Smart Health and Surveillance, Architectures, Security Analysis and Data Transfer: A Review. *International Journal of Software Innovation*, 7(2), 21–40.

[7] Tawalbeh, L., Muheidat, F., Tawalbeh, M., and Quwaider, M. (2020). IoT Privacy and Security: Challenges and Solutions. *Applied Sciences*, 10, 4102.

[8] Insider Intelligence. (2020). Security and Privacy Issues in the Internet of Things Ecosystem – Business Insider. Retrieved from https://businessinsider.com/iot-security-privacy. Accessed 5 September 2021.

[9] Elhoseny, M., Ramírez-González, G., Abu-Elnasr, O. M., Shawkat, S. A., Arunkumar, N., and Farouk, A. (2018). Secure Medical Data Transmission Model for IoT-Based Healthcare Systems. *IEEE Access*, 6, 20596–20608.

[10] Karunarathne, S. M., Saxena, N., and Khan, M. K. (2021). Security and Privacy in IoT Smart Healthcare. *IEEE Internet Computing*, 25(4), 37–48.

[11] Joyia, G. J., Liaqat, R. M., Farooq, A., and Rehman, S. (2017). Internet of Medical Things (IOMT): Applications, Benefits and Future Challenges in Healthcare Domain. *Journal of Communications*, 12(4), 240–247.

[12] Hung, M. (2017). *Leading the IoT – Gartner Insights on How to Lead in a Connected World*. Gartner, Inc, Stamford, CT, 1–29.

[13] Wilkinson, J. S., and Pletcher, I. D. (2016). Internet of Things (IoT). *Communication Technology Update and Fundamentals*, 15th edn, Routledge, Taylor & Francis, Milton Park, eBook ISBN 9781315537245, 157–168.

[14] Schneider-Electric. (2016). IoT 2020 Business Report, 1–20. Retrieved from http://2.schneider-electric.com/documents/presentation/en/local/2016/04/998-19699217_IoT_Report_2016_v2.pdf. Accessed 8 September 2021.

[15] Bhuiyan, M. N., Rahman, M. M., Billah, M. M., and Saha, D. (2021). Internet of Things (IoT): A Review of Its Enabling Technologies in Healthcare Applications, Standards Protocols, Security, and Market Opportunities. *IEEE Internet of Things Journal*, 8(13), 10474–10498.

[16] Höller, J., Tsiatsis, V., Mulligan, C., Karnouskos, S., Avesand, S., and Boyle, D. (2014). *From Machine-to-Machine to the Internet of Things: Introduction to a New Age of Intelligence*. Academic Press, Elsevier Ltd, New York, ISBN 978-0-12-407684-6.

[17] Dhanvijay, M. M., and Patil, S. C. (2019). Internet of Things: A Survey of Enabling Technologies in Healthcare and Its Applications. *Computer Networks*, 153, 113–131.

[18] Li, X., Dai, H. N., Wang, Q., Imran, M., Li, D., and Imran, M. A. (2020). Securing Internet of Medical Things with Friendly-Jamming Schemes. *Computer Communications*, 160, 431–442.

[19] Nazir, S., Ali, Y., Ullah, N., and García-Magariño, I. (2019). Internet of Things for Healthcare Using Effects of Mobile Computing: A Systematic Literature Review. *Wireless Communications and Mobile Computing*, 2019.

[20] Intel. (2018). A Guide to the Internet of Things Infographic. Retrieved from https://intel.co.uk/content/www/uk/en/internet-of-things/infographics/guide-to-iot-new.html. Accessed 8 September 2021.

[21] Yang, X, Fan, D., Ren, A., Zhao, N., and Alam, M. (2019). 5G-Based User-Centric Sensing at C-Band. *IEEE Transactions on Industrial Informatics*, 15, 3040–3047.

[22] Yang, X., Shah, S. A., Ren, A., *et al.* (2018). Wandering Pattern Sensing at S-Band. *IEEE Journal of Biomedical and Health Informatics*, 22(6), 1863–1870.

[23] Hassan, R., Qamar, F., Hasan, M. K., Aman, A. H. M., and Ahmed, A. S. (2020). Internet of Things and Its Applications: A Comprehensive Survey. *Symmetry*, 12(10), 1–29.

[24] Alsubaei, F., Abuhussein, A., and Shiva, S. (2017). Security and Privacy in the Internet of Medical Things: Taxonomy and Risk Assessment. *Proceedings – 2017 IEEE 42nd Conference on Local Computer Networks Workshops, LCN Workshops 2017* (September 2018), 112–120.

[25] Jing, Q., Vasilakos, A. V., Wan, J., Lu, J., and Qiu, D. (2014). Security of the Internet of Things: Perspectives and Challenges. *Wireless Networks*, 20(8), 2481–2501.

[26] Marr, B. (2018). Why The Internet Of Medical Things (IoMT) Will Start To Transform Healthcare in 2018. Retrieved from https://forbes.com/sites/bernardmarr/2018/01/25/why-the-internet-of-medical-things-iomt-will-start-to-transform-healthcare-in-2018/?sh=47f36e6b4a3c. Accessed 8 September 2021.

[27] Maple, C. (2017). Security and Privacy in the Internet of Things. *Journal of Cyber Policy*, 2(2), 155–184.

[28] MedTech Intelligence. (2021). More Cyberattacks in Healthcare, Yet Most MedTech Leaders Unprepared, Says Survey. Retrieved from https://medtechintelligence.com/news_article/more-cyberattacks-in-healthcare-yet-most-medtech-leaders-unprepared-says-survey/. Accessed 15 September 2021.

[29] Fontanazza, M. (2021). IoMT, Connected Devices Introduce More Cyber Threats into MedTech and Healthcare Organizations. Retrieved from https://medtechintelligence.com/news_article/iomt-connected-devices-introduce-more-cyber-threats-into-medtech-and-healthcare-organizations/. Accessed 15 September 2021.

[30] Irdeto. (2019). IoT Cyberattacks Are the Norm, The Security Mindset Isn't. Irdeto Global Connected Industries Cybersecurity Survey. Retrieved from https://go.irdeto.com/connected-industries-cybersecurity-survey-report/.

[31] Alsubaei, F., Abuhussein, A., and Shiva, S. (2019). *A Framework for Ranking IoMT Solutions Based on Measuring Security and Privacy*. Springer Nature Switzerland.

[32] Seliem, M., and Elgazzar, K. (2019). BIoMT: Blockchain for the Internet of Medical Things. *2019 IEEE International Black Sea Conference on Communications and Networking, BlackSeaCom 2019* (3–6 June 2019).

[33] Seničar, V., Jerman-Blažič, B., and Klobučar, T. (2003). Privacy-Enhancing Technologies—Approaches and Development. *Computer Standards & Interfaces*, 25, 147–158.

[34] Ibrahim, H., Liu, X., Zariffa, N., Morris, A. D., and Denniston, A. K. (2021). Health Data Poverty: An Assailable Barrier to Equitable Digital Health Care. *The Lancet Digital Health*, 3(4), e260–e265.

[35] Steger, A. (2020). What Makes IoMT Devices So Difficult to Secure Against Cyberthreats. Retrieved from https://healthtechmagazine.net/article/2020/02/what-makes-iomt-devices-so-difficult-secure-perfcon.

[36] De Meijer, C. R. W. (2021). Blockchain, IoT and 5G: A Marriage a Trois. Retrieved from https://finextra.com/blogposting/20361/blockchain-iot-and-5g-a-marriage-a-trois.

[37] IBM. (2021). Pandemic-Induced Digital Reliance Creates Lingering Security Side Effects. Retrieved from https://newsroom.ibm.com/2021-06-15-IBM-Survey-Pandemic-Induced-Digital-Reliance-Creates-Lingering-Security-Side-Effects.

[38] Sheikh, A., Anderson, M., Albala, S., *et al.* (2021). Health Information Technology and Digital Innovation for National Learning Health and Care Systems. *The Lancet Digital Health*, 3(6), e383–e396.

[39] Taylor, K., Sanghera, A., Steedman, M., and Thaxter, M. (2018). *Medtech and the Internet of Medical Things: How Connected Medical Devices are Transforming Health Care. Deloitte LLP's Life Sciences and Health Care*, Deloitte Centre for Health Solutions, New York, 1–56.

[40] Security, H. N. (2020). Threat Highlight: Analysis of 5+ Million Unmanaged, IoT, and IoMT Devices. Retrieved from https://helpnetsecurity.com/2020/07/24/analysis-of-5-million-unmanaged-iot-and-iomt-devices/.

[41] Jaigirdar, F. T., Rudolph, C., and Bain, C. (2019). *Can I Trust the Data I See?: A Physician's Concern on Medical Data in IoT Health Architectures. In Proceedings of the Australasian Computer Science Week Multi Conference*, Association for Computing Machinery, New York, 1–10.

[42] Lin, Z., and Dong, L. (2018). Clarifying Trust in Social Internet of Things. *IEEE Transactions on Knowledge and Data Engineering*, 30(2), 234–248.

[43] Ng, R. (2019). Privacy and Efficacy of Electronic Health Records (EHRs): A Triangulation Study in Ontario, Canada. Retrieved from https://www.research.manchester.ac.uk/portal/en/theses/privacy-and-efficacy-of-electronic-health-records-ehrs-a-triangulation-study-in-ontario-canada(8fead483-5edf-420e-8f80-6de2564682d0).html.

[44] Musumeci, B. (2020). Medical Devices Are Vital, but Vulnerable. Expert Insights. Armonk, NY: IBM Corporation. Retrieved from https://www.ibm.com/downloads/cas/EQVODWLY.

Chapter 19

Internet of Drones (IOD) in medical transport application

G. Prasad[1], J. Kavya[2] and J. Sahana[3]

Abstract

Internet of Unmanned Aerial Vehicle (IOU) plays an important role in the delivery of emergency medicine to remote locations. Furthermore, it is employed for blood transfer, disaster assistance, missing persons discovering lost hikers in the hill station, and a variety of other emergency services. The use of drones for emergency response services, particularly in medical circumstances, offers up new avenues for life-saving interventions. Using drones to give "eyes" on a risky scenario or to transport medical supplies to stranded patients may increase the capacity of emergency response to physicians to provide care in dangerous conditions. IOU provides several emergency response services that have an influence on daily life. The Federal Aviation Administration conducts completely autonomous missions beyond visual range and flights above people to provide critical medical supplies.

Keywords: Medical product; Transport; Blood; Emergency

19.1 Introduction to unmanned aerial vehicle

The aviation sector has undergone a paradigm shift as a result of rapid technological improvement. Unmanned aerial systems have been an important factor in this. Advancements in unmanned aerial vehicle (UAV) technology have led to benefits in numerous areas, including military operations, civil purposes, agriculture, and research and development. Operators, manufacturers, and businesses are increasingly focusing on UAVs around the world. Without human pilots, UAVs are airplanes. UAVs have been very popular over the last few of years, particularly for use in research and development. The distance and the flight time (endurance) are considered (range). For UAVs, payload and battery power are the most important

[1]Aerospace Engineering, Dayananda Sagar University, Bangalore, India
[2]Biotechnology, ICAR-Sugarcane Breeding Institute, ICAR, Coimbatore, India
[3]Aerospace Engineering, Delft University of Technology, Delft, The Netherlands

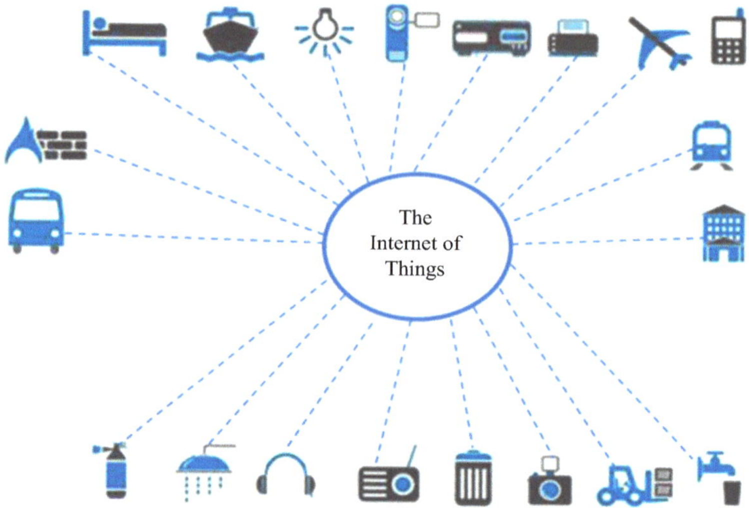

Figure 19.1 Internet of Things

restrictions on an aircraft. To predict UAVs' operational abilities, you have to do real-time experiments. Therefore, the necessary range and endurance for a UAV to accomplish missions may be calculated.

Smaller aircraft, such as UAVs, are now being developed for a variety of uses. The key benefit is that, in comparison to large planes, the cost and training requirements are far lower. These UAVs can also be operated manually or programmed to fly on their own. Depending on the model, the UAV's functional capacity varies significantly.

Figure 19.1 shows the overview of Internet of Things (IoT). Advanced countries are in the initial stages of using drone technology for healthcare. There is a lot of study work that is theoretical and studies the application of drone technology in healthcare systems in Western countries. This piece is geared toward tracking how drone technology is now being applied in the healthcare and other wellness sectors of industry in developed countries [1–3]. The goal of the essay is to outline how UAV are being used in advanced nations for healthcare purposes, synthesize the knowledge base currently being formed from published documents, and identify areas of the existing knowledge base that need more investigation. In this research, we will discuss the prevalence of drone use in healthcare in the industrialized world and provide guidance for the next stage of research.

19.2 Internet of Things in Industry 5.0

Industry 5.0 technologies appear to be suitable for dealing with emergency medical issues. This new industrial revolution will be able to meet the tailored needs of high-quality medical components in order to perform precise and sophisticated treatments.

The fifth industrial revolution has been named Industry 5.0. It is made up of unique technologies that can be used to streamline the manufacturing and healthcare industries by adding wireless connectivity. Machines and humans will be more effective in their collaboration in the face of new technologies that are part of Industry 5.0. It advanced complex systems to help make sustainable, effective, and secure merchandise and services. The concept of Industry 5.0 is gathering traction, thanks to modern innovation, like smart and creative solutions [4,5].

The Internet of Just about everything extends IoT by broadening the idea IoT. In comparison to the device-to-device view, it has a more intricate framework that includes humans and processes. Should the outbreak ever occur, there is a chance that we shall be able to use the invention to deliver healthcare and conduct daily duties (all the while keeping to the principle of social isolation). Medical computer-based systems are assisting in the administration of devices by supporting a collection of devices and software in order to increase patient comfort and simplify operations. Managing multiple ventilators with only a few doctors at COVID-19 pandemic might have been simpler with this strategy.

Artificial intelligence can be used to track the virus's propagation and help isolate patients who are most at danger. Even with prior patient data, determining the risk of death is challenging [6–9]. Unmanned flying devices, commonly referred to as drones, can be utilized for various range of tasks, ranging from monitoring to enforce social separation rules to delivering supplies to afflicted areas.

Figure 19.2 illustrates the Internet of Drones (IOD). All equipment and medical gadgets utilized in human healthcare can now be connected thanks to Industry 5.0 technologies. It is feasible to improve machine-to-machine communication, which aids in the treatment process' efficiency. Robots have been assigned to reduce the workload of healthcare staff, improve their safety, and reduce the danger of infection.

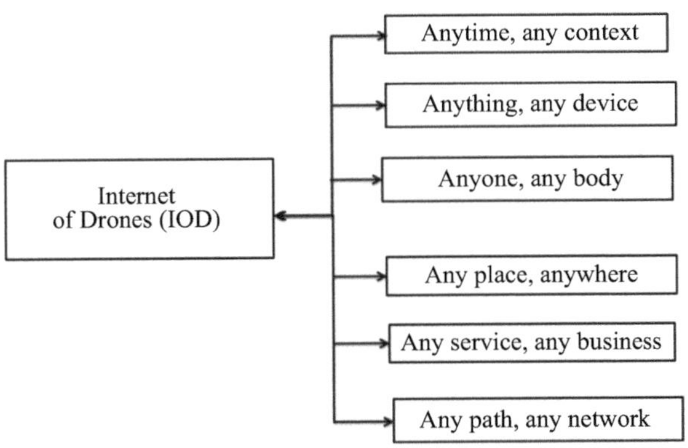

Figure 19.2 Internet of Drones

19.3 Applications in medical transport

Several healthcare industries were investigated, including emergency responders, telemedicine services, and people delivering medical supplies. Patients and the general public were not considered at all while considering what drone technology should be used in the healthcare system. This is because doctors, administrators, and politicians had their own priorities. There are some really big questions being raised right now about who is creating and who is buying drone health applications, and what those people hope to achieve. Only two of the papers were authored by someone in the health sector. Just under a third of the author organizations endorsed working with target communities. Fewer of those who actually get out of their chairs follow on through their calls for this kind of participation. Some may be utilizing the healthcare context to promote surveillance drones and markets, and it appears that they are not very concerned with creating drones to meet a certain health need. This can be an issue when healthcare practitioners who are well informed about the needs of their patients and their facilities—such as frontline employees, users, and administrators—do not have opportunities to gain expertise and autonomy in their respective fields [10–13]. Having interactions with a broader variety of individuals may lead to a greater variety of healthcare drone applications, which would involve considering several kinds of digital literacy and health information.

Figure 19.3 shows the UAV in medical applications. Global Medical Corporation is constantly working to develop and apply new technologies in order to increase efficiency and productivity. Smart machinery and modern technology such as the IoT is referred to as Industry 5.0. Industry 5.0 technologies appear to be suitable for dealing with emergency healing issues. It will be able to meet the tailored needs of high-quality medical components in order to perform precise and sophisticated treatments.

In pandemic situations, telemedicine can assist transform the healthcare system by allowing individuals to seek medical advice while preserving physical distance. Furthermore, after remote patient screening [14–18], it has become really popular to use 3D printing technology to make medical equipment. Modern manufacturing technology can create crucial medical equipment, such as masks, face shields,

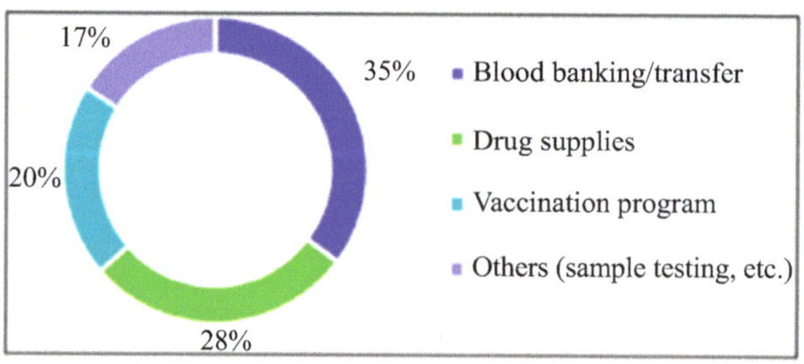

Figure 19.3 UAV in medical applications

respiratory protection, and other similar items swiftly. This new healthcare paradigm has a high chance of succeeding in serving the specific healthcare needs of people affected by the COVID-19 pandemic. With Industry 5.0 technologies in place, a new digital working platform is being built.

19.4 Methodology and approach

Each flight controller has its own set of codes that are maintained by software known as Flight Control Software or Flight Controller Configurator. There is a wide range of flight controller software available. Each one is usually focused on a certain piece of hardware, technology, or goal. A list of the best three flight controller firmware and software options is available, along with some thoughts on each. This will allow you to have a solid idea of what is available so you can decide which you want to use or participate in. Flight controller configurators are utilized in professional drones for industrial applications rather than racing and freestyle software:

- ArduPilot
- PX4 FlightStack
- iNAV

A large-scale technical contribution involves the layers that are implemented with necessary features, and the procedure suites and interfaces are designed. The flaws and redundancies found in the design as it is applied can be taken the advantage of when revisiting the architecture later. Nonprogramming questions arise, like those about routing and delays control, that need to be addressed in order to apply an IOD system. The next projects will feature a main emphasis on this area. A huge undertaking, the IOD involves the collaboration of the entire research community. The design, which is shown in its current state, can be used to begin a dialog with the research community about what protocols will be used to verify the IOD's simulation and physical models. Additionally, the research for IOD can draw from knowledge and research about air traffic control, cellular, and Internet networks and apply that knowledge to IOD.

Figure 19.4 depicts the Skelton of IOD. UAV, sometimes known as quadcopters, are developing as a new medical tool that can assist alleviate logistical issues and improve healthcare distribution. Drones might be used for everything from disaster assistance to transferring transplant organs and blood samples, according to experts. Drones are capable of carrying small payloads and delivering them rapidly to their target [19–21]. Hazardous materials must be delivered safely and in accordance with specialized hazardous materials. Drones can improve access to life-saving pharmaceuticals and vaccines, as well as the speed with which they are delivered. Organ delivery can be made faster, safer, and more cost-effective with the use of drones. Drones can also be used to transport small medical items such as automated external defibrillators (AEDs). Some firms have wondered if our drone can transport AEDs or other minor medical devices from the hospital or emergency medical services to an accident or catastrophe site. The answer is

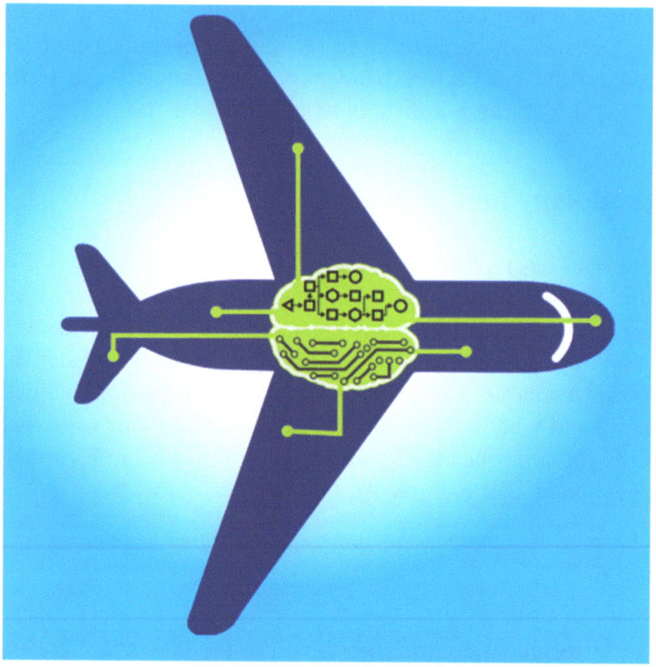

Figure 19.4 The Skelton of IOD

"yes"; unfortunately, aviation officials will not let this at this moment, but it will undoubtedly happen in the future [22,23].

Drone technology has several advantages over conventional modes of transportation, including avoiding traffic in congested locations, avoiding worst road, and safely reaching the destination. Despite the fact that drones are still underutilized in emergency situations and relief efforts, their contributions are becoming more widely recognized.

As demonstrated in Figure 19.5, the TU Delft Ambulance UAVs prototype features a two-way connection radio with video, as well as a cardiac defibrillator. If someone were to have a heart attack, the drone would come to help the patient, and the person's friends and family would be shown how to perform CPR and use an automated defibrillator until the ambulance could arrive.

19.5 Conclusion and future

Drones have many advantages, such as faster help for the injured, shortening the journey time, and fewer complications for patients during floods. Information systems and smart manufacturing are sometimes known as Industry 5.0. In healthcare, the system has significant advantages. It helps to considerably enhance medical gadgets and instruments, which, in turn, makes it possible to improve treatment performance.

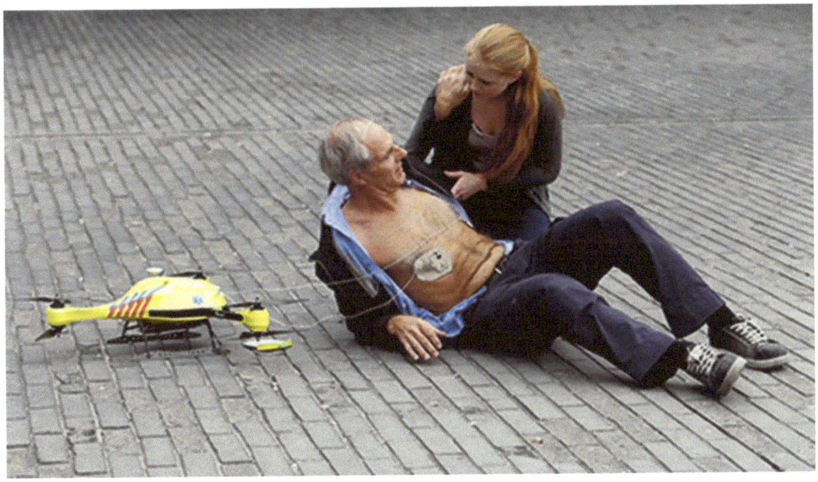

Figure 19.5 TU Delft Ambulance drone

Nevertheless, you should familiarize yourself with the present rules. There are different efforts to increase drone safety, but no rules can protect us from threats posed by the presence of a drone where it was not supposed to be. A global concern for aviation safety has emerged because an unmanned aircraft has flown in regulated airspace. Disrupting an international airport's approach with a drone and getting too close to a passenger plane while filming are two possible scenarios.

This study has discovered many types of healthcare and medical drone use in many industrialized countries; however, further study is required to determine the impact these drones would have on health services. More studies should be conducted to examine how including people in medical device development affects technological and health literacy in patients, healthcare providers, and cultural groups. To increase understanding and support from agricultural, remote, and native groups and gain their approval of outside interventions, ensure that end-user groups are involved in their development and execution, which in turn lets drone developers design technologies that fit their target population's needs. For a more comprehensive assessment of how employing drone technology impacts a whole community, researchers should better study the monetary, human, and quality of healthcare costs that arise from integrating diverse quadcopter applications into existing medical services. Knowing what kind of drones work best for their communities will help the healthcare policymakers, and outcome provide the healthcare and health-related solutions their communities require.

Acknowledgment

We acknowledge all the staff members of Aerospace Engineering, Dayananda Sagar University, Bangalore, India for the constant support and encouragement to carry out the research. I also thank Dr. K.N.B. Murthy (Vice Chancellor), Dr. A. Srinivas (Dean), Dr. BVN Ramakumar (Head of the Department), Dayananda Sagar University, Bangalore, India. I also thank Scientists of ICAR-Sugarcane Breeding Institute, Coimbatore, for the encouragement to the research work. This research received fund from The Institution of Engineers (India) Ref. No. R.4/2/UG/2017-18/RDUG2017026 and Tamilnadu State Council for Science and Technology Ref. No. TNSCST/DIT/03/VR/2017-2018.

References

[1] A. Claesson, L. Svensson, P. Nordberg *et al.*, "Drones may be used to save lives in out of hospital cardiac arrest due to drowning," *Resuscitation*, vol. 114, pp. 152–156, 2017.

[2] M. Balasingam, "Drones in medicine—the rise of the machines," *International Journal of Clinical Practice*, vol. 71, no. 9, Article ID e12989, 2017.

[3] European Commission, Communication from the Commission to the European Parliament and the Council. A New Era for Aviation, European Commission, Brussels, Belgium, 2014.

[4] P. Van de Voorde, S. Gautama, A. Momont, C. M. Ionescu, P. De Paepe, and N. Fraeyman, "The drone ambulance [A-UAS]: golden bullet or just a blank?," *Resuscitation*, vol. 116, pp. 46–48, 2017.

[5] T. Amukele, P. M. Ness, A. A. Tobian, J. Boyd, and J. Street, "Drone transportation of blood products," *Transfusion*, vol. 57, no. 3, pp. 582–588, 2017.

[6] G. Van Berlaer, T. Staes, D. Danschutter *et al.*, "Disaster preparedness and response improvement: comparison of the 2010 Haiti earthquake-related diagnoses with baseline medical data," *European Journal of Emergency Medicine*, vol. 24, no. 5, pp. 382–388, 2017.

[7] M. Mulero-Pázmány, S. Jenni-Eiermann, N. Strebel, T. Sattler, J. J. Negro, and Z. Tablado, "Unmanned aircraft systems as a new source of disturbance for wildlife: a systematic review," *PLoS One*, vol. 12, no. 6, Article ID e0178448, 2017.

[8] J. B. Rosser Jr., B. C. Parker, and V. Vignesh, "Medical applications of drones for disaster relief: a review of the literature," *Surgical Technology International*, vol. 33, pp. 17–22, 2018.

[9] J. Braun, S. D. Gertz, A. Furer *et al.*, "The promising future of drones in prehospital medical care and its application to battlefield medicine," *Journal of Trauma and Acute Care Surgery*, vol. 87, no. 1S, Suppl 1, pp. S28–S34, 2019.

[10] M. Bogle, W. D. Rosamond, K. T. Snyder, and J. K. Zègre-Hemsey, "The case for drone-assisted emergency response to cardiac arrest: an optimized statewide deployment approach," *North Carolina Medical Journal*, vol. 80, no. 4, pp. 204–212, 2019.

[11] Unmanned Aircraft Systems (UAS). (n.d.). ICAO. Retrieved from https://www.icao.int/meetings/uas/documents/circular%20328_en.pdf. Accessed October 10, 2021.

[12] N. Smolyanskiy, A. Kamenev, J. Smith, and S. Birchfield, "Toward low-flying autonomous MAV trail navigation using deep neural networks for environmental awareness," in *Proceedings of the 2017 IEEE/RSJ International Conference on Intelligent Robots and Systems (IROS)*, IEEE, Vancouver, Canada, September 2017.

[13] A. Loquercio, I. Maqueda, C. R. del-Blanco, and D. Scaramuzza, "DroNet: learning to fly by driving," *IEEE Robotics and Automation Letters*, vol. 3, no. 2, pp. 1088–1095, 2018.

[14] D. Palossi, A. Loquercio, F. Conti *et al.*, "Ultra low power deep-learning-powered autonomous nano drones," in *Proceedings of the IEEE/RSJ International Conference on Intelligent Robots and Systems (IROS 2018)*, ETH Zurich, Madrid, Spain, October 2018.

[15] N. Passalis and A. Tefas, "Continuous drone control using deep reinforcement learning for frontal view person shooting," *Neural Computing and Applications*, vol. 32, pp. 4227–4238, 2019.

[16] T. K. Amukele, J. Hernandez, C. L. H. Snozek *et al.*, "Drone transport of chemistry and hematology samples over long distances," *American Journal of Clinical Pathology*, vol. 148, no. 5, pp. 427–435, 2017.

[17] W. Glauser, "Blood-delivering drones saving lives in Africa and maybe soon in Canada," *Canadian Medical Association Journal*, vol. 190, no. 3, pp. E88–E89, 2018.

[18] M. Robakowska, D. Ślęzak, A. Tyrańska-Fobke *et al.*, "Operational and financial considerations of using drones for medical support of mass events in Poland," *Disaster Medicine and Public Health Preparedness*, vol. 13, no. 3, pp. 527–532, 2019.

[19] C. A. Thiels, J. M. Aho, S. P. Zietlow, and D. H. Jenkins, "Use of unmanned aerial vehicles for medical product transport," *Air Medical Journal*, vol. 34, pp. 104–108, 2015.

[20] G. Prasad, P. Abhishek, and R. Karthick, "Influence of unmanned aerial vehicle in medical product transport," *International Journal of Intelligent Unmanned Systems*, vol. 7, no. 2, pp. 88–94, 2019.

[21] G. Prasad, "Performance estimation of twin propeller in unmanned aerial vehicle," *INCAS Bulletin*, vol. 12, no. 2, pp. 143–149, 2020.

[22] G. Prasad, V. Vijayaganth, G. Sivaraj, *et al.*, "*Positioning of UAV using Algorithm for monitoring the forest region*," IEEE Xplore Digital Library, IEEE Conference JCT Coimbatore, pp. 1361–1363, 2018.

[23] K. Naveen Kumar, G. Prasad, K. Rajasekar, P. Vadivelu, S. Gollakota, and S. K. Kavinprabhu, "A study on the forest fire detection using unmanned aerial vehicles," *International Journal of Mechanical and Production Engineering Research and Development (IJMPERD)*, vol. 8, no. 7, pp. 165–171, 2018.

Chapter 20

Blockchain-based Internet of Things (IoT) for healthcare systems: COVID-19 perspective

Anand Sharma[1], *S.R. Biradar*[2], *H.K.D. Sarma*[3] *and N.P. Rana*[4]

Abstract

Blockchain in the Internet of Things (IoT) is a novel development that exhibits with decentralized, scattered, public, dispersed, and continuous record to exchange with IoT centers and hubs. Blockchain is a movement of blocks; each and every block is connected with its previous block. Each block is having the cryptographic hash-code, its data and previous block hash. The transactions in blockchain are the basic units that are being used to propagate data between IoT centers and hubs. The IoT nodes or hub are unambiguous kind of physical yet intelligent devices with implanted sensors, actuators, projects and developed to transact with other IoT nodes or hubs. The key job of blockchain in IoT is to give a method to process ensured about records of data through IoT node points. Blockchain is ensured about advancement that can be used unreservedly, publically and straightforwardly. IoT requires such an advancement to allow secure correspondence among IoT nodes and hubs in heterogeneous condition. The transactions in blockchain could be finished and examined any person who is affirmed to bestow inside the IoT. The blockchain in IoT may help with improving the correspondence security.

It is ordinary that blockchain will change the IoT. The determination of rules is fundamental to the joining of blockchain and the IoT as a segment of government establishments and in healthcare systems. Healthcare system is described as that is prepared for enabling the correspondence between healthcare substances such as specialists, doctors, chaperons, patients, nurse, meds, labs, suppliers and healthcare specialists. Healthcare suppliers can realize unmistakable security endeavors to ensure about the correspondence between different substances. Either their front-end systems that liable for speaking with specialist, doctor or nurse or their back-end structures that has the health-related data can get blockchain-based IoT security.

[1]CSE Department, SET, Mody University of Science and Technology, Laxmangarh, India
[2]ISE Department, SDM College of Engineering and Technology, Dharwad, India
[3]IT Department, Sikkim Manipal Institute of Technology, Rangpo, India
[4]School of Management, University of Bradford, Bradford, UK

Despite pandemics, for instance, the one we are seeing, at this moment, these affiliations necessity to get right and definite information to condemn the best technique: as it has been found throughout ongoing months, solid logical information, quickly, trustworthy sensible data, sharing and declaring or revealing of this data, is the best approach to comprehension, along these lines diminishing overall pandemic. Furthermore, how the sullied cases can be consequently perceived and how the probability of the malady hazard can be assessed or evaluated and foreseen or anticipated by individuals or specialists ceaselessly. In this COVID-19 pandemic, it is critical to consider answers for present blockchain as one of the rising headways as it guarantees health information security, assurance and give legitimate instruments to open minded patient testing, screening, treatment and exchange of defilement anticipation and control information with patients and everyone; fluctuating, appropriate security endeavors for singular security are given.

Blockchain-based IoT application to healthcare business can improve information security; medicinal administrations data can be examined and transmitted while keeping up data security, privacy and protection. This chapter proposes a blockchain-based IoT system that might be applied to healthcare systems to fight against COVID-19 pandemic through consequently recognizing dark tainted cases similarly as predicting and evaluating the risk of COVID-19 pandemic in the networks. Identification, monitoring, reconnaissance, contact tracing and mitigation can bolster and fortify the proposed system with significant highlights if there should arise an occurrence of disease recognition, virus chance expectation and estimation of COVID-19.

Keywords: Internet of Things (IoT); Blockchain; IoT applications; Healthcare systems; COVID-19; Coronavirus; Pandemic

20.1 Introduction

The fast advancements in scaling down and specialized strategies have been added to remarkable progresses in our overall populace. This has achieved an extension in the volume of fitting electronic gadgets for certain regions, a diminishing in their improvement costs and an adjustment in context from this current reality into the progressed computerized world. Along these lines, the way we interface with one another and with the earth has changed, utilizing current progression to extend an overwhelming view of the world. The Internet of Things (IoT) has succeeded as a ton of advances from WSN (wireless sensors networks) to RFID (radio frequency identification) that gives the capacities to recognize sense, influence with and give over the Internet.

The idea of the IoT was presented by Kevin Ashton, a prime supporter of the Auto-ID Center at MIT, in 1998. "Officially characterized, the Internet of Things is a connection between 'objects' of this present reality with the virtual world, along these lines empowering whenever, wherever availability for anything and not just anybody. IoT articles can shift drastically in size from a little wearable gadget to a voyage transport. It alludes to an existence where physical articles and creatures, just as virtual information and situations, all cooperate with one another in a similar reality" [1].

IoT changes common items, for example, vehicles, structures and machines into smart, associated objects that can speak with individuals, applications and one another. So as to empower IoT, every "thing" ought to be able to help three aspects:

- Identifiable
- Communication ability
- Interaction ability

On the off chance that they satisfy those aspects, "things" can be considered "smart object." In an IoT course of action, anything does prepare to pass on to the web at whatever point from wherever and offer organizations to anyone. The IoT is used in pretty much every part of individual life and is being received inside about each industry. IoT arrangements not just include different innovation spaces, for example, portable correspondences, cloud, information, security, media communications, and systems administration; however, they likewise lead to cross-mechanical utilization of information.

The IoT imagines a totally interconnected world, where things can impart assessed data and interface with one another. This makes possible a computerized depiction of this current reality, through which many savvy applications in a grouping of adventures can be created. These include wearables, automotive, smart urban regions, smart homes and healthcare. IoT arrangements are being passed on in various territories, redesigning creation and digitizing organizations. IoT applications are having very certain characteristics; they produce gigantic volumes of information, they require system and force for broad stretches.

IoT systems are working in the assortment of measurements as it is expanding the profitability, improving the effectiveness, creating the new income streams, taking knowledge choices, upgrading the guideline of administration and improving the steadfastness and simplicity of client. Following are a few highlights that are given by IoT (Figure 20.1).

- Scalability
  IoT empowers the assortment and collection of information from tens to thousands of gadgets detecting their condition with network availability.
- Heterogeneity and interoperability
  A system of "things" is essentially a system of "things" that are made by different producers, and these "things" will have certain resistances or bigotries to different "things" to which they interface and convey.

  Interoperability happens at the interface level, implying that when interfaces are comprehended, two particular subsystems can impart through a typical correspondence position without requiring information concerning the usefulness of the subsystems.
- Compatibility and integration

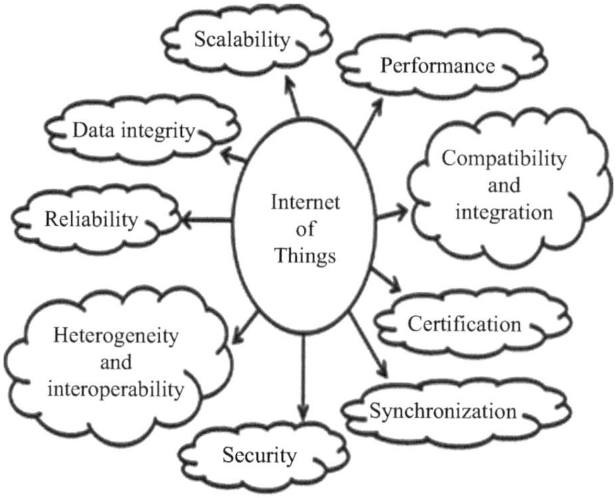

Figure 20.1 Features on IoT

Similarity essentially implies that two subsystems can exist or work related without struggle. Incorporation is a procedure of frequently uniting different subsystems into another system.

- Synchronization
  A system of "things" is a distributed computing system. Distributed systems have various calculations and occasions happening simultaneously. There can be various calculations and occasions (e.g., information sharing) happening in parallel.
- Certification
  On the off chance that thorough IoT certification approaches are in the long run evolved, they ought to decrease a large number of trust worries in this distribution. Be that as it may, building certification approaches is commonly troublesome. One explanation is that confirmation approaches have less viability except if right danger spaces and operational conditions are known. Regularly, these are not known for customary systems, let alone for IoT systems.
- Security
  Security is a worry for all "things." For instance, sensors and their information might be messed with, taken, erased, dropped or transmitted unreliably, permitting them to be gotten to by unapproved parties.
- Reliability
  Reliability is an element of setting and condition. In this way, IoT reliability ought to be founded on the customary definition in [2]. The customary definition is essentially the likelihood of disappointment-free activity of individual segments, gatherings of segments or the entire system over a limited time span and in a fixed domain.

- Data integrity
  The capacity to believe information includes numerous elements: (a) exactness, (b) constancy, (c) accessibility and (d) certainty that the information cannot be adulterated or messed with.
- Performance
  The speed at which calculations and information age can happen in a system of "things" is expanding quickly. Speeding up restrains a system's capacity to log and review any exchanges as the pace of information age surpasses the speed of capacity.

20.2 IoT in healthcare system

Related human administrations yet remain the lethargic monster of the IoT applications. Associated healthcare administrations structure and sharp helpful gadgets bear tremendous potential for associations, yet moreover for the success of people all around. Examination demonstrates that IoT in healthcare systems will be massive in coming years. Healthcare challenges have made new necessities for healthcare suppliers to effectively convey great healthcare administrations. IoT in healthcare systems is away for empowering people to carry on with increasingly valuable life by wearing related gadgets. With the appearance of the advanced era and the plenty of IoT gadgets it brings, there has been a considerable ascent in the measure of information accumulated by these gadgets in various parts like vehicle, condition, diversion, game and health divisions [3].

The accumulated data will help in redid assessment of an individual's prosperity and give altered strategies to fight illness. IoT with its arrangement of advantages, for example, empowering constant monitoring, giving a progressively developed and powerful answer for gather quiet information and following the exercises of patients and staff meet the new prerequisites:

- Advanced health system dealing with present treatment.
- Medical data system to give decision support.
- Get a superior comprehension of patient's ailment in a progression of "stages" and requirement of complex consideration.
- An all-around organized progressing care program premeditated by multidisciplinary group.

A viable model requests IoT applications to be applied for different infections in various healthcare settings. By actualizing IoT in healthcare arrangements, healthcare suppliers get significant information, which give understanding into the indications and example of the sickness, while empowering far off consideration. Additionally, there is growing mindfulness and responsibility of clients concerning their well-being, interest for distant and home possibilities keeps creating, diverse healthcare system players consider novel procedures and associations; and healthcare use decline remains an essential target, close by better quality thought. An undeniably consolidated and IoT-enabled eHealth approach shows central in all of these domains. Notwithstanding, while impending for the information advertise is seen, various issues like security of data, information insurance and sharing, and compulsory necessities of healthcare the executives and checking, among others, are basic. The trust, security and information classification are basic for IoT usage in healthcare systems. Following are some threats in the IoT healthcare systems:

- Physical attacks
  This shows the tempering with components and hardware.
- Environment attacks
  This shows the discovery of device encryption key by the attacker utilizing the recovery of encryption information.
- Cryptanalysis attacks
  This shows the finding ciphertext to break the encryption method.
- Software attacks

This shows exploiting vulnerabilities in the system during its own communication interface and injection of malicious codes.

20.3 COVID-19 outbreak

The world is at present seeing risky movements in the plague of developing SARS-CoV-2, the contributory operator of coronavirus. The contamination, and demise numbers announced by World Health Organization (WHO) about this pandemic estimate expanding dangers to the lives of individuals and the financial aspects of nations. The entire healthcare system will at long last require adjusting to blockchain-based IoT applications for helping and fighting against COVID-19 outbreak. In a globalized world wherein we live, components, for instance, the WHO have set up the protocols to ensure cooperation between different governments on issues related to overall health. Past the part of pandemic readiness and reaction, the instance of COVID-19 infection and its spread give an entrancing contextual analysis to the topical of urban health. The best test that most governments are as of now experiencing is the absence of an exact instrument to recognize obscure tainted cases and anticipate the contamination danger of COVID-19 infection. Following are the preventive estimates one can take for COVID-19:

- Regular hands wash
- Avoid contacting face
- Use of mask
- Practice social distancing
- Avoid party
- Stay home—stay safe

Also, in the current instance of the coronavirus flare-up, this should be maneuvered carefully to abstain from risking endeavors as of now set up to battle the outbreak. On the head, since these cut across different countries, which are a piece of the overall arrange and have remarkable laws and rules regarding issues referred to the previous text, watch them as per the direct of their source country's laws and rules; hereafter, underlining the meaning of moving toward not simply the progressing of data through its usage yet also the necessity for standardized and all around agreed shows.

Aside from these preventive measures, there are an immense rundown of mechanical items [4,5] that can aid early identification of episodes; either through warm cameras or IoT sensors, and early conversations could render endeavors toward a better administration of comparative circumstances in the event of future possible flare-ups, and to improve the health texture of urban areas for the most part.

Here, as innovative devices and labs around the globe share information and on the whole work to devise instruments and fixes, comparable endeavors ought to be considered among IoT and healthcare experts on how community-oriented methodologies could take into account the boost of open health on such and comparative situations.

While thermal sensors cameras are not adequate all alone for discovery of pandemic, like the instance of the COVID-19, the mix of such items with man-made consciousness (AI) can give included advantages. The way that underlying screenings of temperature is being sought after for the instance of the COVID-19 at air terminals and in regions of mass union is a demonstration of its potential in a mechanized manner. Kamel Boulos *et al.* [6] underpin that information from different innovative items can help advance health databases, give increasingly exact, proficient, complete and constant data on flare-ups and their dispersal, in this way supporting in the arrangement of better urban texture hazard the board choices.

Weber and PodnarŽarko [7] recommend that IoT gadgets being used should bolster open conventions, and simultaneously, the gadget supplier ought to guarantee that those designed maintain information honesty and security during correspondence and transmission.

In the previous case, however, significant urban areas are known to set themselves up for likely episodes, their health strategies and conventions are seen to separate from each other. Along these lines, without a worldwide community-oriented methodology, development toward working for a fix and generally satisfactory strategy method can take longer. These feelings of trepidation, of an absence of universal cooperation, were featured by the WHO during a crisis meeting on January 22, 2020 in Geneva to decide if the infection episode had arrived at a level justifying global crisis concern.

20.4 Blockchain

The issue of trust in data systems is incredibly perplexing when neither confirmation nor review components are given, particularly when they need to manage delicate data, such as monetary exchanges with virtual monetary standards. Blockchain is for the most part known as the mechanical stage behind Bitcoin. Bitcoin is virtual cryptographic money that retains its incentives without help from any brought-together power or budgetary element. Blockchain is a system that has authorized exchanges to be checked by a gathering of inconsistent on-screen characters. Blockchain can be characterized as a database that can record exchanges between parties in a safe and perpetual manner [8]. It gives a dispersed, permanent, straightforward, secure and auditable record. Truth be told, its database does not put in a focal area; however, it is circulated over a system of members. Significantly, blockchain is obvious to every part in the system. This decentralized idea gives high strength and security to database put away on blockchain with no single-point disappointment. It can be counseled straightforwardly, permitting access to all exchanges that have occurred since the primary exchange of the system and can be checked and gathered by any substance whenever. Each blockchain comprises three fundamental segments, including information block, circulated record (database) and accord calculations.

The blockchain convention structures data in a chain of blocks. Each block contains three components, a hash; timestamped bunches of ongoing legitimate exchanges and the value of hash of the past block. A participating member necessary to be authorized utilizing an authorization system. The past block hash interfaces the blocks together and keeps any block from being adjusted or a block being embedded between two existing blocks. To help and work with the blockchain, arranged peers need to give the accompanying usefulness: steering, stockpiling, wallet administrations and mining [9]. As indicated by the capacities they give, various kinds of hubs can be a piece of the system. Thusly, each ensuing block fortifies the confirmation of the past block and henceforth the whole blockchain. Blockchain innovation guarantees that put-away records are precise, alter apparent, and from an undeniable source.

In a blockchain-based system, the security components ensure that singular exchanges and messages are cryptographically marked. This guarantees fundamental security and compelling danger the board to handle the present high dangers of hacking, information control and information bargain.

There are two kinds of blockchains:

- Public blockchain
  It is accessible for everyone and anyone can join and cause trades similarly as to participate in the agreement system. The most famous open blockchain applications fuse Bitcoin and Ethereum.
- Private blockchain
  Then again are an invitation-based system oversaw by focal element (Figure 20.2).

The blockchain can be recognized by the going with three phases or periods of the blockchain headway:

- Digital currency (Blockchain 1.0)
  It insinuates the secret development stage (for instance, hashing, mining and the open record), the overlying show (for instance, trade enabling programming) and the high-level money (for instance, Bitcoin or other progressed

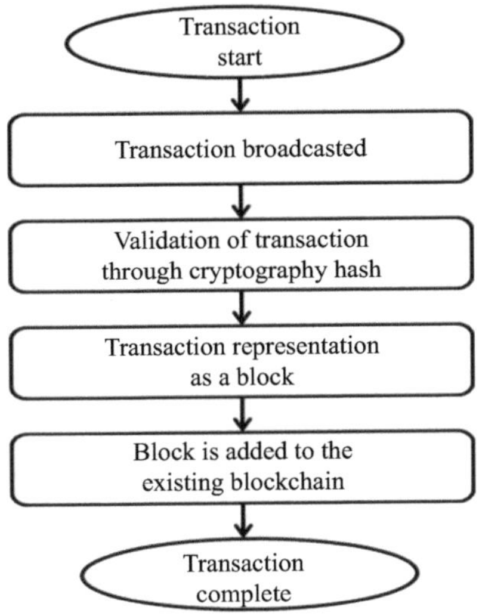

Figure 20.2 Blockchain workflow

coins/tokens) that address a store of huge worth similarly as deal some motivation to the actual show [10]. Bitcoin gives more imperative anonymity than Mastercards. Bitcoin offers the shot at commonly diminished trade costs for on-line purchases. The decentralized design of Bitcoin and other mechanized financial structures guarantees against development. Records are pseudonymous and the show is planned to engage the use of new record numbers for each trade.

- Digital economy (Blockchain 2.0)
  It insinuates the wide extent of financial and cash-related applications that exist past clear portions, moves and trades. Such applications fuse ordinary monetary instruments, for instance, advances and home credits, complex cash-related market instruments, for instance, stocks, protections, possibilities, subordinates, similarly as authentic instruments, for instance, agreements, titles and various assets and property that can be adjusted.
- Digital society (Blockchain 3.0)
  Blockchain 3.0 insinuates gigantic scope of employments that do exclude cash, trade, money related or other monetary development. Such applications join workmanship, well-being, science, character, organization, preparing, open product and various pieces of culture and correspondence. IoT transforms into one more stage for e-business. In any case, old strategies could scarcely fit for the electronic business on the IoT. It is possible to execute the trading of brilliant property and paid data on the IoT with the help of P2P trade subject to the blockchain advancement and shrewd agreement [11]. In the new cyberworld, people oftentimes make trades with somebody that they have not met with. Reputation framework has been comprehensively used in the web as a

feasible strategy to allow people to evaluate the dependability of a logical seller.

Using the blockchain advancement, the possibility of decentralization might be applied to huge extension data the board in an EMR (electronic medical record) framework, giving interoperability, auditability and accessibility through an expansive log. Progressed character enabled by the blockchain development might potentially change lives. With the benefit of modernized person, a significant parcel of the universes 2 billion unbanked individuals could store their characters on blockchain, agree banks to fulfill regulatory necessities, for instance, Know Your Customer and access records, credits and other cash-related organizations currently hard to reach them [12]. Regardless, current reputation frameworks are vulnerable against distortion rating and the acknowledgment of bogus raters is irksome since they can continue purposely to mask themselves. Blockchain development allows new opportunities to upgrading the reputation framework [9].

20.5 Blockchain-based IoT for healthcare systems

Blockchain is forming into a sheltered and productive system for secure information partaking in applications, for example, the money-related industry, tasks the board, food industry, vitality showcase, the IoT and healthcare. The way where standard clinical systems and organizations have been occupied with the healthcare division in the course of the most recent couple of decades is prepared to change. Data and correspondence advances (ICTs) and blockchain are key advances that permit healthcare foundations to be decentralized and digitized and give patients just as specialist co-ops with present day and digitized healthcare ecosystems [13,14]. Blockchain innovation has as of late rose as a key innovation in the healthcare division's advanced change and many examination contemplates [15,16] have recognized potential for blockchain to the healthcare ecosystem. Healthcare-coordinated effort stage can be characterized as the healthcare system that is fit for empowering the correspondence between healthcare elements like doctors, attendants, patients, prescriptions, labs, suppliers and healthcare specialists. Healthcare suppliers can actualize distinctive safety efforts so as to make sure about the correspondences between various substances.

Blockchain innovation is utilized as an intent to share true information, following of pertinent data and help accelerate the treatment procedure. Either their front-end systems that are answerable for speaking with doctor or nurture or their back-end systems that have the electronic health records (EHRs) can embrace blockchain security. Simultaneously, it will safeguard individual's personality. Convenient organization and appropriate usage of the proposed model have the chance to check COVID-19 transmissions and related mortality, particularly in conditions with deficient access to testing offices. This innovation gives patients far reaching, changeless records and access to EHRs liberated from specialist organizations and treatment sites. Blockchain executives systems construct administrations for patients, doctors and healthcare organizations in the fields of patient data access and observing, cases and installment handling, clinical IoT insurance the board and clinical information confirmation and budgetary review transaction, and straightforwardness.

In addition, blockchain can change the way that clinical exchanges happened. It could ensure the quality confirmation for supporting EHRs making, recovering, refreshing, erasing (CRUD) capacities. The board of healthcare during this COVID-19 emergency and as a rule incorporates a few procedures, for example, money-related administration, work force, patients, legitimate issues, coordination, stock, etc. [17].

This likewise concerns individual information assurance, the handling of private data, the evacuation of outsiders, character the executives. In contrast to incorporated systems, the usefulness of the system proceeds despite the fact that solitary hubs separate. It improves certainty, since people do not survey the reliability of the middle person or other system members. At the point when individuals create trust inside the program itself, it is sufficient. Clinical work processes incorporate routine exercises identified with the treatment of patients, which can be portrayed as a grouping of contingent acts. These are intended to give more grounded inward controls; improve quality; consistence, productivity; and decrease hazard, work cycles and overhead in clinics and different suppliers of social insurance (Figure 20.3).

- IoT network
  The initial segment that contains sensors, system and switch speaks to the IoT system for the healthcare system, which is associated with dispersed blockchain through web. The overlay organization is likened to the distributed system in IoT. The constituent sensor hubs could be brilliant gadgets, other high asset gadgets on the patient, some wearable or the client's advanced mobile phone or PC. The sensors are gathering the information and going through system with the various switches sent in the system to the web.
- Data storage
  The subsequent part is for capacity where in the EHRs, disease patter, check information and web-based life information are put away. Ongoing updates to an encoded, mysterious blockchain database are done in these applications to get, track and oversee clinical data. It likewise empowers confining the unapproved individual's entrance to classified data by human services associations. This shows the conceivable utilization of blockchain during the time spent COVID-19. Brief sending and legitimate usage of the proposed model can possibly control COVID-19 transmissions and related mortality, particularly in conditions with inadequate access to test offices. The blockchain innovation with the IoT in healthcare presented in this section has been utilized to create and execute shrewd agreements. This work will advance numerous entertainers keen on controlling the spread of this illness inside the clinical system.
- COVID-19 surveillance
  Most importantly, the IoT framework and data accumulating give a phase that grants general healthcare associations admittance to data for noticing the

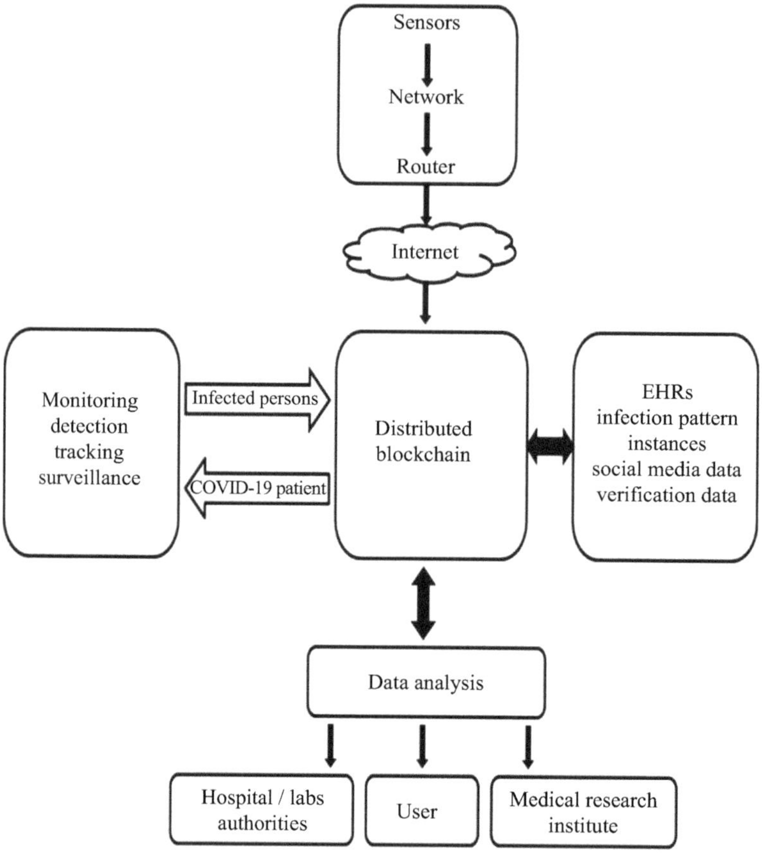

Figure 20.3 Blockchain-based IoT for healthcare system

COVID-19 patient. For example, the "Worldometer" gives a constant update on the real number of people known to have COVID-19 all throughout the planet, including step-by-step new cases of the ailment, affliction apportionment by countries and earnestness of disease. At that point in the wake of getting the total data of COVID-19 patient, the reconnaissance system will screen, identify and track the spread of conceivable COVID-19 patients and contaminated people.

- Data analysis
  In this area, we assess and subjectively break down the gathered information, put away information, and conceivable tainted patients detail. This investigation is worried about the client, healthcare specialists to take appropriate choice and the clinical examination foundations for the improvement of immunization and solutions for the COVID-19 coronavirus.

The basic reaction in various countries is for healthcare workplaces to diminish or even stop various clinical organizations, including finish of offices and postponement of clinical plans or elective operations. This would ensure that patients continue to acknowledge standard clinical thought while diminishing actual pressing of patients into clinical facility premises.

Besides, electronic phone-based programming that distinguishes and records patients' data (e.g., step-by-step temperature and indications) may thwart pointless clinical facility conferences for patients with smooth flu like incidental effects.

Various crisis facilities are collaborating with blockchain associations and pharmacies to pass on patients' medication to their doorsteps. Utilizing blockchain, crisis facilities could ensure advantageous movement of solutions with exact after.

20.6 Advantages of proposed system

The IoT is changing and propelling manual strategies in healthcare frameworks to make them some portion of the electronic time, obtaining volumes of data that gives data at mind-blowing levels. This phenomenal advancement in the IoT has opened up new organization openings, for instance, instruments to access and offer information. This data is empowering the progression of clever medical services frameworks, for instance, the improvement of the organization and the individual fulfillment of patient through the digitization of organizations in the healthcare frameworks. There are giant abilities of blockchain in changing the IoT in healthcare frameworks.

Blockchain can propel the IoT-based medical services framework by offering a trusted in sharing help, where information is strong and can be unmistakable. Data sources can be perceived at whatever point and data stays invariable after some time, extending its security. In the circumstances where the IoT data should be securely divided among various individuals, this mix would address a key change.

A data spill in any piece of the chain could provoke coercion and block the techniques of the journey for infection that can genuinely impact occupant's lives and achieve gigantic money-related costs to associations, divisions and countries by virtue of a COVID-19 erupt. An unrivalled control in these domains would construct understanding data well-being, further developing the data dividing between individuals and diminishing the pursuit time by virtue of a COVID-19 erupt, which can save human lives.

In like manner, the usage of blockchain can enhance the IoT in healthcare framework with strong and secure information. This blockchain development is perceived as the best approach to appreciate flexibility, security and steady quality issues related to the medical care framework.

Following are the potential gains of having blockchain-based IoT healthcare systems:

- Cost saving
  Presumably the best favored situation of blockchain-based IoT in healthcare services is that capable self-administering frameworks will cost less to direct

and utilize as time goes on. Things are far better with respects than open-minded expense speculation reserves in view of less clinical facility voyages similarly as animated diagnostics and treatment.

- Decentralization and scalability
  The move from a joined designing to a P2P disseminated one will clear fundamental issues of dissatisfactions and bottlenecks. It will in like manner assist with preventing circumstances where two or three staggering associations control the taking care of and limit of the information of a tremendous number of people. Various benefits that go with the decentralization of the designing are an improvement of the transformation to nonbasic disappointment and framework adaptability. It would diminish the IoT storage facilities and furthermore add to further developing the IoT flexibility.
- Distributed trust and security
  Data and trades can be ensured about if they are taken care of as trades of the blockchain. Blockchain can treat contraption message exchanges as trades, supported by savvy arrangements, subsequently ensuring about correspondences between devices. Current secure standard shows used in the IoT can be updated with the utilization of blockchain.

  The blockchain is having the instruments for guaranteeing disseminated trust in the IoT organization. In IoT organization, each block keeps up a trust rating for past block that depends on immediate and roundabout proof.
- Safe operation and code deployment
  Taking advantage of blockchain secure-perpetual storing, code can be well-being and securely crashed into medical care contraptions. Makers can track and update with the most imperative assurance. IoT middleware can use this handiness to securely revive IoT devices states.
- User privacy and identity
  Using an ordinary blockchain framework individual can recognize every single device. Data-compromised care into the framework is invariable and curiously recognizes genuine data that was given by a contraption. Besides, blockchain can give trust in passed-on affirmation.

  In addition, the endorsement of devices for IoT applications would address an improvement in the IoT field and its individuals:
- Medical supply chain
  Blockchain can stimulate the creation of an IoT-based healthcare arrangement of organizations and data business focuses, where trades between peers are possible without subject matter experts. Microservices and deftly chain can be helpfully passed on and more limited size portions can be well-being made in a trustless space. It would further develop IoT medical services interconnection and the passageway of well-being related data in blockchain.
- Accessibility and reliability
  The clinic/labs director needs to get to the put-away information for a specific timeframe (e.g., the previous 24 h) or the whole chain of information for a specific patient, so as to execute certain administrations. To get to data, the blockchain makes and signs a multiblock exchange, which should be

approved. Individuals from the framework are prepared for affirming the realness of the data and have the conviction that they have not been screwed with. Likewise, the development enables sensor data perceptibility and obligation. Relentless quality is the vital piece of the blockchain to get the IoT.

20.7 Conclusion and future scope

In the IoT-based healthcare systems with the COVID-19 circumstance, normal gadgets become free, self-ruling and savvy. This vision is changing into a reality by ethicalness of advances being developed, in any case there are still inconveniences to address, especially in the security space, e.g., information unwavering quality, observing and following of patients. Considering the foreseen progression of the IoT-based healthcare system in the COVID-19 flare-up, it is essential to give trust in this gigantic moving toward information source.

While the world continues to rely upon incredible general health measures for dealing with the COVID-19 pandemic, in 2020, there is by and by a wide extent of modernized development that can be used to increment and further develop these overall healthcare methods.

Blockchain has created as a key development that changes the way one can share, store and execute information. Building trust in passed-on conditions without the prerequisite for experts is a creative improvement that can change IoT-based healthcare systems. Starting late, blockchain is considered one of the basic historic techniques in protection and security space for the IoT-based healthcare system. It is considered the ensured security thought for displacing the current third balances confiding in courses of action. The quick utilized and effective use of blockchain in IoT-based healthcare system to handle a significant, worldwide general health challenge in 2020 will most likely expand people in general and administrative acknowledgment of such advances for different territories of healthcare, remembering ceaseless sickness for what's to come.

References

[1] H. Sundmaeker, P. Friess, P. Guillemin, and S. Woelffl, "Visions and challenges for realizing the internet of things," European Commission, Directorate-General for the Information Society and Media, 2010.

[2] S. J. Moore, C. D. Nugent, S. Zhang, and I. Cleland, "IoT reliability: A review leading to 5 key research directions," *CCF Transactions on Pervasive Computing and Interaction*, pp. 1–17, 2020.

[3] Z. Allam, M. Thondoo, and H. Tegally, "Redefining the use of big data in urban health for increased liveability in smart cities," *Smart Cities*, vol. 2, pp. 259–268, 2019.

[4] Z. Allam, *Cities and the Digital Revolution: Aligning Technology and Humanity*, Springer International Publishing: Switzerland, 2020.

[5] Z. Allam, "Data as the new driving gears of urbanization". In *Cities and the Digital Revolution: Aligning Technology and Humanity* Springer International Publishing: Switzerland, 2020; pp. 1–29.

[6] M. N. Kamel Boulos, T. VoPham, and G. Peng, "An overview of GeoAI applications in health and healthcare," *Int. J. Health Geogr.*, vol. 18, no. 7, 2019.

[7] M. Weber and I. PodnarŽarko, "A regulatory view on smart city services," *Sensors*, vol. 19, p. 415, 2019.

[8] "Blockchain" https://en.wikipedia.org/wiki/Blockchain.

[9] Y. Cai and D. Zhu, "Fraud detections for online businesses: A perspective from blockchain technology," *Financ. Innov.*, vol. 2, no. 1, p. 20, 2016.

[10] K. Burgess and J. Colangelo *The Promise of Bitcoin and the Blockchain*. Consumers' Research, Bowerstown, 2015.

[11] Y. Zhang and J. Wen, "The IoT electric business model: Using blockchain technology for the internet of things". *Peer-to-Peer Networking and Applications*, pp. 1–12, 2016.

[12] S. Underwood, "Blockchain beyond Bitcoin," *ACM Commun.*, vol. 59, no. 11, pp. 15–17, 2016.

[13] C. Agbo, Q. Mahmoud, and J. Eklund, "Blockchain technology in healthcare: A systematic review," *Healthcare*, vol. 7, no. 2, p. 56, 2019.

[14] H. D. Zubaydi, Y. W. Chong, S. M. Hanshi, S. Karuppayah, and K. Ko, "A review on the role of blockchain technology in the healthcare domain," *Electronics*, vol. 8, no. 6, pp. 1–29, 2019.

[15] A. Azaria, A. Ekblaw, A. Lippman, and T. Vieira, "MedRec: Using blockchain for medical data access and permission management," *Proc. – 2016 2nd Int. Conf. on OBD 2016*, pp. 25–30, 2016.

[16] B. Shen, Y. Yang, and J. Guo, "MedChain: Efficient healthcare data sharing via blockchain," *Appl. Sci.*, vol. 9, no. 6, 2019.

[17] A. Khatoon, "A blockchain-based smart contract system for healthcare management," *Electronics*, vol. 9, no. 1, p. 94, 2020.

Chapter 21

Artificial intelligence-based diseases detection and diagnosis in healthcare

Said El Kafhali[1] *and Iman El Mir*[2]

Abstract

From the past few decades, the healthcare system depends on the interaction between a doctor and a patient and operates on limited data. The restricted feature of this healthcare system fails to leverage the data. Besides, the healthcare process is time-consuming and tiring resulting in inefficient patient handling. Thus, due to the lack of availability of critical data, many healthcare systems are unsuccessful in providing the needful treatment to patients. Even patients are not in entire control because they have a large number of reports from different doctors that are hard to manage in one place and make the right health decision. Recently, the employ of artificial intelligence (AI) techniques in healthcare can help the healthcare system to overcome the aforementioned challenges and issues. This chapter briefs the different AI algorithms carried out in diverse health disease detection and diagnosis. Further, it provides a review of such used algorithms. By learning this chapter, the readers and investigators will be able to keep the concept of AI on detecting disease and medical diagnosis, as well as to identify the proper and optimized method of research on their field of investigation for further developments.

Keywords: Artificial intelligence; Diseases identification; Healthcare system; Machine learning; Deep learning; Big data

21.1 Introduction

When the population of a country and average age make greater in size every year, there is automatically a strain on its health system. This situation is due to the clinical attention typically required by the elderly and the growing size of the aging population in which many countries in the world faced nowadays. Diseases detection and

[1]Faculty of Sciences and Techniques, Computer, Networks, Mobility and Modeling Laboratory (IR2M), Hassan First University of Settat, Settat, Morocco
[2]Sports Sciences Institute, Hassan First University of Settat, Settat, Morocco

diagnosis is a very severe issue in the healthcare area. The sick person should be diagnosed precisely based on the findings of his medical evaluations and experiments. Many medical centers and hospitals produce enormous data on patient health, keep-ups, medical evaluations, and different drug data. Finding an appropriate method to organize the different types of these data is complex and not at all easy. The mismanagement of these data can affect the disease detection and diagnosis for example. An energetic research area that is gradually gaining in significance in the area of detection and diagnosis of healthcare is computer-aided detection and diagnosis. In the past, before the use of artificial intelligence (AI) in the healthcare field, the potential for medical errors was considerably high. Since the development of AI, it has gradually been integrated into patient care.

The use of decision computer-aided in digital computer systems can be greatly helpful for the effective detection and diagnosis of diseases [1]. Recent study and work in the area of AI technology exhibit that we can improve the accuracy of disease diagnosis that enables computer techniques to think knowledgeably and insightfully as human beings. The people on all sides of the world actually are facing numerous diseases, and many people are dying because of it. From the past few decades, AI becomes the most powerful technology in solving many challenging problems in the healthcare system such as patient monitoring, disease detection, disease diagnosis, and health data management. The most pressing need for AI in healthcare is in the diagnosis and detection of disease. AI enables healthcare professionals to diagnose many types of disease earlier and more accurately [2].

The AI techniques in healthcare are widely used to identify every critical illness and to correctly diagnose it for further alternative treatment. AI performs sophisticated operations using ideally characterized subdomains such as deep learning (DL) and machine learning (ML) to provide rapid healing with the greatest satisfaction of patient and physician. ML and DL use different algorithms for an accurate decision on disease detection and diagnosis. ML is a set of data mathematical methods programmed to learn patterns from datasets. Using statistical assumptions and analytical rules, ML algorithms develop a model among the features of the datasets. Different measured features in the dataset express the input of the ML algorithms. To train patient datasets in healthcare applications, ML algorithms typically use the concept of supervised learning (SL). Therefore, AI would optimize predictive capabilities and improve efficiency by using structured or unstructured datasets. Many researchers have suggested different ML and DL algorithms to implement healthcare identification and diagnostic systems such as AI-based oncology, AI-based ophthalmology, AI-based radiology, AI-based neurology, AI-based cardiology, and recently AI-based system for COVID-19 identification and treatment.

The contributions of this chapter are as follows:

- We present an overview of identifying and diagnosing existing diseases in healthcare, in which a complete taxonomy is used to sort them into different classes based on the AI techniques.
- We identify a set of actual studies and describe new perspectives regarding the disease detection and diagnosis schemes.

- We derive future perspectives for utilizing AI for disease detection and diagnosis in healthcare.

The rest of this chapter is organized as follows. Section 21.2 presents an overview of disease detection and diagnosis techniques. SL models are presented in Section 21.3. Section 21.4 presents unsupervised learning (USL) models. Section 21.5 presents reinforcement-learning (RL) models. Some critical analysis and discussion about disease detection and diagnosis schemes are presented in Section 21.6. Section 21.7 presents open research challenges concerning some new emerging ideas of disease detection and diagnosis schemes. Finally, Section 21.8 concludes the chapter.

21.2 Overview of diseases detection and diagnosis techniques

This section describes existing disease identification and diagnosis methods based on AI algorithms. Researchers have developed algorithms that are three main learning techniques: SL models, USL models, and RL models. In SL, the task is to deduce a method that maps input to output based on instances of pairs of inputs and outputs. In USL, the task is to learn from a test dataset that has not been labeled to identify common features in the dataset. In RL, the task is to act within the given environment to minimize penalties as specified by some accumulative nature form. In Figure 21.1, we illustrate the proposed taxonomy of disease detection and diagnosis techniques in healthcare.

21.3 Supervised learning models

SL technique is the most popular method of learning used when the dataset is labeled. SL focuses on two types of problems: classification and regression that involve the training datasets to estimate the output parameters. It necessitates a dataset established in advance to learn and enhance the performance of the system. Several algorithms like naïve Bayes (NB), support vector machines (SVM), neural networks (NN), *K*-nearest neighbor (*K*NN), decision trees (DT), a belief Bayesian network (BBN), logistic regression, and Bayesian networks are categorized under SL technique. In this section, we briefly explain the studies that used SL models for disease identification and diagnosis.

21.3.1 Deep learning models

Classical ML techniques can make use of the data volume to some magnitude. Their performance will not improve further even we add more data. DL methods can use big data by building a complex model to learn nonlinear relationships between data. With many digitized activities, such as electronic health records [3], data is recorded and available [4]. This available big data can be used using DL techniques to give more precision compared to classical ML methods. Advances in

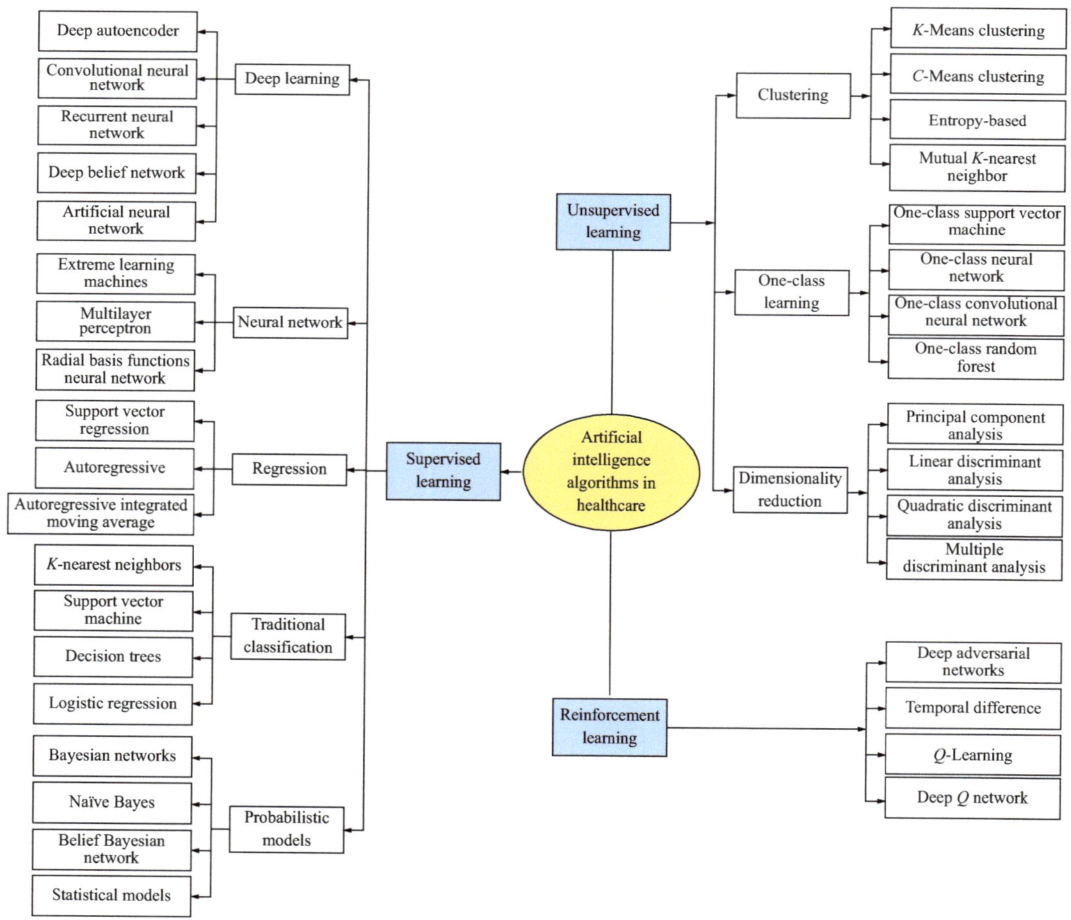

Figure 21.1 Taxonomy of the artificial intelligence algorithms in healthcare

computing power have made great strides in the development of more complex techniques such as convolutional neural networks (CNN) and recurrent neural networks (RNN) that show significant performance improvements in many healthcare applications. DL is to automatically build this relevant representation of data through the learning phase, thus avoiding human intervention. We, therefore, speak of learning by representation. A DL algorithm holds increasingly complex hierarchical representations of data. This type of algorithm is, therefore, suitable for signal data (images, texts, sounds, etc.), because they are very hierarchical.

The use of DL is found in radiomics or the clinical detection of the various features relevant to imaging data that goes beyond things seen via the human eye. DL and radiomics are often used in oncology-focused image review. The combined use of these two technologies allows for increased accuracy in disease diagnosis compared to other invented automated tools for image analysis. Usually, DL is applied in the healthcare field for the recognition of the cancerous lesions related to the radiological images. CNN is one of the well-known DL techniques that are especially designed for image recognition and computer vision applications. Recently, DL has achieved great success in disease detection and diagnosis. For instance, RNN to predict Alzheimer's disease progression [5], CNN to diagnose chest disease [6], artificial neural network (ANN) as a diagnostic tool in tuberculosis [7], deep belief networks to track the progress of Parkinson's disease remotely [8], and deep autoencoder to the diagnosis of heart diseases [9].

21.3.2 Neural networks models

NNs are a forceful implement to assist physicians model, process, analyze, and interpret more complicated clinical data in a wide variety of medical diagnosis exercises. This technology has been around since the 1960s and is used for the categorization of applications such as determining aspects of patient health relating to disease acquisition [10]. It considers the complexities associated with the input and output of disease, and the characteristics that associate the input to output. NN is a computational tool that seeks to account for the parallel manner of the human brain in which a network of extremely interconnecting processing units is run in parallel. A typical NN is presented in Figure 21.2 in which the initial layer is the input layer of NN, the final layer is the output layer of NN, and between the two layers, there can be many hidden layers.

Deep NNs are not just a stack of layers of neurons. Indeed, to solve increasingly complex problems, it is not enough to add more and more layers. The two considerable problems of NNs, which are the difficulty of learning and the increasing computational complexity with the number of layers, are indeed still present. The solutions provided by current research make it possible to limit these problems but not to solve them completely. The RNNs have notably revolutionized the recognition of speech by machines (speech recognition) or the comprehension and generation of text natural language processing (NLP). This later includes two techniques, such as statistical NLP and semantic NLP. Computer language helps as the underlying support for statistical NLP (including deep NNs), which has

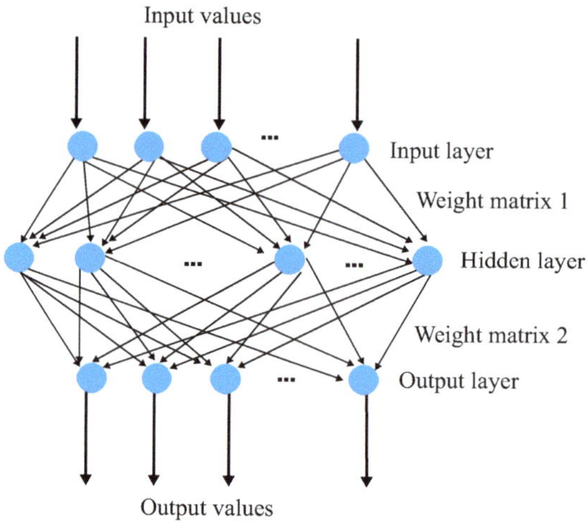

Figure 21.2 A typical neural network

increased the level of accuracy in recognizing the disease. This usually requires an expanded "corpus" as well as a body of language from which doctors learn. NLP in health services creates, understands, classifies clinical documents as well as published health problems. NLP can also review different unstructured patient notes, formulate reports such as X-rays, transcripts of patient interactions, and conversations related to AI.

In [11], the heart disease diagnosis is handled by using the extreme learning machine (ELM) technique. The latter consists of a three-layered NN together with a function of sigmoid activation. The simulation results from real data around 300 patients showed that this technique has an accuracy of 80% in detecting heart disease. The work in [12] examines various approaches that use a multilayered technique based on CNN and perceptron NN (MLP) to detect and diagnose breast cancer in terms of accuracy of diagnosis and detection. In [13], a new hybrid approach based on a self-organization map using radial basis function NN is proposed to automate epileptic disease diagnosis.

21.3.3 Regression models

The regression method for diagnostic calculates how well the models characterize the underlying relationships among predictors' variables and patient results existing in the health data, whether the health data that the model was built on or the health data from another population. Several regression methods have been proposed in the exiting works to detect and diagnose disease in healthcare, which includes support vector regression, linear regression (LR), regression fitting, regression trees, autoregressive (AR), and autoregressive integrated moving average (ARIMA) [14]. For example, the authors in [15] used an SVM classification algorithm to diagnose chronic kidney disease. This classification algorithm has been used with two feature selection techniques such as filter and wrapper approaches for dataset dimensionality reduction. The obtained results showed that the SVM by using filtered has a higher accuracy rate up to 98.5% in the diagnosis compared to other studied methods. The authors of [16] presented a model based on the AR model to predict and diagnose the human immunodeficiency virus (HIV). Specifically, they focused on the forecast of the diagnosis rates of novel HIV at the local government level by using openly available and observed data. The ARIMA model could serve as a useful technique to model, control, and predict malaria in some African countries. It, therefore, played an important role in shaping malaria control in KwaZulu-Natal, South Africa [17].

21.3.4 Traditional classification models

SVM, DT, LR, and *K*NN are the most famous classical classification models; they have been commonly used for disease detection and diagnosis applications or other research applications. In [18], SVM provides the highest accuracy of 94.60% for the heart disease diagnosis in diabetic patients using a dataset of 500 patients that bring together from the Chennai Research Institute. On the other side, a hybridization technique in which DT and ANN are hybridized is proposed for a better prediction of heart disease [19]. LR models are often used for predicting the results of prospective patients based on the predictor variables of every patient. The accuracy of an LR model is primarily judged by taking into account calibration and discrimination. Calibration is the capability of the model to allocate the reasonable mean absolute risk level, while discrimination is the capability of the model to properly allocate a greater risk of a result to patients who are actually at higher risk [20]. Furthermore, in [21], the authors developed an ensemble *K*NN classifier to detect Parkinson's disease with an accuracy of 98.46%.

21.3.5 Probabilistic models

Probabilistic methods are considered the more of great significance ML techniques for describing the existing issues of disease detection and diagnosis in healthcare. These methods use variables generated in a random way, such as the construction of ML models represented by probabilistic relations. A disease progression modeling–based probabilistic way to quantize the diagnostic incertitude of Alzheimer's disease seriousness in a clinical scenario is presented in [22]. The proposed model is considered a hopeful tool for clinical trial data analysis that can account for every missing data patterns and quantify the incertitude related to the absent information. In [23], an NB algorithm is used to detect pressure ulcers from intensive care unit electronic healthcare records. Similarly, in [24], the authors use a BBN model to detect and predict the dependency among chronic obstructive pulmonary disease symptoms.

21.4 Unsupervised learning models

Data used for training is not categorized or labeled in the dataset. The goal is to find patterns hidden in the data. The model is trained to easily predict the hidden patterns for any new input dataset. It concludes from the datasets to describe the hidden patterns. In the USL technique, no response in the dataset is visible. The USL methods are generally used to classify systems by detecting helpful clusters in the input dataset. The important USL methods used are *K*-means clustering (KMC), mutual nearest neighbor, principal component analysis (PCA), one-class classification (OCC), and maximum likelihood learning [25].

21.4.1 Clustering models

Clustering models are the most common USL techniques that could help the healthcare staff to schedule patients in a better way to have good treatment. For example, in [26], clustering technique is used to identify four groups of patients with interstitial lung disease and demonstrated that grouping patients could enhance the effectiveness of therapeutic interventions in future clinical trials. Clustering consists of grouping the identical characteristic data into classes or clusters. KMC method is one of the fastest and easiest clustering methods that works excellently if the clusters are spherical. The *K*-means algorithm comes to be an excellent way for pre-clustering that reduces the space into smaller disjoint subspaces whereabouts other clustering methods can be applied [27]. In [28], the Fuzzy *C*-mean clustering method has been used with morphological operators for the detection of primary glaucoma. Authors in the paper [29] have used entropy-based features from the flexible analytic wavelet transform to automatically detect nonfocal and focal electroencephalogram (EEG). Finally, mutual-*K*NN methods that are dedicated to graph-based semi-SL can be used for disease detection and diagnosis [30].

21.4.2 One-class classification models

OCC techniques aim to build classification models when the other class (negative) has no or very few instances or can be either absent, poorly representative, or unclear [31]. For example, for disease diagnosis, it is comparatively facile to assemble positive instances (all patients have a common disease) but negative instances can be difficult to obtain because other patients in the dataset cannot be considered negative if they have not at all been tested and these tests can be expensive, especially if the disease does not occur very often. Different techniques have been proposed in the literature for disease detection and diagnosis based on OCC. There are many OCC models proposed in the literature for disease diagnoses such as the one-class neural network model, one-class support vector machine model (OCSVM), one-class conventional neural network model, and one-class random forest model. In [32], a classifier based on OCSVM model is proposed for an epilepsy diagnosis. The model requires epilepsy and natural data for training, although it recognizes epilepsy data, natural data, and alike other disorders that were not considered in training samples. Authors in [33] proposed a simple and efficient OCC based on the ELM algorithm, which leads to much faster learning speed and superior generalization performance. The proposed algorithm is built for cases where solely the positive class is well described. The paper [34] proposes a novel OCC scheme for medical images based on kernel principle component analysis (KPCA). The proposed scheme is constructed with the feature subset strategy in which each one-class classifier is trained with one category of features extracted from the training medical images. The proposed scheme obtained promising results on the UCI breast cancer dataset (diagnostic).

21.4.3 Dimensionality reduction models

In different ML algorithms, the dimensionality reduction method could be utilized as a classification model with a poor compute cost because the input data can be expressed with fewer variables without a significant error. Various techniques are proposed for disease detection and diagnoses, such as linear discriminant analysis (LDA) [35], PCA [36], multiple discriminant analysis (MDA) [37], and quadratic discriminant analysis (QDA) [38]. Although PCA has been introduced primarily to minimize the initial data dimensionality while keeping relationships between data, it has been evenly employed as a classifier. In the case of disease detection, which is well respected as a two-class classification problem, the PCA calculates the principal components of the positive and negative classes. Moreover, PCA could also be used for the case of when the data contains missing values for the different features, as is the case with the feature extraction for heart disease diagnosis approach described in [39]. The proposed approach extracts the projection vectors that contribute to the utmost covariance and these projection vectors are used to minimize the dimension of the features. In [35], LDA is used to build a hybrid model for automated Parkinson's disease detection to achieve better classification accuracy. The accuracy obtained by this intelligent system using entirely the extracted features is 95% on the training dataset and 100% on the testing dataset. MDA is used in [37] for the classification of clinical pain descriptions. Finally, QDA was used in [38] as an automatic seizure detection method capable of analyzing EEG data and detecting epileptic seizures with high accuracy.

21.5 Reinforcement learning models

RL model does not use a labeled dataset nor the outcomes are associated with data, so the model learns from the experiment. In RL, the model enhances its presentation based on its combination with the environment and determines how to discuss its flaws and achieve the right result by evaluating and testing diverse perspectives. In recent years, RL models have been successfully applied in many healthcare services. Generally, these services can be classified into three main categories: dynamic treatment of critical care, automated disease diagnosis, and other general services such as health resource allocation and planning, drug discovery and development, and health management [40]. There are also several RL models used for disease diagnoses such as *Q*-learning (QL), deep *Q*-network (DQN), the temporal difference, and deep adversarial networks (DAN). In this regard, in [41], QL is used as a pretreatment of automatic extraction of a kidney region. In [42], the authors have used DAN to construct a framework to predict brain graph change over time. The obtained results from the experiment showed that the proposed model could remarkably reinforce the prediction accuracy compared to the baseline methods. The authors of [43] have proposed an RL framework with multilayer perceptron deep Q networks (MLP-DQN) to build a dialog system for automatic diagnosis. The proposed framework has also been extended by enhancing the DQN with craft features among diseases and symptoms, generated from the training set [44]. The new framework incorporates a knowledge-driven graph branch and a relational refinement branch, taking full advantage of medical information has and doctor experience (historical diagnostic cases). Finally, an RL-based evolutionary fuzzy rule-based approach is proposed for a diabetes diagnosis [45]. Two different datasets are used to evaluate the performance of the proposed system. The obtained evaluation results showed that the proposed system has high accuracy that makes it suitable for many diabetes diagnoses.

21.6 Summary of some applications for disease diagnosis in healthcare

The rapid development of AI technology reflects the need for urgent techniques that can aid in the diagnosis of many types of chronic and dangerous diseases. Several studies and research articles have taken place in this area to give an accurate and early diagnosis of all types of diseases. ML models, as techniques of dynamically computer-guided health data analysis and interpretation, are more important in AI. Automatic and dynamic clinical decisions establish a better patient–doctor relationship and reduce healthcare costs. Table 21.1 summarizes the research papers with the best reported performance models for disease detection and diagnosis in healthcare.

Furthermore, there are many health applications actually in which ML is highly being applied to early detection and diagnosis of some diseases like cancers, diabetic retinopathy, chronic disease, cardiovascular diseases, vascular dementia, osteoporosis, heart disease, Alzheimer's disease, and epilepsy. The applications of AI for the different types of diseases can be categorized as follows:

- **Cancer disease diagnosis:** the cancer cells are tortuous cells with extra pulps and nodulous that can be seen and defined by various types of medical imaging. With the up-to-date techniques of AI, these cancer cells can be fixed by the new technology that can be missed by the human intervention due to human errors.
- **Cardiovascular disease diagnosis:** AI can help to prevent and reduce heart attacks by defining the places and sites of the thrombus in the blood before it attains closed veins in the human body.
- **Medical imaging:** AI can do the ECG and define the sites and any abnormalities in the reports quickly and without error instead to lose the doctor's time.
- **Gene expression:** AI plays a greatly important role in interrupting the microarray of the genes to detect any types of abnormalities.
- **COVID-19 detection and monitoring:** AI has been recently involved in the management, monitoring, and diagnosis of the new viral pandemic COVID-19 that has been affecting the whole world since the beginning of 2020.

Table 21.1 Summary of important existing AI models for disease detection and diagnosis

Authors	Application	The efficient model	Performance
Książek *et al.* [46]	Hepatocellular carcinoma cancer detection	Support vector machine (SVM)	Accuracy = 88.49% $F1$-score = 87.62%
Abdar *et al.* [47]	Wart disease classification	Improved adaptive particle swarm optimization (IAPSO)	Precision = 89.08% Recall = 89.43% F-measure = 89.16% Accuracy = 90.0%
Acharya *et al.* [48]	Coronary artery disease classification	K-Nearest neighbors (KNN)	Specificity = 99.34% Sensitivity = 94.57% Accuracy = 98.17%
Abdar *et al.* [49].	Coronary artery disease detection	NuSVM algorithm	Accuracy = 93.08% $F1$-score = 91.51%
Patro *et al.* [50]	ECG data classification	Selection operator statistical learning method and least absolute shrinkage using K-nearest neighbors (KNN)	Accuracy = 99.1379%
Ahmed *et al.* [51]	Heart disease prediction	Optimal real-time model based on random forest classifier	Accuracy = 94.9%
Luo *et al.* [52]	Asthma disease detection in children	Random forest (RF)	Accuracy = 75.8% Specificity = 82.0%
Sharma [53]	Cervical cancer disease prediction	Decision tree	Accuracy = 67.5%
Prerana *et al.* [54]	Patient's disease prediction on Google App Engine	Naïve Bayes	Accuracy = 93.4%
Rahman *et al.* [55]	COVID-19 epidemic diagnosis	Deep learning	Accuracy = 98.17% Sensitivity = 84.00% Specificity = 100.00%
El-Rashidy *et al.* [56]	COVID-19 detection and monitoring	Convolutional neural network	Accuracy = 97.95% Specificity = 98.85%

21.7 Some open research problems

AI provides a large number of approaches that aid in diagnostic and prognostic challenges faced in healthcare. While AI models for healthcare have many advantages in detecting and diagnosing disease, unfortunately, they are not standard perfect models. Several research problems are encountered when we want to develop AI models for healthcare disease detection and diagnosis. Some issues are summarized in the following:

- The analysis of medical data faces some problems such as limited availability of data due to confidentiality concerns, restricted specialists availability for labeling the data, the existence of unbalanced datasets for diseases such as cancer and rare diseases, variability in genes, change in experts' opinion in decision-making, environment, and lifestyle of patients.
- There are significant challenges related to data satisfaction, which should influence any decision related to the execution of AI models. The majority of health data is unstructured data and comes in the form of diverse types, such as output summaries, images, reports, and audio or video recordings. It is therefore very difficult to measure the quantity of this data and to categorize it. Besides, the amount of data generated by patients is growing exponentially and becoming increasingly difficult to manage in the period necessary to be clinically useful.
- Different AI models are suitable for a certain health problem for a specific health dataset and may not work well on another dataset. Therefore, selecting suitable and efficient AI models for a particular dataset is a very big challenge in healthcare.
- AI models for disease detection and diagnosis need high quality and large datasets to be trained. However, these types of datasets need more time to be collected. The availability of data is considered to be one of the biggest challenges for the development and evaluation of AI models for disease detection and diagnosis in healthcare.
- Some AI models for healthcare disease detection and diagnosis enquire time, resources, and hardware to generate highly reliable results. It is very difficult to prove that the performance made by these models works properly for all possible scenarios. It depends on the IT resources and equipment used.
- The purpose of OCC models is to induce generalized classifiers when a single class is well characterized by the training data and the negative class is absent, badly sampled or the negative class is not well defined. The limited data availability makes the issue of OCC models more difficult and interesting as a research field [31].
- Methods for integrating total patient data such as clinical notes, test values, patient disease indicators, gene expression data, and medical images are required to develop a complete model. There is a need to build many datasets on various diseases and make them available for researchers. Researchers need to create generative models to perform to increase the size of the dataset than simple methods of data augmentation. This makes it possible to develop complex models on small datasets and to avoid the overfitting issue.
- Finding methods to meet the challenges of processing medical data for disease detection and diagnosis. The challenges include handling small datasets, missing data, noisy labels, and unbalanced datasets.

21.8 Conclusions

The chapter discusses the challenges in healthcare for detecting and diagnosing diseases. Various methods deal with the challenges like SL, USL, and RL. We have presented an overview of diagnosing existing diseases in healthcare, in which a complete taxonomy is used to sort them into different classes based on the AI techniques. We have identified and described new perspectives concerning the disease detection and diagnosis schemes. Furthermore, we have focused on the type of AI technique we can use for the type of disease a patient is currently facing in healthcare. Readers and researchers can benefit from this chapter by understanding the opportunities of AI for healthcare, especially for disease diagnosis. The chapter concludes with open research problems to be explored in utilizing AI to provide robust disease diagnosis solutions.

References

[1] Rong, G., Mendez, A., Assi, E. B., Zhao, B., and Sawan, M. (2020). Artificial intelligence in healthcare: review and prediction case studies. *Engineering*, 6(3), 291–301.

[2] Sajda, P. (2006). Machine learning for detection and diagnosis of disease. *Annual Review of Biomedical Engineering*, 8, 537–565.

[3] El Kafhali, S., and Salah, K. (2018). Performance modelling and analysis of Internet of Things enabled healthcare monitoring systems. *IET Networks*, 8(1), 48–58.

[4] El Kafhali, S., Salah, K., and Alla, S. B. (2018, November). Performance evaluation of IoT-fog-cloud deployment for healthcare services. In *2018 4th International Conference On Cloud Computing Technologies and Applications (CloudTech)* (pp. 1–6). IEEE.

[5] Nguyen, M., He, T., An, L., Alexander, D. C., Feng, J., Yeo, B. T., and Alzheimer's Disease Neuroimaging Initiative. (2020). Predicting Alzheimer's disease progression using deep recurrent neural networks. *NeuroImage*, 222, 117203.

[6] Abiyev, R. H., and Ma'aitah, M. K. S. (2018). Deep convolutional neural networks for chest diseases detection. *Journal of Healthcare Engineering*, 2018.

[7] Dande, P., and Samant, P. (2018). Acquaintance to artificial neural networks and use of artificial intelligence as a diagnostic tool for tuberculosis: a review. *Tuberculosis*, 108, 1–9.

[8] Nilashi, M., Ahmadi, H., Sheikhtaheri, A., *et al.* (2020). Remote tracking of Parkinson's Disease progression using ensembles of Deep Belief Network and Self-Organizing Map. *Expert Systems with Applications*, 159, 113562.

[9] Deperlioglu, O., Kose, U., Gupta, D., Khanna, A., and Sangaiah, A. K. (2020). Diagnosis of heart diseases by a secure Internet of Health Things

system based on Autoencoder Deep Neural Network. *Computer Communications*, 162, 31–50.

[10] Davenport, T., and Kalakota, R. (2019). The potential for artificial intelligence in healthcare. *Future Healthcare Journal*, 6(2), 94.

[11] Ismaeel, S., Miri, A., and Chourishi, D. (2015, May). Using the Extreme Learning Machine (ELM) technique for heart disease diagnosis. In *2015 IEEE Canada International Humanitarian Technology Conference (IHTC2015)* (pp. 1–3). IEEE.

[12] Desai, M., and Shah, M. (2021). An anatomization on breast cancer detection and diagnosis employing multi-layer perceptron neural network (MLP) and convolutional neural network (CNN). *Clinical eHealth*. 4, 1–11.

[13] Osman, A. H., and Alzahrani, A. A. (2018). New approach for automated epileptic disease diagnosis using an integrated self-organization map and radial basis function neural network algorithm. *IEEE Access*, 7, 4741–4747.

[14] Fatima, M., and Pasha, M. (2017). Survey of machine learning algorithms for disease diagnostic. *Journal of Intelligent Learning Systems and Applications*, 9(01), 1–16.

[15] Polat, H., Mehr, H. D., and Cetin, A. (2017). Diagnosis of chronic kidney disease based on support vector machine by feature selection methods. *Journal of Medical Systems*, 41(4), 55.

[16] Shand, L., Li, B., Park, T., and Albarracín, D. (2018). Spatially varying autoregressive models for prediction of new human immunodeficiency virus diagnoses. *Journal of the Royal Statistical Society: Series C (Applied Statistics)*, 67(4), 1003–1022.

[17] Ebhuoma, O., Gebreslasie, M., and Magubane, L. (2018). A seasonal autoregressive integrated moving average (SARIMA) forecasting model to predict monthly malaria cases in KwaZulu-Natal, South Africa. *South African Medical Journal*, 108(7), 573–578.

[18] Parthiban, G., and Srivatsa, S. K. (2012). Applying machine learning methods in diagnosing heart disease for diabetic patients. *International Journal of Applied Information Systems (IJAIS)*, 3(7), 25–30.

[19] Maji, S., and Arora, S. (2019). Decision tree algorithms for prediction of heart disease. In *Information and Communication Technology for Competitive Strategies* (pp. 447–454). Springer, Singapore.

[20] Meurer, W. J., and Tolles, J. (2017). Logistic regression diagnostics: understanding how well a model predicts outcomes. *JAMA*, 317(10), 1068–1069.

[21] Gök, M. (2015). An ensemble of k-nearest neighbours algorithm for detection of Parkinson's disease. *International Journal of Systems Science*, 46(6), 1108–1112.

[22] Lorenzi, M., Filippone, M., Frisoni, G. B., Alexander, D. C., Ourselin, S., and Alzheimer's Disease Neuroimaging Initiative. (2019). Probabilistic disease progression modeling to characterize diagnostic uncertainty: application to staging and prediction in Alzheimer's disease. *NeuroImage*, 190, 56–68.

[23] Kaewprag, P., Newton, C., Vermillion, B., Hyun, S., Huang, K., and Machiraju, R. (2017). Predictive models for pressure ulcers from intensive care unit electronic health records using Bayesian networks. *BMC Medical Informatics and Decision Making*, 17(2), 81–91.
[24] Mcheick, H., Saleh, L., Ajami, H., and Mili, H. (2017). Context relevant prediction model for COPD domain using Bayesian belief network. *Sensors*, 17(7), 1486.
[25] Carnevale, L., Celesti, A., Fiumara, G., Galletta, A., and Villari, M. (2020). Investigating classification supervised learning approaches for the identification of critical patients' posts in a healthcare social network. *Applied Soft Computing*, 90, 106155.
[26] Adegunsoye, A., Oldham, J. M., Chung, J. H., *et al.* (2018). Phenotypic clusters predict outcomes in a longitudinal interstitial lung disease cohort. *Chest*, 153(2), 349–360.
[27] Babu, S., Vivek, E. M., Famina, K. P., *et al.* (2017, April). Heart disease diagnosis using data mining technique. In *2017 International Conference of Electronics, Communication and Aerospace Technology (ICECA)* (Vol. 1, pp. 750–753). IEEE.
[28] Pavithra, G., Manjunath, T. C., and Lamani, D. (2018, November). Detection of primary glaucoma using fuzzy C mean clustering and morphological operators algorithm. In *International Conference On Computational Vision and Bio Inspired Computing* (pp. 1407–1419). Springer, Cham.
[29] You, Y., Chen, W., Li, M., Zhang, T., Jiang, Y., and Zheng, X. (2020). Automatic focal and non-focal EEG detection using entropy-based features from flexible analytic wavelet transform. *Biomedical Signal Processing and Control*, 57, 101761.
[30] Tan, M., Zhang, S., and Wu, L. (2020). Mutual kNN based spectral clustering. *Neural Computing and Applications*, 32(11), 6435–6442.
[31] Khan, S. S., and Madden, M. G. (2014). One-class classification: taxonomy of study and review of techniques. *The Knowledge Engineering Review*, 29 (3), 345–374.
[32] Chen, Z., Lu, G., Xie, Z., and Shang, W. (2020). A unified framework and method for EEG-based early epileptic seizure detection and epilepsy diagnosis. *IEEE Access*, 8, 20080–20092.
[33] Leng, Q., Qi, H., Miao, J., Zhu, W., and Su, G. (2015). One-class classification with extreme learning machine. *Mathematical Problems in Engineering*, 2015, 1–11.
[34] Zhang, Y., Zhang, B., Coenen, F., Xiao, J., and Lu, W. (2014). One-class kernel subspace ensemble for medical image classification. *EURASIP Journal on Advances in Signal Processing*, 2014(1), 1–13.
[35] Ali, L., Zhu, C., Zhang, Z., and Liu, Y. (2019). Automated detection of Parkinson's disease based on multiple types of sustained phonations using linear discriminant analysis and genetically optimized neural network. *IEEE Journal of Translational Engineering in Health and Medicine*, 7, 1–10.

[36] Sell, S. L., Widen, S. G., Prough, D. S., and Hellmich, H. L. (2020). Principal component analysis of blood microRNA datasets facilitates diagnosis of diverse diseases. *PLoS One*, 15(6), e0234185.

[37] Dubuisson, D., and Melzack, R. (1976). Classification of clinical pain descriptions by multiple group discriminant analysis. *Experimental Neurology*, 51(2), 480–487.

[38] Bari, M. F., and Fattah, S. A. (2020). Epileptic seizure detection in EEG signals using normalized IMFs in CEEMDAN domain and quadratic discriminant classifier. *Biomedical Signal Processing and Control*, 58, 101833.

[39] Shah, S. M. S., Batool, S., Khan, I., Ashraf, M. U., Abbas, S. H., and Hussain, S. A. (2017). Feature extraction through parallel probabilistic principal component analysis for heart disease diagnosis. *Physica A: Statistical Mechanics and its Applications*, 482, 796–807.

[40] Peng, Y. S., Tang, K. F., Lin, H. T., and Chang, E. (2018). Refuel: exploring sparse features in deep reinforcement learning for fast disease diagnosis. *Advances in Neural Information Processing Systems*, 31, 7322–7331.

[41] Kubota, Y., Mitsukura, Y., Fukumi, M., Akamatsu, N., and Yasutomo, M. (2004, November). Automatic extraction of a kidney region by using the Q-learning. In *Proceedings of 2004 International Symposium on Intelligent Signal Processing and Communication Systems, 2004. ISPACS 2004* (pp. 536–540). IEEE.

[42] Gürler, Z., Nebli, A., and Rekik, I. (2020, October). Foreseeing brain graph evolution over time using deep adversarial network normalizer. In *International Workshop on PRedictive Intelligence in MEdicine* (pp. 111–122). Springer, Cham.

[43] Wei, Z., Liu, Q., Peng, B., *et al.* (2018, July). Task-oriented dialogue system for automatic diagnosis. In *Proceedings of the 56th Annual Meeting of the Association for Computational Linguistics* (Vol. 2: Short Papers, pp. 201–207).

[44] Xu, L., Zhou, Q., Gong, K., Liang, X., Tang, J., and Lin, L. (2019, July). End-to-end knowledge-routed relational dialogue system for automatic diagnosis. In *Proceedings of the AAAI Conference on Artificial Intelligence* (Vol. 33, No. 01, pp. 7346–7353).

[45] Mansourypoor, F., and Asadi, S. (2017). Development of a reinforcement learning-based evolutionary fuzzy rule-based system for diabetes diagnosis. *Computers in Biology and Medicine*, 91, 337–352.

[46] Książek, W., Abdar, M., Acharya, U. R., and Pławiak, P. (2019). A novel machine learning approach for early detection of hepatocellular carcinoma patients. *Cognitive Systems Research*, 54, 116–127.

[47] Abdar, M., Wijayaningrum, V. N., Hussain, S., *et al.* (2019). IAPSO-AIRS: a novel improved machine learning-based system for wart disease treatment. *Journal of Medical Systems*, 43(7), 1–23.

[48] Acharya, U. R., Sudarshan, V. K., Koh, J. E., *et al.* (2017). Application of higher-order spectra for the characterization of coronary artery disease using

electrocardiogram signals. *Biomedical Signal Processing and Control*, 31, 31–43.

[49] Abdar, M., Książek, W., Acharya, U. R., Tan, R. S., Makarenkov, V., and Pławiak, P. (2019). A new machine learning technique for an accurate diagnosis of coronary artery disease. *Computer Methods and Programs in Biomedicine*, 179, 104992.

[50] Patro, K. K., Reddi, S. P. R., Khalelulla, S. E., Kumar, P. R., and Shankar, K. (2020). ECG data optimization for biometric human recognition using statistical distributed machine learning algorithm. *The Journal of Supercomputing*, 76(2), 858–875.

[51] Ahmed, H., Younis, E. M., Hendawi, A., and Ali, A. A. (2020). Heart disease identification from patients' social posts, machine learning solution on Spark. *Future Generation Computer Systems*, 111, 714–722.

[52] Luo, G., Stone, B. L., Fassl, B., *et al.* (2015). Predicting asthma control deterioration in children. *BMC Medical Informatics and Decision Making*, 15(1), 1–8.

[53] Sharma, S. (2016). Cervical cancer stage prediction using decision tree approach of machine learning. *International Journal of Advanced Research in Computer and Communication Engineering*, 5(4), 345–348.

[54] Prerana, T. H. M., Shivaprakash, N. C., and Swetha, N. (2015). Prediction of heart disease using machine learning algorithms-Naïve Bayes, introduction to PAC algorithm, comparison of algorithms and HDPS. *International Journal of Science and Engineering*, 3(2), 90–9.

[55] Rahman, M. A., Hossain, M. S., Alrajeh, N. A., and Guizani, N. (2020). B5G and explainable deep learning assisted healthcare vertical at the edge: COVID-I9 perspective. *IEEE Network*, 34(4), 98–105.

[56] El-Rashidy, N., El-Sappagh, S., Islam, S. M., El-Bakry, H. M., and Abdelrazek, S. (2020). End-to-end deep learning framework for coronavirus (COVID-19) detection and monitoring. *Electronics*, 9(9), 1439.

Index